Anthracycline Antibiotics

Academic Press Rapid Manuscript Reproduction

Based on the Symposium on Anthracyclines
Sponsored by the Carbohydrate and Medicinal Chemistry Divisions
of the American Chemical Society Held in New York, August 24–25, 1981

Anthracycline Antibiotics

Edited by

Hassan S. El Khadem

Presidential Professor
Department of Chemistry and Chemical Engineering
Michigan Technological University
Houghton, Michigan

1982

ACADEMIC PRESS

A Subsidiary of Harcourt Brace Jovanovich, Publishers
New York   London
Paris   San Diego   San Francisco   São Paulo   Sydney   Tokyo   Toronto

ACADEMIC PRESS, INC.
111 Fifth Avenue, New York, New York 10003

United Kingdom Edition published by
ACADEMIC PRESS, INC. (LONDON) LTD.
24/28 Oval Road, London NW1 7DX

Library of Congress Cataloging in Publication Data
Main entry under title:

Anthracycline antibiotics.

"Papers presented in the symposium on anthracyclines,
held in New York on August 24-25, 1981, and sponsored by
the Carbohydrate and Medicinal Chemistry divisions of the
American Chemical Society"--P.
Includes index.
1. Cancer--Chemotherapy--Congresses. 2. Anthracyclines
--Testing--Congresses. 3. Structure-activity relation-
ships (Pharmacology)--Congresses. I. El Khadem, Hassan
Saad, Date.   II. American Chemical Society.
Division of Carbohydrate Chemistry. III. American
Chemical Society. Division of Medicinal Chemistry.
[DNLM: 1. Antibiotics, Antineoplastic. QV 269 A626]
RC271.A63A567   1982   615'.329   82-11548
ISBN 0-12-238040-1

PRINTED IN THE UNITED STATES OF AMERICA

82 83 84 85   9 8 7 6 5 4 3 2 1

Contents

Contributors

Numbers in parentheses indicate the pages on which the authors' contributions begin.

Edward M. Acton (119), *Life Sciences Division, SRI International, Menlo Park, California 94205*

Federico Arcamone (59), *Ricerca and Sviluppo Chimico, Farmitalia Carlo Erba, Milan, Italy*

J. Boivin (225), *Institut de Chimie, des Substances Naturelles, 91190 Gif-sur-Yvette, France*

Giuseppe Cassinelli (59), *Ricerca and Sviluppo Chimico, Farmitalia Carlo Erba, Milan, Italy*

R. Cermak (253), *Department of Chemistry and Chemical Engineering, College of Engineering, Michigan Technological University, Houghton, Michigan 49931*

H. S. El Khadem (253), *Department of Chemistry and Chemical Engineering College of Engineering, Michigan Technological University, Houghton, Michigan 49931*

John M. Gruber* (119), *Life Sciences Division, SRI International, Menlo Park, California 94205*

Derek Horton (197), *Department of Chemistry, The Ohio State University, Columbus, Ohio 43210*

Andrew S. Kende (141), *Department of Chemistry, University of Rochester, Rochester, New York 14627*

Margaret Logan King (141), *Department of Chemistry, University of Rochester, Rochester, New York 14627*

A. Martin (225), *Institut de Chimie, des Substances Naturelles, 91190 Gif-sur-Yvette, France*

*Present address: *Zoecon Corporation, Palo Alto, California 94302.*

vii

D. Matsuura (253), *Department of Chemistry and Chemical Engineering, College of Engineering, Michigan Technological University, Houghton, Michigan 49931*

C. Monneret (225), *Institut de Chimie, des Substances Naturelles, 91190 Gif-sur-Yvette, France*

Carol W. Mosher (119), *Life Sciences Division, SRI International, Menlo Park, California 94205*

M. Benton Naff (1), *Developmental Therapeutics Program, Division of Cancer Treatment, National Cancer Institute, National Institutes of Health, Silver Spring, Maryland 20910*

V. L. Narayanan (1), *Developmental Therapeutics Program, Division of Cancer Treatment, National Cancer Institute, National Institutes of Health, Silver Spring, Maryland 20910*

Toshikazu Oki† (75), *Central Research Laboratories, Sanraku-Ocean Company, Ltd., Fujisawa, Japan*

M. Pais (225), *Institut de Chimie, des Substances Naturelles, 91190 Gif-sur-Yvette, France*

Sergio Penco (59), *Ricerca and Sviluppo Chimico, Farmitalia Carlo Erba, Milan, Italy*

Jacqueline Plowman (1), *Developmental Therapeutics Program, Division of Cancer Treatment, National Cancer Institute, National Institutes of Health, Silver Spring, Maryland 20910*

Waldemar Priebe (197), *Department of Chemistry, The Ohio State University, Columbus, Ohio 43210*

James P. Rizzi (141), *Department of Chemistry, University of Rochester, Rochester, New York 14627*

D. L. Swartz (253), *Department of Chemistry and Chemical Engineering, College of Engineering, Michigan Technological University, Houghton, Michigan 49931*

John S. Swenton (167), *Department of Chemistry, The Ohio State University, Columbus, Ohio 43210*

Paul F. Wiley (97), *Cancer Research, The Upjohn Company, Kalamazoo, Michigan 49001*

†Present address: *Nagoya Biochemistry Laboratory, Pfizer-Taito Co., Ltd., Taketoyo, Japan, and School of Pharmaceutical Sciences, Kobe-Gakuin University, Kobe, Japan.*

Foreword

This symposium, organized by The Division of Carbohydrate Chemistry in conjunction with The Division of Medicinal Chemistry of the American Chemical Society, focuses on a topic of high relevance to cancer therapy—the chemistry of anthracycline antibiotics. Both adriamycin (doxorubicin) and daunomycin (danorubicin) have been extensively studied clinically and have been rapidly accepted as major therapeutic tools in the treatment of cancer. They play a significant role in the effective treatment of acute leukemia, breast cancer, Hodgkins disease, non-Hodgkins' lymphomas, and sarcomas.

However, their extensive use is limited by the rather narrow spectrum of activity and dose-limiting toxicities. For example, the parent anthracyclines are not clinically useful against lung and colon tumors. The dose-limiting toxicity for these drugs is a cumulative cardiotoxicity. In addition, these exhibit conventional toxicities; for example, myelo-suppression, alopecia, and nausea and vomiting. Therefore, there is wide interest in developing new broad spectrum anthracyclines of low toxicity.

The present symposium is devoted to a survey of the recent international developments in the chemistry of anthracycline antibiotics. The topics include the following: new anthracycline analogs modified in both the aglycon and sugar portion of the molecule, total synthesis, microbial transformations, semisynthetic modifications, and "nonclassical" anthracyclines like aclacinomycins and nogalamycin.

These new developments in the chemistry of anthracyclines make feasible the synthesis of a wide variety of novel compounds for structure-activity/toxicity optimization. These widely divergent structural types might exert their antitumor activities by different mechanisms. Hence, it is reasonable to expect a separation of antitumor activity from toxicity, leading to drugs of enhanced therapeutic effectiveness.

V.L. Narayanan

Preface

Ten of the major papers presented in the symposium on anthracyclines held in New York on August 24 – 25, 1981, and sponsored by the Carbohydrate and Medicinal Chemistry Divisions of the American Chemical Society are published in this volume. Most of the authors have included in their papers data that had not been presented in the sessions to render the book more up-to-date.

The ten chapters comprising the present volume are authored by recognized authorities in the field of anthracycline chemistry, both in the United States and abroad. Their order follows roughly the logical order of presentation of the papers in the symposium.

Ven L. Narayanan, director of the Drug Synthesis and Chemistry Branch of NCI, who chaired the first session of the symposium, wrote an overview of the symposium for this volume. The first chapter gives an overview of the structure–antitumor activity relationships in anthracyclines as correlated by Naff, Plowman, and Narayanan. This is a very valuable chapter since it summarizes the extensive screening data available at the National Cancer Institute, an organization that runs the largest screening program in the world. Because of their unique position in the NCI, these authors were able to correlate the effect of the various structural changes that have been made in the hundreds of anthracycline molecules screened. As might be expected, this chapter is the longest in the book.

The following three chapters describe work carried out by major pharmaceutical companies working in the anthracycline area. The chapter by Arcamone, Cassinelli, and Penco describes the recent developments in the chemistry of doxorubicin and related anthracycline glycosides. This work reviews research carried out in Farmitalia of Milan, following the development of the clinically successful doxorubicin. In his chapter Oki deals with the microbial transformation of anthracycline antibiotics and the development of new families of anthracyclines related to aclacinomycin. It will be recalled that the latter drug was developed by Sanraku–Ocean Company of Fujisawa, Japan, and has shown a great promise clinically in Japan. Wiley of the Upjohn Company discusses the research carried out by this company on nogalamycin and its analog.

The chapter by Acton, Mosher, and Gruber of SRI International discusses the development of several N-substituted anthracyclines with enhanced activity.

The next two chapters deal with the synthesis of the aromatic moieties of anthracyclines, namely, the anthracyclinones, and discuss various strategies developed toward their total synthesis. The first, by Kende, Rizzi, and King, deals with the total synthesis of deoxyanthracyclinones, while the second, by Swenton, deals with regiospecific conversion strategies for anthracyclinone synthesis using quinone bis- and monoketals.

The next three chapters deal with modifications in the sugar moiety of anthracyclines. The first, by Horton and Priebe, is on glycon- and C-14 -modified doxorubicin analogs having enhanced activity. This is followed by the chapter of Monneret, Boivin, Martin, and Pais on the synthesis of disaccharide analogs of aclacinomycins, and then the chapter by El Khadem, Matsuura, Swartz, and Cermak dealing with anthracycline analogs having monosaccharide and disaccharide moieties.

This volume includes the most comprehensive and up-to-date study of the structure – antitumor activity relationships in the area of anthracyclines, and although by its nature it does not attempt to cover all aspects of present day research in anthracyclines, it does offer the reader an insight on the recent developments in ten very active centers in the world.

Hassan S. El Khadem

Houghton, Michigan
April 1982

ANTHRACYCLINES IN THE NATIONAL CANCER INSTITUTE PROGRAM

M. Benton Naff
Jacqueline Plowman
V. L. Narayanan

Developmental Therapeutics Program
Division of Cancer Treatment
National Cancer Institute
National Institutes of Health

The intense interest shown by researchers in the chemistry and biological activity of anthracyclines is illustrated by the wide variety and large numbers of these compounds submitted to the National Cancer Institute (NCI). Over a period of fifteen years, approximately four hundred anthracyclines became part of the program effort to develop agents superior to the clinically used adriamycin.

This paper presents and correlates chemical structures with anticancer data obtained in the in vivo P388 leukemia system for all anthracyclines screened by NCI*. The outcome of this testing was the selection of several anthracyclines for more extensive antitumor evaluation.

DEFINITIONS

For the purpose of this chapter an anthracycline is defined as an aglycone of four fused six-membered rings attached to at least one sugar moiety. The numbering pattern and letter designation of the rings in the aglycone are shown below:

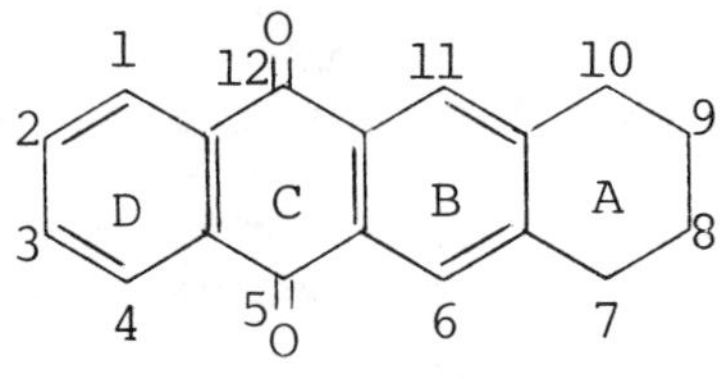

*This excludes about 10% of the anthracyclines which are still classified.

Rings B and D are aromatic, ring C quinoid and ring A non-aromatic. Two carbons in a side chain attached at the 9-position are numbered 13 and 14 proceeding along the chain away from the A-ring.

The aglycone core (rings BCD) of the anthracyclines tested by NCI differ in the number and/or the distribution of the phenolic hydroxyls (or methoxyls) on rings B and D. Only two anthracyclines had a change on the quinoid ring; in both, the 5-position oxygen was replaced by the isoelectronic NH group.

TESTING INFORMATION

Most of the anthracyclines were evaluated for antitumor activity against the i.p. implanted murine P388 lymphocytic leukemia*. Mice received an i.p. inoculum of 10^6 cells on day 0 and i.p. treatment with the anthracycline was initiated at least 24 hours later. Anthracyclines entering the program early in its history were administered daily for nine days starting on day 1 (Q01DX9,D-1). Later a more stringent delayed intermittent treatment schedule was employed with the anthracycline administered on days 5,9, and 13 (Q04DX3, D-5). Four or five doses of each anthracycline covering an 8-16 fold dosage range were initially evaluated. Median survival times of treated mice and non-treated controls were deter-mined and the results expressed as a percent T/C where

$$\% \ T/C = \frac{\text{median survival time of test animals X 100}}{\text{median survival time of control animals}}$$

A T/C value $\geq$ 120% is considered necessary to demonstrate activity, whereas a T/C value < 85% indicates toxicity. Depending on compound availability, experiments in which the compound demonstrated initial activity were confirmed and inactive, non-toxic experiments were repeated using higher doses of the anthracycline. Acceptable median survival time range for control animals was 9-13 days. Experiments were terminated on day 30 if any test mice were still alive on that day.

The tables of this chapter show the highest % T/C obtained in the two experiments and the dosage level (optimal dose) which produced this value.

*CANCER CHEMOTHERAPY REPORTS PART 3, Vol. 3, No. 2, p. 9 (1972).

COMPARISON OF ACTIVITIES

Adriamycin was selected as the parent for comparisons of activities. The % T/C of an anthracycline analog was divided by the average % T/C of adriamycin (determined in over 200 experiments) to provide a number referred to as the analog to parent ratio (A/P ratio). An A/P ratio >1.00 indicates that the analog is superior to adriamycin.

Data on two of the best known anthracylines are shown in Table I:

TABLE I

NSC	COMPOUND	Daily Schedule Q01DX9 D-1			Intermittent Schedule Q04DX3 D-5		
82151	daunomycin	0.79^a	179^b	1.00^c	0.82^a	143^b	8.00^c
123127	adriamycin	1.00	226	1.00	1.00	174	8.00

These are average values from many tests of daunomycin and adriamycin.

    a. A/P   analog to parent ratio

    b. % T/C test animal survival divided by control animal survival both measured in days and the fraction multiplied by 100.

    c. optimum dose (mg/kg/injection).

The same order for A/P ratio, % T/C, and optimum dose is used for all the tables in this chapter.

Note, that the term activity refers to the A/P ratio, throughout the discussions to the tables.

SYMBOLS FOR TABLES

R's are hydrogen unless another group is indicated in the table column. The designation of the orientation of a group as above or below the plane of the aglycone is indicated by a wedge ━■(above) and by a dotted line ..... (below). Haworth projection formulas are used for sugars.

A cartwheel ⊕ by the dose means that of the two experiments run on the same schedule the highest T/C of the first experiment differed from that of the second by at least 20%.

An ↑ alongside the dose indicates the optimum T/C was not attained in the experiment.

Special designations are interpreted in table footnotes as necessary.

The NSC symbol is an abbreviation identifying the National Cancer Institute acquisition number.

APPROACH TO STUDY AND ORGANIZATION OF CONTENTS

All the anthracyclines in the NCI program were categorized into tables according to structural types. Screening data were added and each table analyzed. Proprietary compounds were then eliminated and the truncated tables became the basis for discussion.

The organization of the main body of this chapter is under the heading of "Structure-Activity Correlations". It consists of a series of structural formulas each followed by an applicable table and an appropriate statement or discussion of the table. A summary encompassing the main points of the discussion concludes the chapter.

STRUCTURE-ACTIVITY CORRELATIONS

Figure 1 is the structural formula for Tables II through VIII.

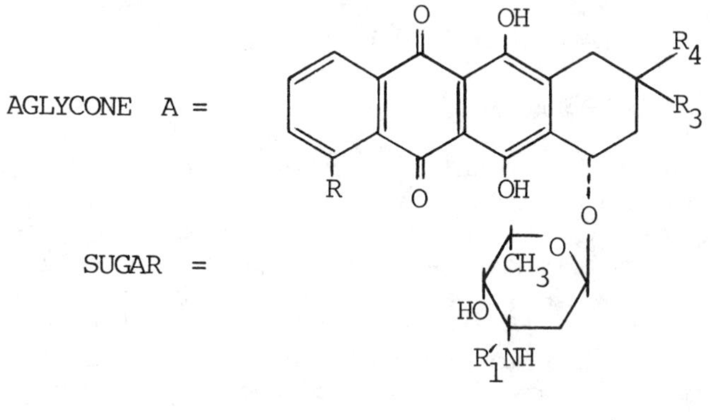

FIGURE 1

TABLE II   HETEROATOM MONOSUBSTITUTION ; A-RING 9-POSITION

refer to figure 1. R=OCH$_3$

NSC	R$_1'$	R$_3$,R$_4$	Q01DX9	D-1		Q04DX3	D-5	
268708		... OH,H	1.04	236	12.50	1.04	181	75.00
268709		◀ OH,H	0.76	173	6.25			
281634		$-OCH_3$ (a)				0.61	107	50.00↑
265493 TFA(b)		= O	0.46	104	1.56			
272678 TFA		= NHOH	0.56	128	25.00			
272679 TFA		∿∿NHOH,H	0.51	116	25.00↑			

Table II emphasizes the importance of the 9-hydroxyl group. Note that the best A/P ratio results if the hydroxyl lies below the plane of the aglycone as in NSC-268708.

(a) NSC-281634 has a 9,10 position double bond.
(b) TFA is the trifluoroacetyl group.

TABLE III   HYDROXYL AND ALDEHYDE DERIVATIVES AS SUBSTITUENTS ; A RING 9-POSITION

refer to figure 1. $R=OCH_3$ $R_1'=H$ ....$R_3=OH$

NSC	►R4	Q01DX9	D-1		Q04DX3	D-5	
272681	$-CH_2OH$	0.80	183	1.56	0.82	143	9.00
274882	$-CH(OH)_2$	0.74	168	2.00	0.87	153	50.00
281633	$-CH=NOH$				0.93	163	50.00
272677	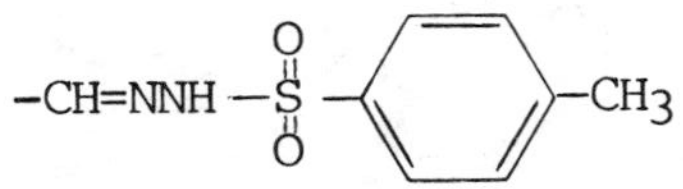 $-CH=NNH-S(=O)(=O)-$C$_6$H$_4$-CH_3	0.78	178	12.50			
235816	$-COOH$	0.72	163	25.00			
237638	$-COOCH_3$	0.65	149	75.00			
252929	$-CONH_2$	0.66	151	6.25↑			

It is apparent from Table III that the presence of a carbon attached to the 9-postion bearing a double bond to the nitrogen (i.e. C=N) confers good activity e.g. NSC-281633. A strong electron withdrawing group on one of the nitrogens of a pair reduces this enhance—ment (see NSC-272677).

6

TABLE IV   THE CONTRIBUTION OF A 9-HYDROXYL

refer to figure 1. $R_1'=H$

NSC	R	....R₃	▲R₄	Q01DX9		D-1	Q04DX3		D-5
294827	CH₃O-	H-	COCH₃				0.78	136	25.00
298225	CH₃O-	H-	COCH₂OH				0.78	136	5.00
256439	H-	HO-	COCH₃	0.90	205	0.40	1.00	174	2.40
82151	CH₃O-	HO-	COCH₃	0.79	178	1.00	0.82	143	8.00
256438	H-	HO-	COCH₂OH	1.15	261	0.20⊕	1.05	183	1.00
123127	CH₃O-	HO-	COCH₂OH	1.00	226	1.00	1.00	174	8.00
301478*	H-	HO-	COCH₂OH				1.09	190	6.25
268708	CH₃O-	HO-	H-	1.04	236	12.50	1.04	181	75.00

The comparison in Table IV shows that (1) Compounds without the 9-hydroxyl (i.e. R_3=H) are less active. (2) With the daunomycin (NSC-256439 and NSC-82151) and adriamycin (NSC-256438 and NSC-123127) pairs where R=H or OCH₃, the compounds with R=H are somewhat more active. (3) The compound with the highest A/P ratio (Schedule Q04DX3 D-5) in Table IV is NSC-301478 where R=H and methyl groups are substituted at the 2- and 3-positions. (4) A striking difference in activity is seen when either NSC-294827 or NSC-298225 where R_3=H and R_4=COCH₃ or COCH₂OH, respectively, are compared to NSC-268708 where R_3=OH and R_4=H. This comparison points out that the combination of a 9-OH and 9-H is better than a 9-acetyl or 9-hydroxyacetyl and a 9-H. Thus the hydroxyl function appears to be the most important group at the 9-position.

Also D-ring is substituted by methyl at both the 2- and 3-positions.

TABLE V EFFECT OF INCREASING SIZE OF ACYL GROUP AT 9-POSITION

refer to figure 1. $R=OCH_3$ $R_1'=H$ ....$R_3=OH$

NSC	R_4	Q01DX9	D-1	Q04DX3	D-5
82151	$-\overset{O}{\overset{\|}{C}}CH_3$	0.79 178	1.00	0.82 143	8.00
279509	$-\overset{O}{\overset{\|}{C}}CH_2CH_3$			0.78 136	25.00
282178	$-\overset{O}{\overset{\|}{C}}CH(CH_3)_2$	0.51 117	6.25	0.73 128	37.50
287498	$-\overset{O}{\overset{\|}{C}}(CH_2)_2Ph$			0.77 135	50.00

Table V presents data which suggests a trend towards lower
A/P ratios and lower potency as the size of the 9-acyl group
increases. It is interesting that in NSC-287498 compared to
NSC-279509 a phenyl (a relatively large group) has replaced
a hydrogen at the end of an ethylene unit with little change
in the A/P ratios of the two compounds.

TABLE VI

HYDRAZIDES, 13-POSITION

refer to figure 1.　　R=OCH₃　R₁'=H　....R₃=OH　$R_4 = -C=NNHR_4'$ with CH_2R_4'

NSC	R₄'	R₄''	Q01DX9	D-1		Q04DX3	D-5	
211391	H	$-CO(CH_2)_3CH_3$	1.09	247	8.00			
233853	OH	$-CO(CH_2)_6CH_3$	0.98	222	3.12	1.02	179	80.00
164011	H	$-COPh$	1.26	287	4.00	1.33	233	32.00
216071	OH	$-COPh$	1.72	390	8.00	1.60	279	48.00⊕
221266	H	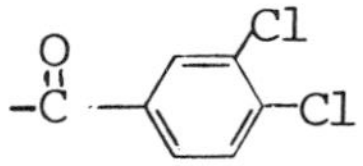 3,4-dichlorobenzoyl ($-C(=O)-$ with two Cl)	1.30	295	4.00			
237672	OH	same moiety as above	1.06	241	8.00	1.04	181	16.00⊕
273429	H	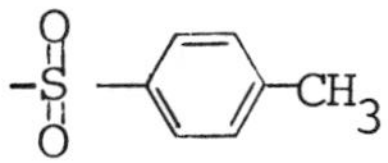 p-toluenesulfonyl ($-S(=O)(=O)-$ with CH_3)	0.79	179	25.00			
269436	OH	same moiety as above	0.75	171	6.25			

The hydrazides in Table VI contain a 9-position C=N group. The effect on activity of the C=N group was first noted in Table III. It is apparent from the data of Table VI that hydrazides of daunomycin have high A/P ratios except when substituted by the powerful electron withdrawing toluenesulfonyl group.

TABLE VII   HETEROCYCLIC RING AND HYDROXYL AT 9-POSITION

refer to figure 1.

R=OCH$_3$ ....R$_3$=OH

NSC	R$_1'$	R$_4$	Q01DX9	D-1		Q04DX3	D-5	
273428	-H	-CH$_2$CH$_3$	0.74	169	1.56	0.80	140	18.80
82151	-H	-COCH$_3$	0.79	179	1.00	0.82	143	8.00
286636	-H	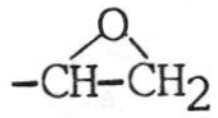				0.69	120	50.00
286635	TFA	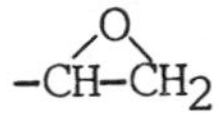				0.64	111	25.00
275650	-H	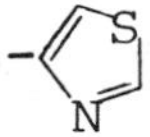				0.90	157	50.00
265490	-H	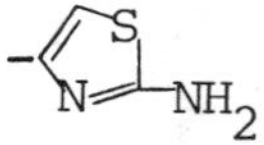	0.78	178	25.00	0.72	127	50.00
268705	-H	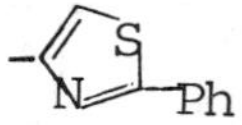	0.80	182	6.25			
275651	-H	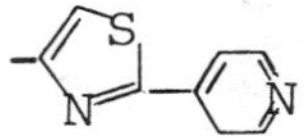				0.77	135	100.00
268706	-H	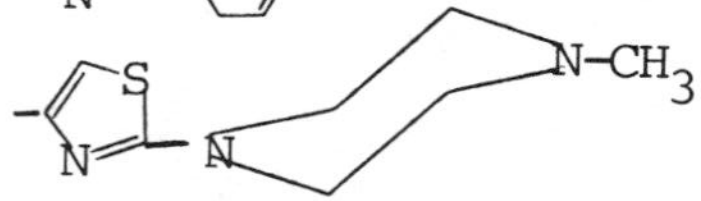	0.69	158	3.13	0.61	107	37.50↑

10

It is postulated that perhaps the high A/P ratio observed for NSC-275650 in this group of compounds in Table VII is due to the contribution of the C=N bond from one of the resonance forms of the thiazolo group at the 9-position. The attachment of a substituent to the 1,3-thiazole ring would influence this resonance contribution. Furthermore, protonation of a basic substituent should decrease activity through delocalization of charge (e.g. NSC-265490 was used as a dihydrochloride salt in the tests).

TABLE VIII

EIHERS AND ESTERS, 14-POSITION

refer to figure 1.   R=OCH$_3$ ....R$_3$=OH   R$_4$= $\overset{O}{\overset{\|}{C}}CH_2R_4'$

NSC	R$_1'$	R$_4'$	QO1DX9	D-1		QO4DX3	D-5	
123127	H	-OH	1.00	226	1.00	1.00	174	8.00
275647	H	-OCH$_3$				0.72	127	50.00
272687	H	-OCH$_2$CH$_3$	0.72	163	3.13			
280412	H	-OCH(CH$_3$)$_2$				0.68	119	25.00
268704	H	-OPh	0.82	186	6.25			
268703	TFA	-OPh	0.69	157	6.25$^{\oplus}$			
263465	H	-SPh	0.61	138	6.25			
149581	H	-O-COCH$_3$	0.88	200	0.08			
271940	Ac	-O-COCH$_3$	0.57	131	12.50↑			
263463	H	-S-COCH$_3$	0.64	146	12.50			

11

TABLE VIII (Cont'd)

ETHERS AND ESTERS; 14-POSITION

NSC	R_1'	R_4'	Q01DX9	D-1		Q04DX3	D-5	
149586	H	$-O-COCH_2CH_3$	1.11	252	2.00			
246131	TFA	$-O-COCH_2CH_2CH_2CH_3$	1.34	303	30.00	1.27	221	150.00
149584	H	$-O-CO(CH_2)_6CH_3$	1.37	311	2.00$^{\oplus}$			
149585	H	$-O-COPh$	0.84	190	2.00↑			
149582	H	$-O-COCH_2Ph$	0.93	212	4.00$^{\oplus}$			
203768	H	$-O-\overset{O}{\overset{\|}{C}}CH_2-$	1.22	277	4.00$^{\oplus}$			
263464	H	$-S-COPh$	0.63	144	3.13			

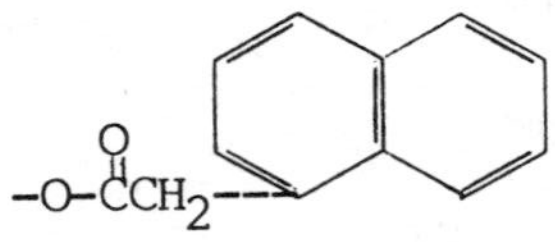

The ethers relative to adriamycin (NSC-123127) have low
A/P ratios while the esters show both low and high A/P
ratios. The contrast in activity of the phenyl and thio-
phenyl ethers (NSC-268704 and NSC-263465) suggests that the
14-position sulfur has a deleterious effect on activity.
This effect is also apparent when two pairs of esters are
compared. Thus the thioacetyl and thiobenzoyl esters
(NSC-263463 and NSC-263464) demonstrate less activity than
the acetyl and benzoyl esters, respectively (NSC-149581 and
NSC-149585).

The difference in the A/P ratios of the two classes of
compounds, the ethers and the esters, undoubtedly is due to
a difference in the ease with which the 14-position group is
removed. Indications are that the more lipophilic the
14-ester group the greater the activity. This appears true
in the alkanoyl ester group (NSC-149581 through NSC-149584)
and the aroyl and ara-alkanoyl group (NSC-149585 through
NSC-203768).

There is a major point of uncertainty in this analysis
since NSC-149585, was not tested at sufficiently high dose
levels. However, the A/P ratio of 0.84 for NSC-149585 must
be very close to its actual value, on the assumption that
there is a parallel in the difference in activities between
NSC-149581 and NSC-263463 and between NSC-149585 and
NSC-263464.

Of special interest in Table VIII is NSC-246131 (AD-32),
a clinical drug, which was developed because it demonstrated
greater antitumor activity than adriamycin.

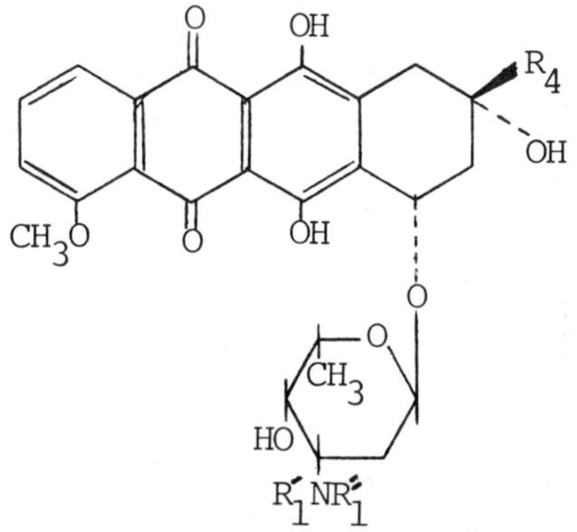

FIGURE 2

TABLE IX   9–POSITION SIDE CHAIN "OL" AND "KETO" ANTHRACYCLINES

refer to figure 2.

NSC	R_1'	R_1''	R_4(ol)	R_4(keto)	Q01DX9	D-1		Q04DX3	D-5	
273428(a)			$-CH_2CH_3$		0.74	169	1.56	0.80	140	18.80
286637(b)			$-CHOHCH_3$					0.60	104	6.25
180510			$-CHOHCH_3$		0.86	195	5.00			
82151				$-COCH_3$	0.79	179	1.00	0.82	143	8.00
268238			$-CHOHCH_2OH$		1.17	266	8.00	1.44	252	25.00$^{\oplus}$
123127				$-COCH_2OH$	1.00	226	1.00	1.00	174	8.00

(a) NSC–273428 is included for comparison purposes only
(b) NSC–286637 has a 9,10 double bond.

TABLE IX (Cont'd)   9–POSITION SIDE CHAIN "OL" AND "KETO" ANTHRACYCLINES

NSC	R_1'	R_1''	R_4(ol)	R_4(keto)	Q01DX9	D-1		Q04DX3	D-5	
273430	CH_3	CH_3	$-CHOHCH_3$		0.92	209	6.25	0.79	138	18.80
258812	CH_3	CH_3		$-COCH_3$	1.01	228	2.00	0.83	145	10.00
282181	$CH_3(CH_2)_9-$	$CH_3(CH_2)_9-$	$-CHOHCH_3$					0.63	110	37.50
282179	$CH_3(CH_2)_9-$	$CH_3(CH_2)_9-$		$-COCH_3$	0.50	113	50.00	0.80	140	150.00↑
292686	$CH_3(CH_2)_9-$	$CH_3(CH_2)_9-$	$-CHOHCH_2OH$					0.59	103	25.00
271937	$-CH_2CH_2CH_2CH_2CH_2-$		$-CHOHCH_2OH$		0.69	157	1.56	0.87	152	18.80

15

TABLE IX (Cont'd)   9-POSITION SIDE CHAIN "OL" AND "KETO" ANTHRACYCLINES

NSC	R_1'	R_1''	R_4(ol)	R_4(keto)	Q01DX9	D-1		Q04X3	D-5	
268240		PhCH$_2$-	-CHOHCH$_3$		1.00	226	6.25	1.15	201	18.80
268241		PhCH$_2$-		-COCH$_3$	0.82	187	6.25	1.29	226	37.50$\oplus$
269434		PhCH$_2$-	-CHOHCH$_2$OH		0.86	196	1.56	0.82	143	37.50
269433		PhCH$_2$-		-COCH$_2$OH	0.99	224	6.25	1.14	200	18.80
278170	PhCH$_2$-	PhCH$_2$-	-CHOHCH$_3$		1.03	233	12.50	1.08	187	25.00
268242	PhCH$_2$-	PhCH$_2$-		COCH$_3$	1.19	271	25.00	1.30	227	37.50
316162	PhCH$_2$-	PhCH$_2$-	-CHOHCH$_2$OH					1.21	212	100.00
269435	PhCH$_2$-	PhCH$_2$-		-COCH$_2$OH	0.79	175	6.25↑			
263466		TFA	-CHOHCH$_3$		0.83	189	25.00↑			
268711		TFA	-CHOHCH$_2$OH		0.69	158	3.13			

Table IX compares the data for the daunomycin and adriamycin analogs possessing a 13-position hydroxyl group (ol series) with the data for the most closely related keto compound.

Interesting facts about Table IX are:

1. The presence of an oxygen function in the 9-position side chain contributes to higher activity, - compare NSC-180510 and NSC-82151 with NSC-273428.

2. The lack of activity of NSC-286637, even though it possesses a side chain oxygen function, is possibly due to the change in stereochemistry of the A-ring resulting from conjugation of the double bond with the adjacent aromatic ring (ring B).

3. The "ol" derivatives (NSC-180510 and NSC-268238) are more active than the corresponding "keto" parent compounds (daunomycin, NSC-82151 and adriamycin, NSC-123127). In contrast, keto compounds with one or more substituent(s) on the amino group of the sugar generally are more active than the corresponding "ol" derivatives. In addition, the "ol" forms with dialkyl and piperidino groups (e.g. NSC-282181 and NSC-271937) on the sugar are less active (A/P $\leq$ 0.92) than the benzyl substituted compounds which have A/P ratios equal to or greater than 1.00 with the exception of the adriamycin analog, NSC-269434.

4. The trifluoroacetyl group reduces the A/P ratio of the "ol" form of adriamycin, see NSC-268238 versus NSC-26711. It is questionable whether this is true in the case of the daunomycin analogs (NSC-180510 versus NSC-263466) because NSC-263466 was not tested at sufficiently high dose levels.

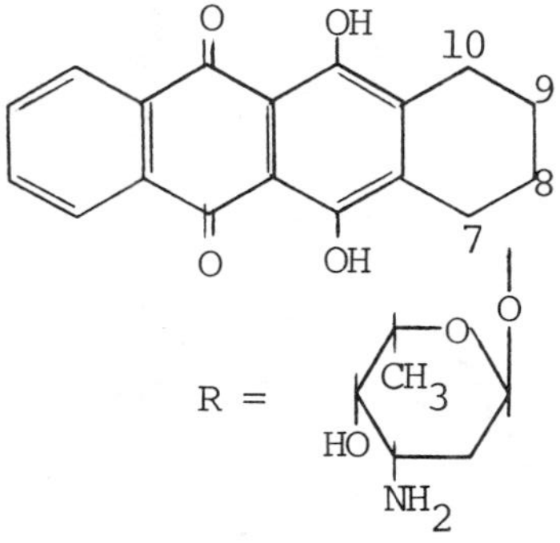

FIGURE 3

TABLE X

SUGAR AS SOLE SUBSTITUENT ON A-RING
NO SUBSTITUENTS ON D-RING

refer to figure 3.

NSC NO.	7-POSITION	8-POSITION	Q01DX9 D-1	Q04DX3 D-5	Q04DX3 D-1
200682	◢R ; H	H ; H			0.61 106 2.50
200681	....R ; H	H ; H			0.56 98 2.50
221267*	◢R ; H ....R ; H	H ; H	0.50 113 4.00	0.64 112 3.13	
262635	H ; H	◢R ; H	0.52 118 4.00		
262634	H ; H	....R ; H	0.48 109 1.00		

None of the compounds in Table X show antitumor activity. Thus the influence that the position of the sugar, daunosamine, has on activity cannot be determined. The level of activity of these compounds also is lower than that of the only aglycone (no sugar) bearing a 9-position hydroxyl and acetyl which has been tested NCI program (NSC-10935l, see figure 5 where R_1=OH and R_4'=H Q01DX9 D-1 0.53 119 100.00). Thus Table X emphasizes the need for both a sugar and 9-functional group(s) such as OH, $COCH_3$, or an alternative like OH and CH_2CH_3 for activity.

* mixture of stereoisomers

Figure 4 is the structure for Tables XI and XII.

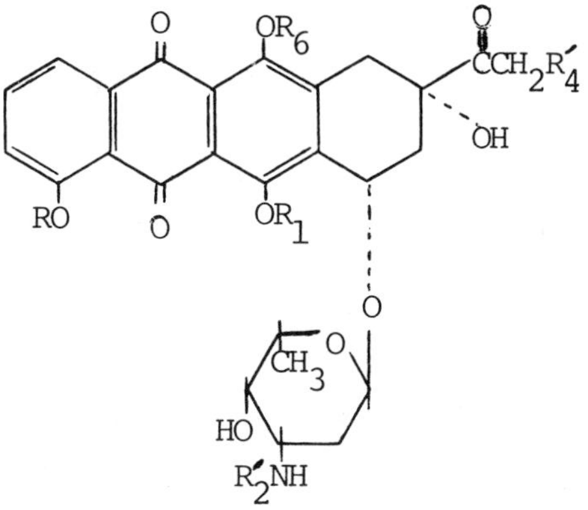

FIGURE 4

TABLE XI   ALKYL & ARA-ALKYL DERIVATIVES; D-RING 4-POSITION

refer to figure 4 for structure $R_1=R_6=H$

NSC NO.	R	R_2'	R_4'	Q04DX3	D-5	
82151	CH_3-			0.82	143	8.00
272330*	CH_3-			0.84	147	8.00
281629	CH_3CH_2-			0.78	136	25.00
298231	$CH_3(CH_2)_2-$			0.85	149	25.00
283161	$(CH_3)_2CH-$			0.93	162	12.50
302671	$CH_3(CH_2)_3-$			0.81	141	25.00
302672	$(CH_3)_2CHCH_2-$			0.73	128	12.50

* As a dodecyl sulfate salt.

ALKYL & ARA-ALKYL DERIVATIVES: D-RING 4-POSITION

TABLE XI (Cont'd)

NSC NO.	R	R_2'	R_4'	Q04DX3	D-5
286631	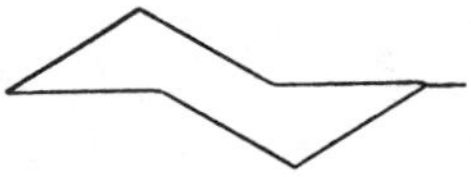			0.70	122	50.00↑
286628	PhCH$_2$-			0.89	155	50.00$^\oplus$
286629	PhCH$_2$-	TFA		0.59	104	12.50↑
314641	PhCH$_2$-		OH	0.75	131	12.50

The average of the A/P ratios in Table XI is 0.82, the same as the A/P ratio for daunomycin. NSC-286631 and NSC-286629 were not tested at sufficiently high doses and were excluded from the calculation. Only the isopropyl ether, NSC-283161, gave an A/P ratio significantly better (10% or greater) than the average. The adriamycin analog NSC-314641 is considerably less active than adriamycin NSC-123127.

TABLE XII AROMATIC HYDROXYLS AND THEIR ETHERS

refer to figure 4 for structure $R_4' = H$

NSC	R	R_1	R_6	R_2'	Q01DX9	D-1		Q04DX3	D-5	
258813	CH_3	CH_3	CH_3		0.74	169	128.00			
82151	CH_3	H	H		0.79	179	1.00	0.82	143	8.00
291097	H	CH_3	H					0.74	129	12.50
294399	H	H	CH_3					0.72	125	50.00
180024[a]	H	H	H		0.78	177	0.14	0.95	166	1.00
275649[b]	H	H	H					1.02	179	$3.13^{\oplus}$
275648	H	H	H	TFA				1.22	214	$200.00^{\oplus}$
286629	$PhCH_2$	H	H	TFA				0.59	104	12.50↑

On the more stringent schedule the ethers in Table XII are less active than the analogs having free hydroxyl groups.

[a] Free Base
[b] HCl Salt

FIGURE 5

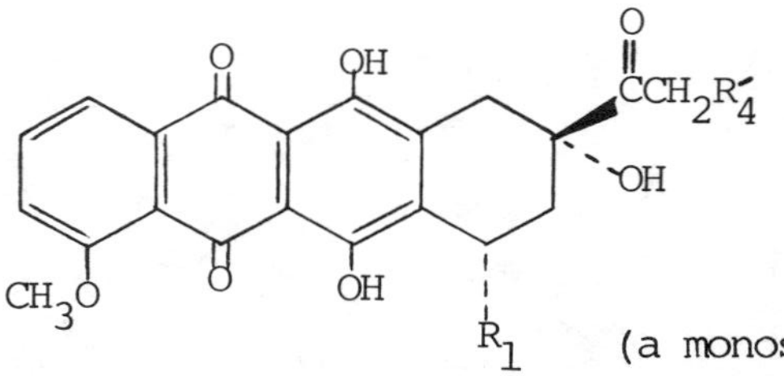

(a monosaccharide)

TABLE XIII   THE 3'-DESAMINO L-FAMILY   DAUNOMYCIN AND ADRIAMYCIN ANALOGS
refer to figure 5

R_4'	R_1
H 284682 1.10 192 200.00	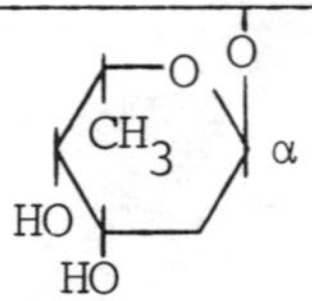
Br 307989 0.62 109 25.00	OH 307990 1.54 269 50.00
H 283158 1.06 186 200.00⊕	
H 327472 0.65 113 25.00	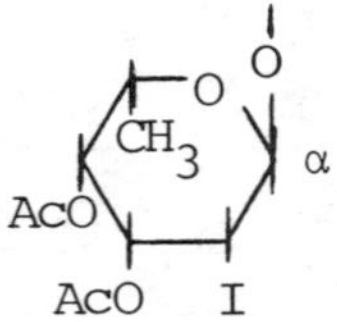
H 331962 1.42 247 50.00	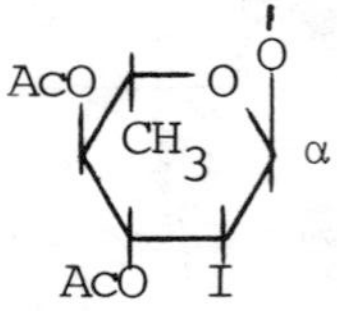

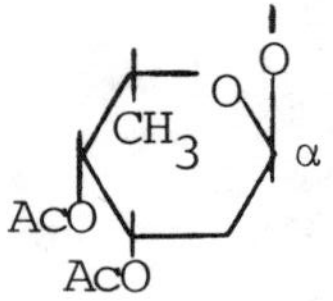

*In each data set corresponding to a sugar structure (R_1):
line (1) is an R_4' atom or group, (2) is the NSC number of the compound,
(3) is schedule Q04DX3 D-5 data.*

22

The 3′-desamino-L-family of daunomycin and adriamycin analogs evaluated are shown in Table XIII. The data illustrate that some of the most active compounds contain a desaminosugar as the only sugar. Thus replacement of a 3′-amino group in daunomycin by a 3′-hydroxyl group as in NSC-284682 has produced a daunomycin analog with greater P-388 activity than that shown by adriamycin. Acetylation of the hydroxyl groups of the sugar makes little difference in activity; compare NSC-284682 and NSC-283158.

As a general rule substituted adriamycins show decreased activity while substituted daunomycins exhibit increased activity. NSC-307990 presents an interesting exception to this phenomenon.

Examination of NSC-327472 and NSC-331962 reveals that a change in the configuration of only the 4-acetoxy group on the sugar causes an impressive change in activity. High activity associated with the iodo group on the sugar 2-position is very unusual.

Table XIII deemphasizes the early contention that an aminosugar is necessary for activity.

TABLE XIV   THE 3′-DESAMINO D-FAMILY   DAUNOMYCIN ANALOGS
refer to figure 5

R4′	R1	R4′	R1
H		H	
299555		298498	
0.58 100 50.00↑		0.64 112 50.00	
		H	
		294987	
		0.58 101 50.00↑	
		H	
		297279	
		0.58 102 50.00	

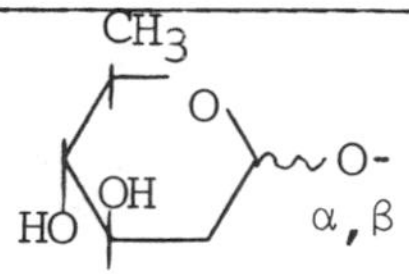

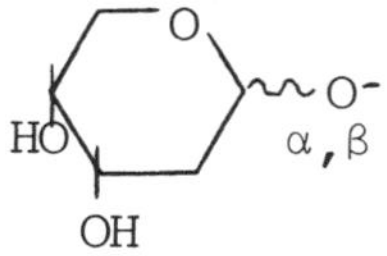

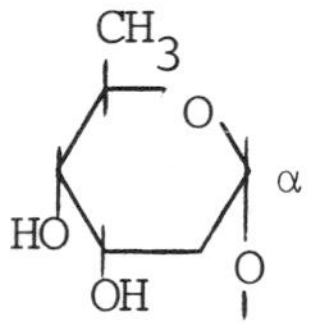

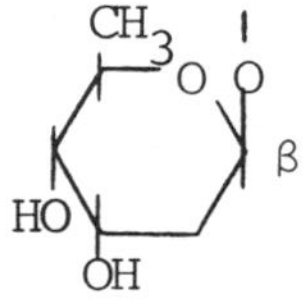

See Table XIII footnotes for explanation of data sets

23

THE DISCUSSION FOR TABLES XIV AND XV FOLLOWS TABLE XV.

TABLE XV   THE 3'-AMINO D-FAMILY   DAUNOMYCIN ANALOGS
refer to figure 5

R_4	R_1	R'_4	R'_1
H	CH₃ sugar (NH₂, HO) α		
275272			
0.71 125 100.00			
H	CH₃ sugar (NH₂, HO) β		
302648			
0.66 115 25.00			
		H	H₂NCH₂ sugar (HO, NH₂) α
		302048	
		0.59 103 50.00	

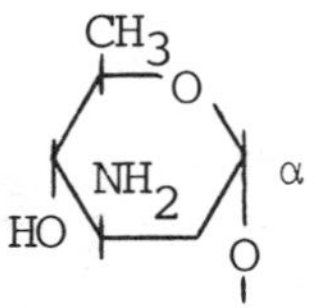

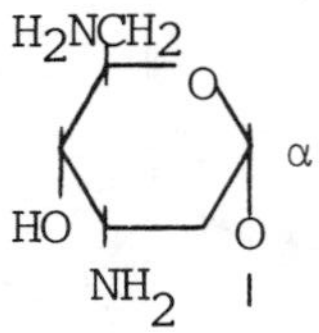

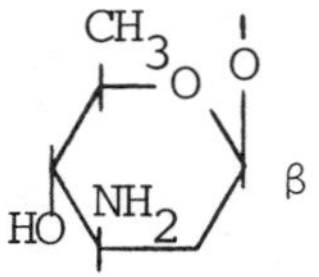

Obviously the 3'-desamino D-Family daunomycin analogs have very low activity although some were not available in sufficient quantity to complete testing. The 3'-amino D-family analogs are not much better. The highest A/P ratio is given by the compound of α-D-arabino configuration, NSC-275272. The comparison of NSC-275272 with NSC-302048 is hardly justified on a configurational basis since NSC-302048 exists in vivo as a diprotonated species.

In the D-family, the anomeric form appears to make little difference in activity as the difference in the A/P ratios of NSC-275272 and NSC-302648 is small.

Note the sugar of NSC-275272 has the arabino configuration, see also NSC-256942 in Table XVII.

See Table XIII footnotes for explanation of data sets.

TABLE XVI   THE 3′-AMINO L-FAMILY   DAUNOMYCIN ANALOGS

refer to figure 5

R4′	R1	R4′	R1
H 82151 143 8.00 0.82 178 (0.79 1.00)	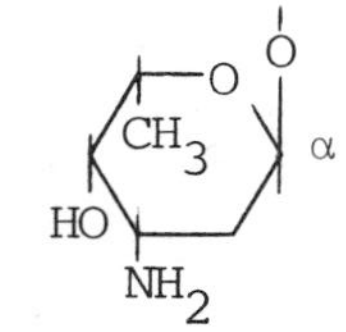	H 257457 (1.02 231 25.00)	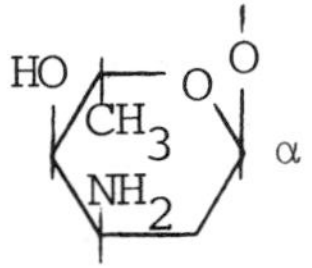
		H 249334 0.87 197 25.00	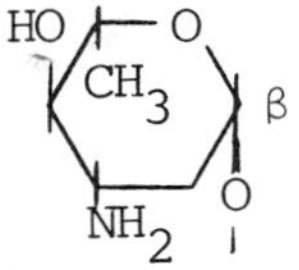
H 314333 0.58 101 3.13	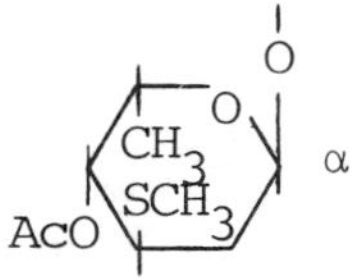	H 314332 0.63 110 50.00	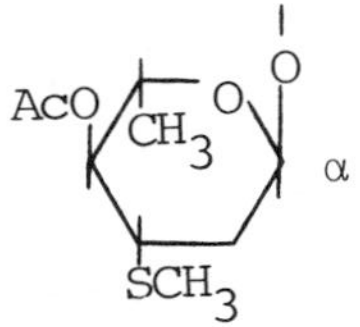

In each data set corresponding to a sugar (R1) structure:
*   line (1) is an R4′ atom or group*
*   (2) is the NSC number of the anthracycline*
*   (3) are data for schedule Q04DX3 D-5 unless enclosed in parenthesis. Data enclosed*
*   in parenthesis are for the Q01DX9 D-1 schedule.*

25

Comparison of the A/P ratios obtained on the intermittent schedule for the daunomycin analog containing the D-sugar(NSC-302648, Table XV) and that containing the L-sugar (NSC-249334, Table XVl) indicates that the L-sugar provides the more active anthracycline. The thio analogs of daunomycin, NSC-314333 and NSC-314332, are essentially devoid of activity as noted previously for the thio ethers and esters (Table VIII).

TABLE XVII   THE 3´-AMINO L-FAMILY   ADRIAMYCIN ANALOGS

refer to figure 5

$R_4´$			R_1	
OH				
267469				
1.00	175	3.13		
(1.38	314	0.90)		
OH				
256942				
1.11	194	16.00		
(1.09	248	1.20)		
OH				
123127				
1.00	174	8.00		
(1.00	226	1.00)		
OH				
301477				
0.98	172	3.13		
(1.43	324	1.08)		

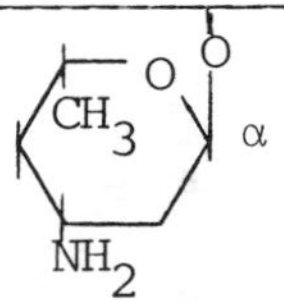

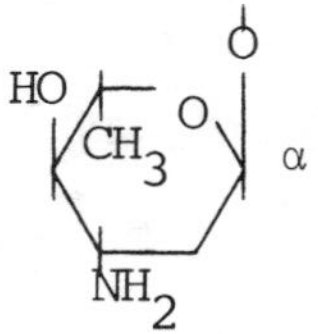

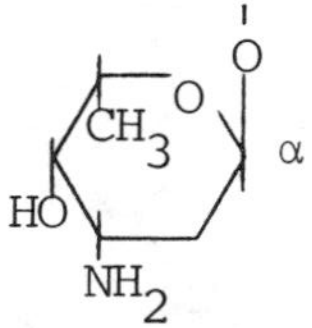

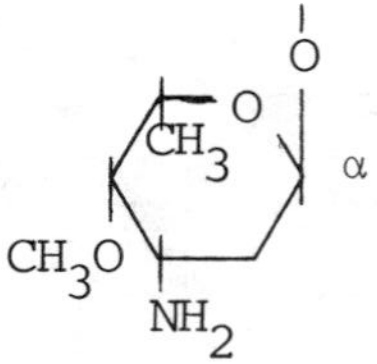

See Table XVII footnotes for explanation of data sets.

The sugar moieties in Table XVII have identical groups and configuration at positions 1, 3 and 5; the distinguishing difference is at position 4. On the more stringent treatment schedule (Q04DX3 D-5) three of the compounds, including adriamycin, have an A/P ratio of about 1.00. The fourth compound, NSC-256942, is about 10% more active than the others and suggests that the arabino configuration confers greater activity. However, the daily schedule (Q01DX9 D-1) fails to confirm the overall superiority of the α-L-arabino configuration. Nevertheless this analog is clearly an improvement over adriamycin.

TABLE XVIII   SUBSTITUTIONS ON AMINOSUGAR NITROGEN

refer to figure 5 for structure $R_4' = H$ unless indicated otherwise

$R_1 =$

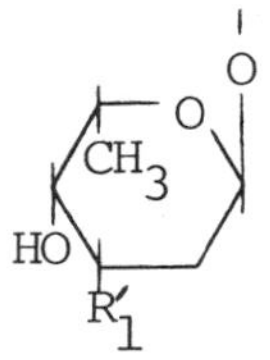

R_1 for NSC-304944 =

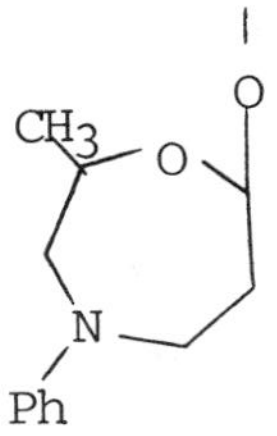

TABLE XVIII (Cont'd)   SUBSTITUTIONS ON AMINOSUGAR NITROGEN
refer to previous page for structural details.

NSC	R_1'	R_4'	Q01DX9	D-1	Q04X3	D-5
304944					0.60 105	50.00
267211	$(CH_3)_2CHNH$		0.88 199	12.50	0.85 148	75.00
269741	$CH_3(CH_2)_3NH$		0.60 136	32.00↑		
282180	$CH_3(CH_2)_9NH$		0.47 108	3.13	0.60 106	18.80
258812	$(CH_3)_2N$		1.00 228	2.00	0.83 145	10.00
261045	$(CH_3)_2N$	OH	0.71 160	0.50	0.72 125	6.00
265205	$(CH_3CH_2)_2N$		0.80 183	4.00	0.81 141	24.00
268239	$(CH_3CH_2)_2N$	OH	0.78 178	3.13		
282179	$[CH_3(CH_2)_9]_2N$		0.50 113	50.00	0.80 140	150.00$^{\oplus}$

28

TABLE XVIII (Cont'd) SUBSTITUTIONS ON AMINOSUGAR NITROGEN

NSC	R₁'	R₄'	Q01DX9	D-1	Q04X3	D-5
245426	$(CH_3)_3N^+$		0.53	120 25.00		
249335	$(CH_3)_3N^+$	OH	0.82	187 12.50		
268241	$PhCH_2NH$		0.82	187 6.25	1.29	226 18.80⊕
269433	$PhCH_2NH$	OH	0.99	224 6.25	1.14	200 18.80
339278	$(Ph)_2CHCH_2NH$				0.85	147 200.00↑
322100	$PhCH_2NCH_3$				0.98	172 25.00⊕
268242	$PhCH_2NCH_2Ph$		1.19	271 25.00	1.30	227 37.50
269435	$PhCH_2NCH_2Ph$	OH	0.77	175 6.25↑		
344822	$PhCH_2NCH_2CH_2OH$				1.38	240 128.00↑

29

TABLE XVIII (Cont'd)   SUBSTITUTIONS ON AMINOSUGAR NITROGEN

NSC	R$_1$	R$_4$	Q01DX9	D-1	Q04DX3	D-5
319094	NH				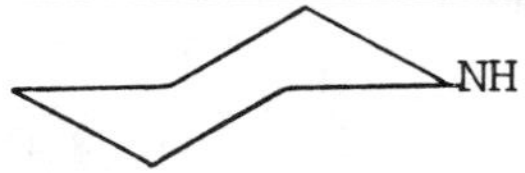 0.62 108	200.00
271936	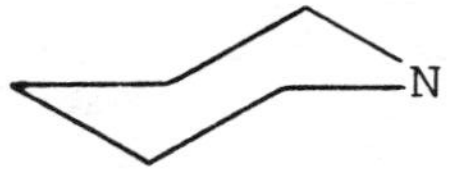 N	OH	0.75 171	6.25$^{\oplus}$		
334353	N, CH$_3$O				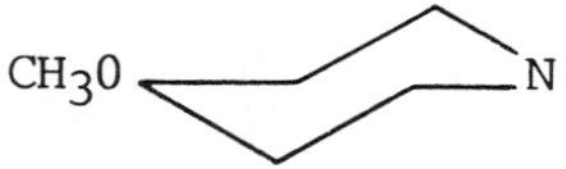 1.25 217	6.25
343492	N, (CH$_3$OCH$_2$)$_2$				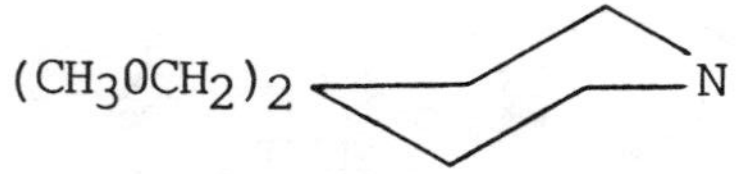 1.22 212	12.50
328399	NH				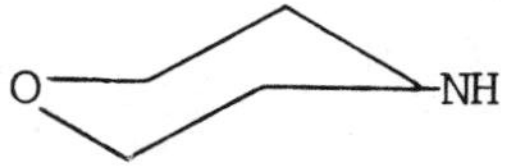 0.78 136	100.00
321826	N				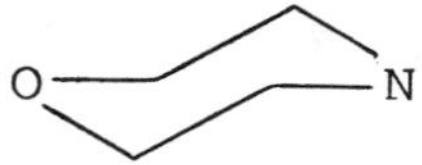 1.02 178	0.80 ↑
332304	N, CN				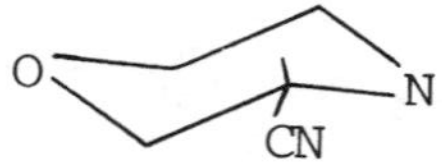 1.19 207	0.39

Analysis of Table XVIII:

1. Monoalkyl substituted sugar.

   The data suggest that the activity of daunomycin analogs decreases with increase in the size of alkyl group attached to nitrogen. Unfortunately, NSC-269741 was not tested at sufficiently high dose levels.

2. Dialkyl substituted sugar.

   On the Q01DX9 D-1 schedule the A/P ratio for daunomycin analogs drops from 1.00 to 0.50 as the size of the dialkyl substituents increase. In contrast, on the Q04DX3 D-5 schedule the A/P ratios for the same analogs appear insensitive to a change in chain length. However, the value for the didecyl compound was not confirmed and the true activity may be lower than indicated. In the case of the adriamycin analogs, dialkyl substitution of the sugar decreases the A/P ratio compared to that of the parent.

3. Quaternary salt forms.

   The quaternary salts of daunomycin (NSC-245426) and adriamycin (NSC-249335) are less active than the parents. The change in A/P ratio from the parent to the quaternized adriamycin is roughly the same as that from parent to the dialkylamino adriamycin.

4. Puckered rings.

   Comparison of NSC-319094 with NSC-328399 shows an improvement in activity that may be attributed to an oxygen in the ring opposite a secondary amino nitrogen. opposite an amino nitrogen. An even more dramatic increase in the A/P ratio above that of NSC-319094 is observed for the methoxy (NSC-334353) and bis-methoxymethyl piperidino (NSC-343492) compounds. In view of this result it is not surprising to see NSC-321826 and NSC-332304, where oxygen is opposite nitrogen and both elements are in the same six membered puckered ring, exhibit high activity.

5. Ara-alkyl substitutions.

In contrast to the daunomycin analogs with mono-and di-alkyl substituted sugars, those with ara-alkyl substituted sugars tested on the Q04DX3 D-5 schedule were significantly more active than daunomycin. In fact several were more active than adriamycin, particularly NSC-268242 and NSC-344822; the two most active anthracyclines in Table XVIII. The one example of an adriamycin analog containing an ara-alkyl substitution tested on the delayed intermittent schedule (NSC-269433) also was more active than adriamycin.

6. Polarizability.

The contrast in A/P ratio between NSC-319094 and NSC-268241 or NSC-269433 is probably the result of the greater polarizability of the phenyl ring (of the benzyl group). This idea has support from the comparison of NSC-258812 with NSC-322100 (although the A/P value of NSC-322100 is equivocal) and NSC-268242. For obvious structural reasons the effect is not evident in NSC-304944.

Substitution on the aminosugar nitrogen by relatively large non-polar or non-polarizable groups as in NSC-282180 and NSC-319094 appears to give inactive compounds (the data for NSC-282179 on the Q04DX3 D-5 schedule is uncertain). In these cases the effect of substitution is as deleterious as the replacement of the sugar by a pseudo-sugar, - see NSC-304944.

7. Synergism.

The most active compound in Table XVIII is NSC-344822. Structurally NSC-344822 combines a polarizable phenyl group (as part of a benzyl group) and an oxygen atom separated by an ethylene unit (refer to NSC-321826 and NSC-332304).

32

TABLE XIX

ACYL SUBSTITUTED AMINOSUGAR NITROGEN

refer to figure 2 for structure $R_1'' = H$

NSC	R_1'	R_4	Q01DX9 D-1	Q04DX3 D-5
227012	CHO	$COCH_3$	0.90 205 4.00⊕	
239738	CHO	$COCH_2OH$	0.88 200 25.00	
118714	$COCH_3$	$COCH_3$	1.06 240 12.50	
269432	$COCH_3$	$COCH_2OH$	0.88 201 100.00	0.91 159 400.00
283464	$COCF_3$	$COCH_2OH$		1.18 206 200.00
256955	$CO(CH_2)_6CH_3$	$COCH_3$	0.66 149 12.00↑	0.81 140 200.00
264072	$CO(CH_2)_6CH_3$	$COCH_2OH$	0.81 184 25.00	0.82 142 150.00

TABLE XIX (Cont'd) ACYL SUBSTITUTED AMINOSUGAR NITROGEN

NSC	R_1'	R_4	Q01DX9 D-1			Q04DX3 D-5		
256956	$CO(CH_2)_{10}CH_3$	$COCH_3$	0.69	158	12.00↑	0.76	133	64.00
264071	$CO(CH_2)_{10}CH_3$	$COCH_2OH$	1.06	240	12.50	0.96	167	150.00
256957	$CO(CH_2)_{14}CH_3$	$COCH_3$	0.55	125	12.00↑			
264073	CO 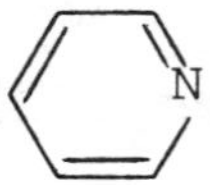	$COCH_3$	0.70	159	12.50	0.68	120	150.00

The data on the daily schedule (Q01DX9 D-1) include many compounds which were not tested at a sufficiently high dose. However, in general it can be stated that:

(1) Daunomycin analogs with fatty acid substitution on the sugar nitrogen (except formyl and acetyl) are less active than daunomycin.

(2) Adriamycin analogs, are all less active than the parent except for NSC-283464 on the Q04DX3 D-5 schedule and NSC-264071 on the Q01DX9 D-1 schedule.

34

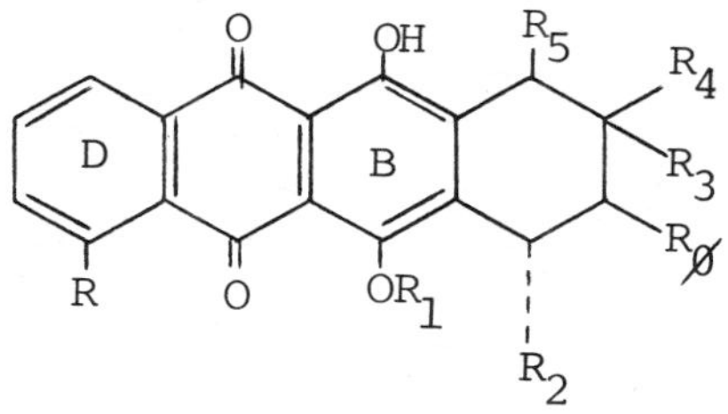

FIGURE 6

TABLE XX   TWO IDENTICAL SUGARS SEPARATELY LOCATED ON A-RING

refer to figure 6; $R_\emptyset$=H.

R=OCH$_3$ R$_5$= H   R=OH

R$_1$=H   R$_2$ and ...R$_3$=   R$_1$=CH$_3$

R$_4$= $\overset{O}{\overset{\|}{C}}CH_3$

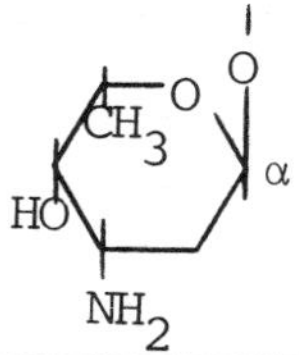

	Common To Both Compounds	

NSC	Q01DX9	D-1		NSC	Q04DX3	D-5
272682	0.60	137	25.00	286633	0.57	99	50.00

35

Table XX (Cont'd)

R=OH   R1=H   R₂   and   ──►R₅= HO...N(CH₃)₂   ...R₃=OH   ──►R₄= CH₂CH₃

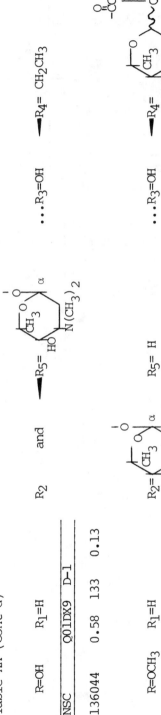

NSC	Q01DX9	D-1	
136044	0.58	133	0.13

R=OCH₃   R₁=H   R₂=   R₅= H   ...R₃=OH   ──►R₄=   α,β

NSC	Q04DX3	D-5	
311156*	0.57	100	50.00

The difference between NSC-272682 and NSC-286633 is the location of a methoxy group. The A/P ratios are low whether the methoxy is on ring D or B. The substitution of a daunosaminyl group for the OH at the 9-position has a large deleterious effect on the A/P ratios (e.g. NSC-272682 versus NSC-82151 and NSC-286633 versus NSC-291097 Table XII). Similarly the substitution of the 14-hydroxy by a sugar as in NSC-311156 lowers the activity (compare to NSC-307990 Table XIII).

Anthracycline NSC-136044 with the second sugar at the 10-position (R₅) has a poor A/P ratio when compared to the closest analog that NCI has evaluated i.e. NSC-258812 Table XVIII.

From the four examples in Table XX, it would appear that a second sugar attached to the A-ring in either the 9- or 10- position reduces the activity of the anthracycline, possibly through interference with transport.

* *Mixture of Isomers.*

36

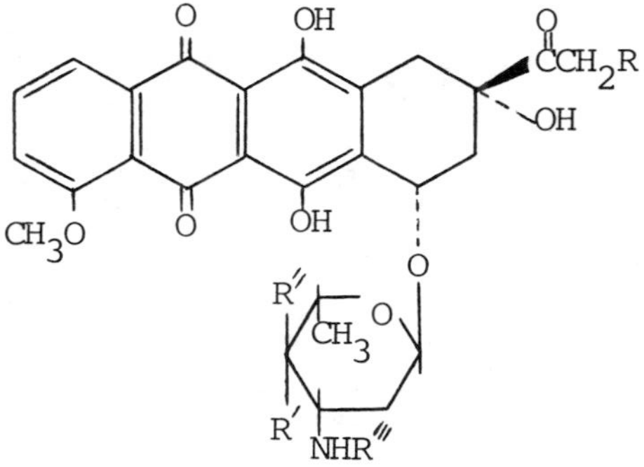

FIGURE 7

DISACCHARIDE ANALOGS

TABLE XXI
refer to figure 7.   Note: A hydrogen atom substitutes for an undesignated position under any R group.

NSC	R'	R''	R	Q01DX9	D-1	Q04DX3	D-5
Section 1							
268712	(sugar structure: CH3, HO, NH2)			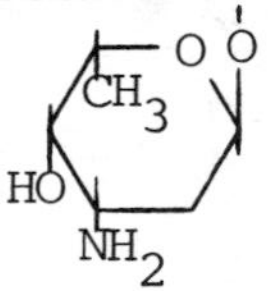 0.86 196 $3.13^{\oplus}$			
82151	HO			0.79 178 1.00		0.82 143 8.00	
123127	HO		OH	1.00 226 1.00		1.00 174 8.00	

TABLE XXI (Cont'd)

DISACCHARIDE ANALOGS

NSC	R'	R''	R	Q01DX9 D-1	Q04DX3 D-5
Section 2					
304946	(α-pyranose; O; CH$_3$; CH$_3$O; NH$_2$)				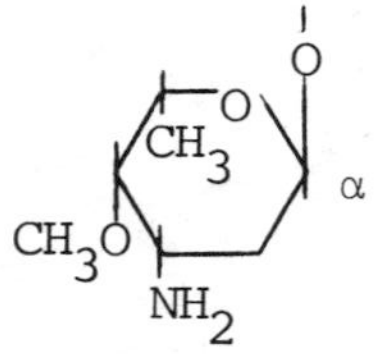 0.83 146 25.00
301477	CH$_3$O		OH	1.43 324 1.08	0.98 172 3.13
Section 3					
286634	(α-pyranose; O; HO; CH$_3$; NH$_2$; CH$_3$O)		OH		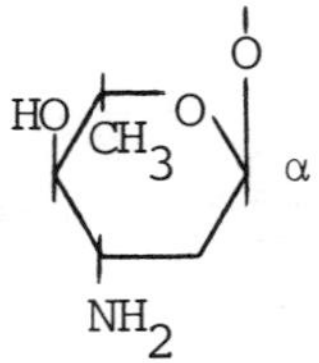 0.89 156 100.00$^{\oplus}$
256942	H		OH	1.09 248 1.20	1.11 194 16.00
Section 4					
312889	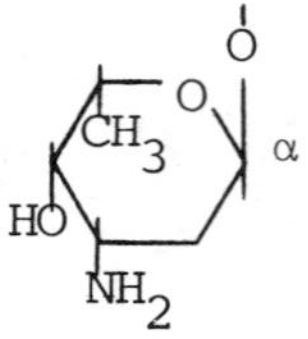 (α-pyranose; O; HO; CH$_3$; NH$_2$)	TFA	OH	0.55 125 6.25	
283464	HO	TFA	OH	0.65 148 50.00↑	1.08 189 100.00

The first compound in each section of Table XXI is a disaccharide anthracycline. The terminal sugar of the disaccharide in a given section of the table is the same as the sugar of the mono-saccharide analog or analogs listed in that section.

In the first section the disaccharide analog of daunomycin, NSC-268712, appears slightly more active than daunomycin. One might surmise on the basis of the trisaccharide-monosaccharide comparisons of both the aclacinomycin and bohemic acid families, that a longer sugar chain is partly responsible for higher activity. Note also that the adriamycin monosaccharide analog in every section shows greater activity than the corresponding daunomycin disaccharide.

Comparison of NSC-312889 and NSC-268712 carrying the same disaccharide units show an unexpected reverse in the normal order of activity; the daunomycin analog is more active than the adriamycin analog. Thus substitution on the sugar moiety directly attached to the aglycone in a disaccharide anthracycline may influence activity to an important extent.

TABLE XXII
Refer to figure 6.

OTHER ANTHRACYCLINES

R= OCH₃; H for NSC-320299   R₁=H   R₂'=H; TFA for NSC-291098   R₂=

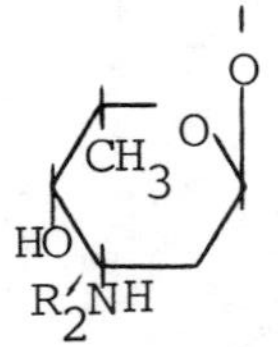

NSC	Rφ	R₄	R₃	R₅	Q01DX9 D-1	Q04DX3 D-5
294827	H-	CH₃C(=O)▲	H-	H-		0.78 136 25.00
320299	CH₃C~	CH₃C(=O)▲	HO....	H-	0.67 118 9.60	
320300	CH₃O▲	CH₃C(=O)▲	HO....	H-		0.79 138 9.60
304942	H-	CH₃C....(=O)	HO▲	CH₃O....		0.66 115 50.00
298227	H-	CH₃C(=O)▲	HO....	CH₃O▲		0.76 133 12.50
312888	H-	CH₃C(=O)▲	HO....	N₃▲		0.78 136 25.00
302669	H-	CH₃C(=O)▲	HO....	CH₃O▲		0.81 141 6.25
294401	H-	HOCH₂C(=O)▲	⎫ —CH₂— ⎭			0.58 100 50.00↑
291098	H-	CH₃C(=O)~	⎫ —N₂CH₂— ⎭			0.58 100 200.00↑

On the intermittent schedule (Q04DX3 D-5), daunomycin, NSC-294827 and NSC-320300 demonstrate equivalent activity (the average A/P ratio for daunomycin is 0.82). Thus the 8-position methoxy group appears to have little effect on the A/P ratio. However an 8-position methyl group apparently reduces the activity as suggested by comparison on the daily (Q01DX9 D-1) schedule of NSC-320299 and daunomycin (average A/P = 0.79).

Both the 8- and 10-methoxy substituted analogs (NSC-320300 and NSC-298227), as well as the 10-azido substituted NSC-312888, show comparable activity suggesting that small or linear polar groups at the 8- or 10-position whether strongly or weakly electron withdrawing have essentially no influence on activity.

The unnatural configuration at the 9-position causes a definite drop in the A/P ratio (see NSC-304942). A similar effect occurs when the 9, 10-positions are bridged as in NSC-294401 and NSC-291098. In these compounds there is no 9-position hydroxy group and the A-ring is locked into an unfavorable conformation.

The 10-methoxy adriamycin analog, NSC-302669, has low activity in comparison to adriamycin. However, this is not unexpected since in many cases substitution on adriamycin at other positions also causes a drop in the A/P ratio.

AGLYCONE A$_2$ =

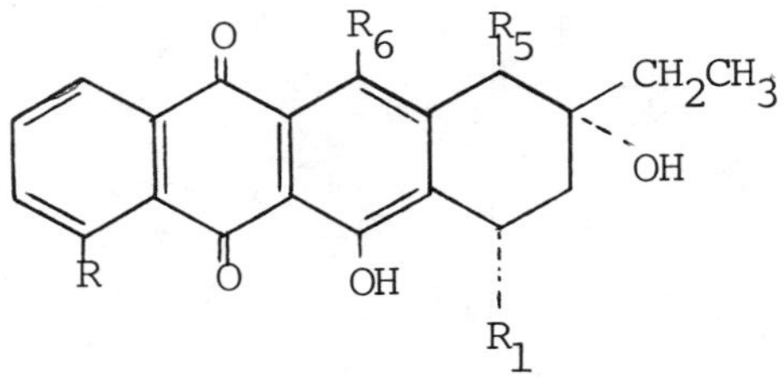

SUGAR =

FIGURE 8

TABLE XXIII   10–CARBOMETHOXY ANTHRACYCLINES
refer to figure 8 for aglycone

R$_6$=OH

R$_1$= (sugar structure)

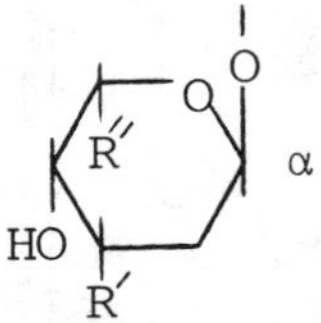

NSC	R	R'	R''	R$_5$	Q01DX9	D-1	Q04DX3	D-5
271883	-OH	-OH	-H	-COOCH$_3$	0.50	115	12.50	
278011	-OH	-OH	-CH$_3$	-COOCH$_3$			0.68 119	100
263854	-OH	-NH$_2$	-CH$_3$	-COOCH$_3$	0.64	145	8.00	
273428	-OCH$_3$	-NH$_2$	-CH$_3$	-H	0.74	169	1.56	

42

The A/P ratio for NSC-278011 is 0.14 of a unit below that of daunomycin on the intermittent (Q04DX3 D-5) schedule, and on the daily (Q01DX9 D-1) schedule the ratios for NSC-271883 and NSC-263854 fall 0.29 and 0.15 lower, respectively. Only the anthracycline without the 10-carbomethoxy group, NSC-273428, has an A/P value close to that for daunomycin.

Hydrogen bonding between the 11-hydroxy (R_6) and the 10-carbomethoxy groups may influence the activity of the compounds. The observed drop in activity is most likely due to some spatial effect of the carbomethoxy group on the 9-position substituents.

TABLE XXIV

THE ACLACINOMYCINS

refer to figure 8 for aglycone A_2 structure

$R=OH$ $R_6=H$ $R_5= \overset{O}{\overset{\|}{C}}OCH_3$

$R_1 =$

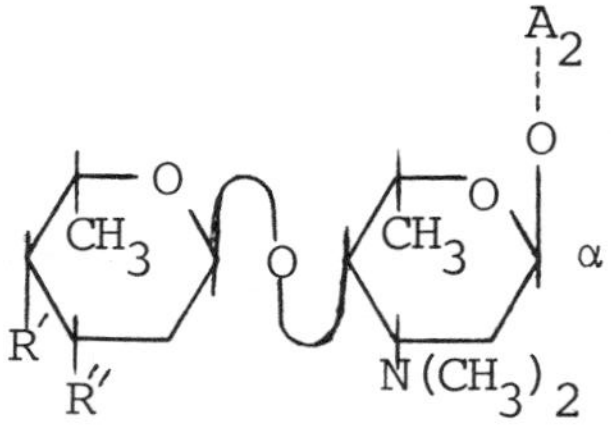

NSC	R'	R''	Q01DX9 D-1			Q04 DX3 D-1*			Q04DX3 D-5		
208734	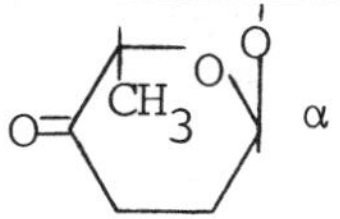	OH	1.04	236	8.00	0.74	203	9.00	1.05	184	9.40
208735	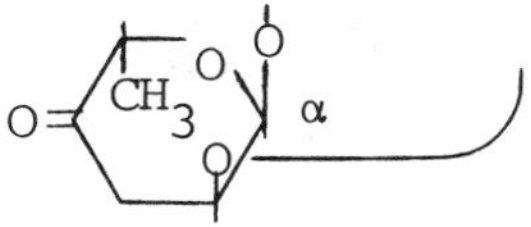		0.71	162	4.00						

*Adriamycin average values for schedule Q04DX3 D-1 are A/P=1.00, %T/C=273, dose=4.5 mg/kg/injection.

43

The A/P ratio for aclacinomycin A (NSC-208734) is close to that for adriamycin. The two compounds differ in the nature of the substituents on their aglycones. Especially noticeable is the 10-carbomethoxy group and the attached trisaccharide.

The lower activity (A/P=0.71) of aclacinomycin B (NSC-208735) may result from the nature and resistance to cleavage of the terminal sugar of the trisaccharide chain. Some support for this argument is found in the fact that the removal of the terminal sugar of aclacinomycin A would produce a compound similar in structure to NSC-219941, a bohemic acid disaccharide derivative (see Table XXV), which exhibited activity equivalent to that of aclacinomycin A on the daily (Q01DX9 D-1) schedule.

AGLYCONE A$_3$ =

SUGAR =

FIGURE 9

TABLE XXV   THE BOHEMIC ACID COMPLEX

refer to figure 9 for aglycone A$_3$ structure

R$_1$ sugar for section 1 of Table XXV

R$_1$ sugar for section 2 of Table XXV

45

TABLE XXV   (Cont'd)   THE BOHEMIC ACID COMPLEX

NSC	R'	R''	Q01DX9 D-1	Q04DX3 D-5 or D-1[b]
Section 1				
272352	OH	CH_3	0.64 145 12.00	0.65 114 18.80 (D-5)
219941	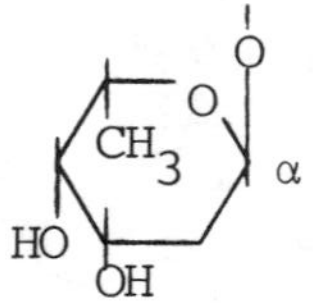 (sugar structure: CH_3, HO, OH, α, O)	CH_3	0.98 222 1.60	0.80 217 5.76 (D-1)
304416[a]	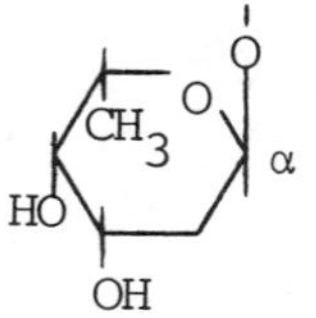 (sugar structure: CH_3, HO, OH, α, O)	CH_3		0.74 129 25.00 (D-5)

(a) *The configuration of the groups in the 10-position are reversed i.e. the carboxymethyl group is below the aglycone ring and hydrogen above.*

(b) *Adriamycin average values for schedule Q04DX3   D-1 are A/P=1.00, %T/C=273, dose=4.5mg/kg/injection.*

Footnotes (a) and (b) to Section 1 of this Table also apply to Section 2.

TABLE XXV (Cont'd)

THE BOHEMIC ACID COMPLEX

NSC	R'	R''	R'''	Q01DX9 D-1			Q04DX3 D-5 or D-1(b)		
Section 2									
304415(a)	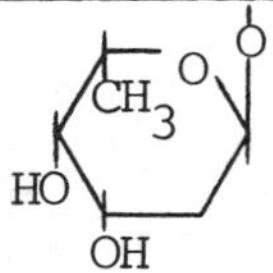	OH	H				0.77	134	25.00(D-5)
265211	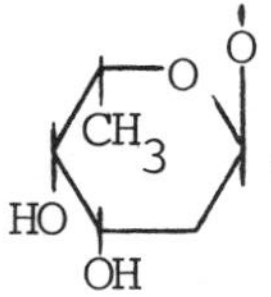	OH	CH$_3$	0.74	169	1.00	0.71	194	1.80(D-1)
304417(a)	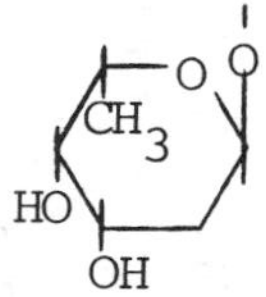	OH	CH$_3$				0.77	134	50.00(D-5)
243022	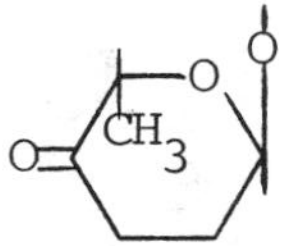	OH	CH$_3$				0.68	186	2.88(D-1)
293858	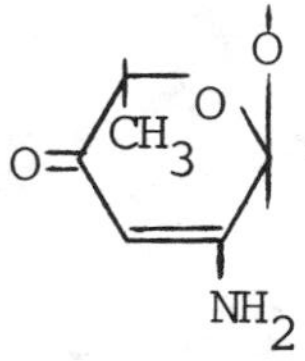	OH	CH$_3$	0.80	182	1.50			
243023	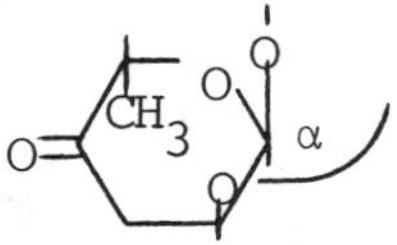		CH$_3$				0.69	191	2.16(D-1)

47

A bohemic acid aglycone has an additional hydroxy group located at the 1-position that is not present in the aclacinomycin aglycone. A comparison of the relative contribution of the two aglycones to anticancer activity is possible. Since aclacinomycin A, NSC-208734, A/P=0.74 and the bohemic acid, NSC-243022, A/P=0.68 (Q04DX3 D-1) have identical sugars, the aclacinomycin aglycone shows slight improvement over the bohemic acid aglycone.

The aglycone of bohemic acid is inferior to that of daunomycin. Thus the daunomycin analog, NSC-258812 (Table XVIII), and the bohemic acid analog, NSC-272352 (section 1 Table XXV), with the same dimethylamino sugar give A/P ratios of 0.83 and 0.65, respectively (Q04 DX3 D-5 schedule).

The addition of a 2'-deoxy-L-fucose unit to NSC-272352 (Table XXV) results in NSC-219941, apparently the most active of the bohemic acids. Since the addition of 2'-deoxy-L-fucose to daunomycinone also gives a more active analog (NSC-284682 Table XIII), it appears that the increase in sugar chain length and nature of the terminal sugar in the disaccharide, NSC-219941, is the reason for the enhancement in activity.

If the nature of the terminal sugar, or its linkage to the disaccharide unit, is important to activity (as it appeared to be in the aclacinomycins of Table XXIV) then NSC-265211, NSC-243022 and NSC-243023 should demonstrate activities different from each other. Perhaps the reason the data are contraindicating is that the intermittent treatment schedule compared to the daily schedule does not differentiate between the pharmacokinetic parameters of the analogs.

Compounds having the same terminal sugar NSC-304415, NSC-304416 and NSC-304417 show equivalent A/P ratios on the more stringent schedule. Also of interest is the fact that monomethyl and dimethylamino compounds have the same activity (NSC-304415 and NSC-304417).

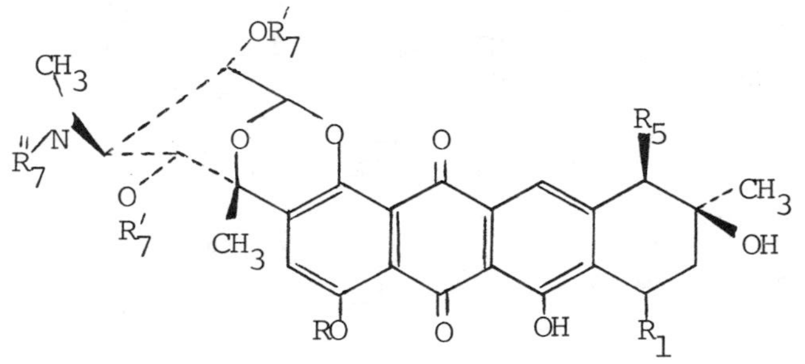

FIGURE 10*

The structure in Figure 10 is based on a composite of X-ray crystallographic and circular dichroism studies. There is some uncertainty in this representation and the actual structure may be a mirror image of all parts except the sugar nogalose.

The nogalamycins screened by the National Cancer Institute are divided into three groups: nogarols, nogamycins, and nogalarols. Nogamycins, in contrast to nogarols, have a sugar at the 7-position; neither has a substituent at the 10-position. The nogalarols have both a 7-position sugar and a 10-position substituent.

*Paul F. Wiley et. al. J. Org. Chem. 44,4034 (1979).

49

TABLE XXVI
refer to figure 10 for structure

THE NOGAROLS

NSC	R_1	R=R$_5'$=R$_7$=H Q01DX9 D-1			R$_7''$=CH$_3$ Q04DX3 D-5		
269148	CH$_3$O—	1.31	297	12.50	1.06	184	150.00
314249	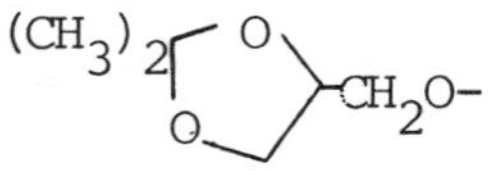 (CH$_3$)$_2$ CH$_2$O—	0.54	123	16.00			
308327	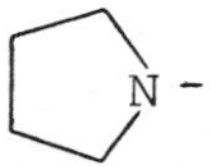 N— (pyrrolidine)	0.61	140	50.00			
308328	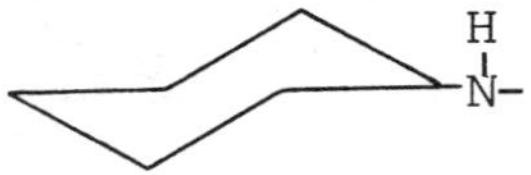 cyclohexyl—NH—N—	0.58	133	20.00			

Three of the four nogarols in Table XXVI have low A/P ratios, the exception is NSC-269148. A possible explanation for the high activity is that a readily cleavable group at the 7-position is necessary for metabolic activation. Also the hydrophobic nature of the group at the position undoubtedly plays a role in the degree of activity.

TABLE XXVII
refer to figure 10 for structure

THE NOGAMYCINS

R5=H

R1 =

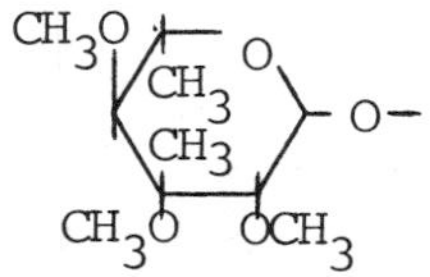

NSC	R	...R1;►R	R_7'	R_7''	Q01DX9 D-1	Q04DX3 D-1*
314246	H-	α	H-	H-		0.45 124 33.00↑
265450	H-	α	H-	CH3-	0.85 193 5.00	
293864	CH3-	α	H-	CH3-	0.74 168 20.00	
308326	H-	β	H-	CH3-	0.65 147 12.50	
321245	H-	α	Ac-	CH3-		0.51 141 50.00↑

The good but not exceptional A/P ratio of NSC-265450 may be due to a balance of effects, the hydrophobic nature and the unique structure of the L-sugar, nogalose (nogalose has the manno-configuration as in NSC-331962 Table XIII).

As noted previously (see Table XII) the change from a hydroxy to methoxy at the 4-position results in a decrease in activity due to the loss of an ionizable hydroxy group (compare NSC-265450 to NSC-293864).

* Note: Change in day of the injection. The average adriamycin value for calculating the A/P ratio is given as a footnote to Table XXIV.

51

The low activity of NSC–308326 (compared to NSC–265450) is attributable to the β-form of nogalose. That the compound has some activity probably is the result of the same side location of the A-ring 7-oxygen and 9-OH.

TABLE XXVIII
refer to figure 10 for structure

THE NOGALAROLS

$R_5 = \overset{O}{\overset{\|}{C}}OR_5'$

$R_1 =$

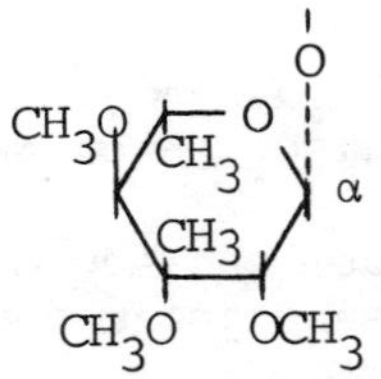

NSC	R	R5'	R7'	R7"	Q01DX9 D-1			Q04X3 D-1*		
314241	H	CH₃–	H–	H–				0.58	160	25.00
314242	H	CH₃–	H–	CHO–				0.41	112	25.00
265449	H	H–	H–	CH₃–	0.61	138	10.00			
70845	H	CH₃–	H–	CH₃–	0.66	150	1.00	0.53	147	1.80
314244	H	CH₃–	Ac–	CH₃–				0.53	147	3.12

The nogalarols possess in addition to the sugar, nogalose, a 10-position carbomethoxy group (R₅). Table XXVIII illustrates the low A/P ratios of these compounds. A comparison of the A/P ratios of the nogamycin, NSC–265450, and the nogalarol, NSC–70845, supports the earlier observation with the anthracyclines of Table XXIII that the 10-position carbomethoxy group is not favorable to good activity.

* Note: change in day of injection.

SUPPLEMENT

There are four additional types of anthracyclines which were tested in the NCI program but are not discussed in the main body of this chapter mostly for proprietary reasons. They are the metal salt complexes, polymer complexes, bishydrazide derivatives of daunomycin and the 5-imino-daunomycin and -adriamycin (NSC-254681 and NSC-332988). Of the small number of metal complexes tested only one (NSC-267703) represented as $[ADR\ Fe_3Cl_{10}H]^+$ has activity which is better than that of adriamycin on the more stringent P-388 schedule.

Many complexes of adriamycin and daunomycin have been synthesized with various polymers including DNA and some show excellent antitumor activity in P-388 on the Q04DX3 D-5 schedule.

The linkage of two daunomycin units through a dicarboxy-dihydrazide unit generally yields compounds with A/P ratios (Q04DX3 D-5) of 1.29 to 0.83 whereas the A/P for daunomycin on the same schedule is 0.82.

Imino-daunomycin and -adriamycin represent an interesting structural change in which a quinone oxygen has been replaced by an isosteric NH group at the 5-position. Such a modification has little effect on the activity of the dauno-mycin (A/P=0.78,%T/C=136,dose=3.0, Q04DX3 D-5 for NSC-254681), but increases the activity of the adriamycin (A/P=1.24,%T/C= 217,dose=100.00, Q04DX3 D-5 for NSC-332988).

Summary

A wide variety of anthracyclines have been evaluated by NCI in the P-388 lymphocytic leukemia test system. These data were used to calculate an analog/parent ratio (A/P ratio) using the maximum T/C values obtained with the analog and the average historical maximum T/C value for adriamycin. This ratio numerically minimizes all but relatively significant differences in activity of the tested compounds.

An alternative approach would have been to calculate an A/P ratio using data for adriamycin and the analog obtained in the same experiment. This approach was not employed as direct comparative data were not available for every analog and also any unusual T/C value for adriamycin would have skewed the analysis.

Key structural features that were discussed in their
relationship to anticancer activity of an anthracycline are
sumarized below:

Sugars, Position of Attachment on Aglycone

The sugar may be attached either to ring A or ring D or
to both rings. The sugar (or sugar chain) is attached to
ring A in daunomycin, adriamycin, aclacinomycin, rhodomycin,
carminomycin and bohemic acid analogs, to ring D in the
nogarol analogs and to both rings in the nogamycin and
nogalarol analogs. Most of these classes contain at least
one compound with significant antitumor activity.

Type of Sugar

One of the most active anthracyclines, at least in the
daunomycin and adriamycin series, has a 7-position
desaminosugar rather that an aminosugar. Even more
surprising is the fact that an iodo desaminosugar analog
(NSC-331962) shows excellent activity. The order of
activity based on the sugar family increases from D to L.
Based on the configuration in the L-family, the activity
increases in the order: lyxo, ribo*, arabino.

1. Substituent(s) on the amino group of the sugar.
   An N-benzyl group substituted on the daunosaminyl
   group of daunomycin or replacement of the amino group
   of daunomycin by an appropriately polar substituted
   piperidino ring (in which the ring nitrogen and the
   daunosaminyl nitrogen are one and the same) provide
   for excellent activity relative to both the unsubstituted and alkyl substituted aminosugar analogs of
   daunomycin.

2. Sugar Chain
   Daunomycin disaccharide analogs whose terminal sugar
   corresponds to the sugar in the monosaccharide parent
   are more active than the parent. The enhanced activity
   is apparently dependent on either the terminal sugar
   configuration or substitution. Trisaccharide anthracyclines provide additional evidence in support of this
   phenomenon. In the trisaccharides apparently two factors
   are involved: 1) attachments between the terminal sugar
   and the rest of the molecule, 2) the configuration and
   substitution of the terminal sugar.

*Position in sequence somewhat uncertain due to insufficient
 test data.*

It is interesting that substitution on the amino group of the aminosugar directly attached to the aglycone in a sugar chain may or may not influence the activity of the anthracycline. Thus a trifluoroacetyl group drastically reduces activity. However, removal of a methyl group from a dimethyl substituted aminosugar in the chain has little effect on activity.

A-Ring Substitution

1. Minimum Requirements.
It is reasonably clear from the data in the tables that both the 7- and 9- positions (A-ring) must be substituted by appropriate groups to obtain compounds of good to excellent antitumor activity. For example, little if any activity is shown when a sugar or sugar chain is missing from the molecule, even when the prerequisite group is on the 9-position. In addition, the compound is inactive if the sugar (daunosamine) at the 7- or 8- position is the only group on ring A. In the case of the nogalamycins, where a sugar is attached to the 1- and 2- positions of ring D, the substituent at the 7-position of ring A, whether a sugar or non-sugar, needs to be relatively readily cleaved in vivo for activity. Thus in the nogarol series, only 7-Omen, NSC-269148, shows good anticancer activity.

2. Stereochemistry; A-Ring.
It is possible that the absolute chirality at the 7- and 9-positions is unimportant to activity as long as the attached groups are on the same side of the aglycone plane. However, some nogalamycins, based on the presently available structure, seem to violate the same side requirement and still show significant activity (e.g. the nogamycins). Perhaps for nogamycins the stabilizing effect of a possible hydrogen bond between the 9-hydroxyl and the 7-position sugar is not needed due to the additional strongly attached sugar on the D-ring.

3. Effect of Adjacent Groups on A-Ring.
Substituting a small or linear polar group at either the 8- or 10- position in an active anthracycline appears to have little effect on activity. The situation is different for a carbomethoxy group at the 10-position which reduces activity. A double bond between the 9,10 positions or a bridge encompassing these positions also reduces the anticancer activity. The altered conformation of the A-ring may account for this reduction in activity.

4. Nature of the 9-Substituents.
The 9-position may carry a variety of groups. A hydroxyl
group alone, or an acetyl group alone, provide active
compounds. However, most of the active compounds have
both a hydroxyl and a group like acetyl, hydroxyacetyl,
1-hydroxy ethyl, 1,2-dihydroxyethyl, methyl, or ethyl at
the 9-position. Also some very active compounds are
esters of the hydroxyacetyl group and others are daunomycin hydrazides. It is probable that activition of the
hydrolyzable derivatives occurs through metabolic cleavage
to yield the original anthracycline.

D-Ring Substitution

Two types of anthracycline analogs provide an indication
of the effect of small groups on the D-ring towards overall
activity. In the daunomycin analogs the activity increases
as the 4-position substituent is changed from OCH_3 to OH to
H. In the adriamycin series the activity increases from the
parent adriamycin to 4-demethoxyadriamycin to 2,3-dimethyl-4-
demethoxyadriamycin. The D-ring sugar in the nogalamycins
also may contribute analogous effects towards the activity
of this parent and its derivatives.

Aglycones-Relative Contribution to Anticancer Activity.

It would be interesting to compare the relative contributions towards antitumor activity of different aglycones in
a series of anthracyclines. Available data allows a comparison of one bohemic acid analog with a corresponding
daunomycin analog (NSC-272352, NSC-258812) and a second
bohemic acid analog with aclacinomycin A (NSC-243022,
NSC-208734). However, data are not available to make a
direct comparison of the aclacinomycin and daunomycin
aglycones.

ACKNOWLEDGMENTS

The assistance of the following is appreciated:

DR. FREDERICO ARCAMONE.........Institute Ricerca Farmitalia
For declassification of many Farmitalia anthracyclines.

DR. EDWARD ACTON and DR. THOMAS SMITH.....SRI International
DR. HASSAN EL KHADEM......Michigan Technological University
For furnishing stereochemical information on several
compounds.

DR. RUTH GERAN................ Drug Evaluation Branch, NCI
For comments regarding test systems.

DR. PAUL WILEY..........................The Upjohn Company
For stereochemistry of the nogalamycin analogs.

MS. EDNA GOODMAN...Drug Synthesis and Chemistry Branch, NCI
For typing manuscript and drawing of structures.

MS. EVELYN WALL ....Information Technology Branch, NCI
For computer searches.

RECENT DEVELOPMENTS IN THE CHEMISTRY
OF DOXORUBICIN-RELATED ANTHRACYCLINE
GLYCOSIDES

Federico Arcamone
Giuseppe Cassinelli
Sergio Penco

Ricerca & Sviluppo Chimico
Farmitalia Carlo Erba
Milan, Italy

I. INTRODUCTION

This presentation represents an account of work recently performed within the frame of a program concerning the development of new and clinically useful antitumor anthracyclines related to doxorubicin (1). The objectives of doxorubicin analogues development are (i) new agents with lower toxicity thus allowing higher dosages with consequent enhanced efficacy of treatment, (ii) new agents active by the oral route, (iii) new agents endowed with diminished cumulative cardiotoxicity thus allowing prolongation of treatment, and (iv) new agents with wider antineoplastic spectrum or effective towards tumors not responsive to doxorubicin.

The approaches used for doxorubicin analogues development were the following:

(a) Simple derivatization of the biosynthetic antibiotics.
(b) Synthesis of glycosides with different sugar residues.
(c) Total synthesis and glycosidation of new aglycones.
(d) Chemical modification of the biosynthetic glycosides.
(e) Semisynthesis by chemical modification and glycosidation of the biosynthetic aglycones.
(f) New biosynthetic compounds produced by *S. peucetius* mutant strains.

In this account we shall deal with topics related with points
(b), (d), (e) and (f) as defined above. In addition, the synthesis of the enantio form of 4-demethoxydaunorubicin and data concerning the biological activity of the new compounds will be
shown.

II. NEW SEMISYNTHETIC GLYCOSIDES

Approach (b) has been one of the most important fields of
the investigation in our laboratory. This because the presence
of the sugar moiety is a strict structural requirement for bioactivity and because of the known dependence of enzymic and bio
logical transport processes from structure and absolute configuration of carbohydrate derivatives. Daunosamine related ami-
nosugars are also known constituents of the molecule of other
antibiotics. This approach, leading to new semisynthetic glycosides, has resulted in a number of biologically active analogues, among which 4'-epidoxorubicin and 4'-deoxydoxorubicin
are presently developed as less toxic agents and hopefully endowed with a wider spectrum of activity (1,2). Other daunorubicin and doxorubicin analogues modified at the 4' position are
represented by the new C-4'-methyl glycosides Ia-d, IIa-d, obtained by coupling of daunomycinone with the suitably protected
target sugar halides in the presence of silver triflate according to a general method developed in our laboratory (3).

*SCHEME 1. Synthesis of 4-C-Methyl Analogues of Daunosamine
and Acosamine*

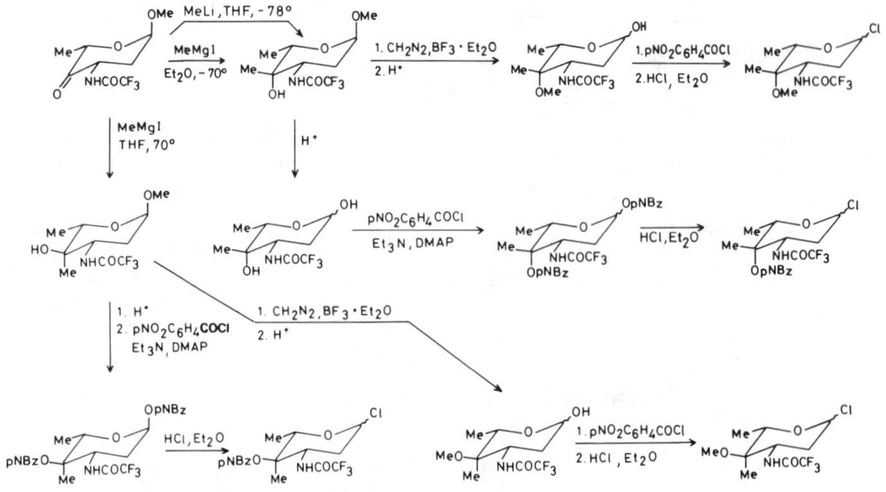

Scheme 1 reports the sequence of reactions followed for the synthesis of 1-chloro 4-C-methyl protected analogues of daunosamine and acosamine using, as starting material, methyl N--trifluoroacetyl-α -daunosamide, *via* the corresponding 4-keto derivative (4,5). The doxorubicin analogues Ic-d, IIc-d are obtained from the corresponding daunorubicins *via* bromination at C-14 and hydrolysis (6).

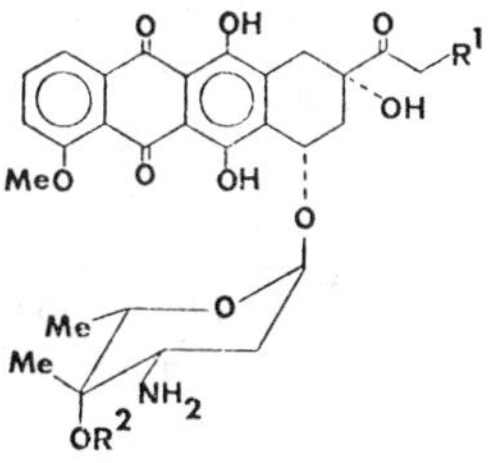

Ia,IIa : $R^1 = R^2 = H$
Ib,IIb : $R^1 = H$, $R^2 = Me$
Ic,IIc : $R^1 = OH$, $R^2 = H$
Id,IId : $R^1 = OH$, $R^2 = Me$

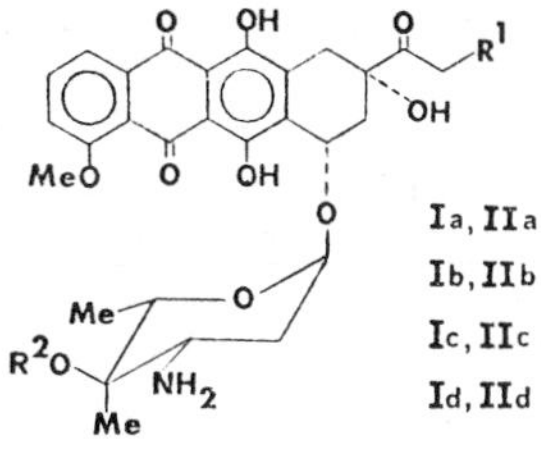

I   II

The chemistry of the new branched-chain analogues of daunosamine has been extended as shown in Scheme 2. In fact the me

SCHEME 2 . Synthesis of New Branched Sugar Derivatives Related to Daunosamine

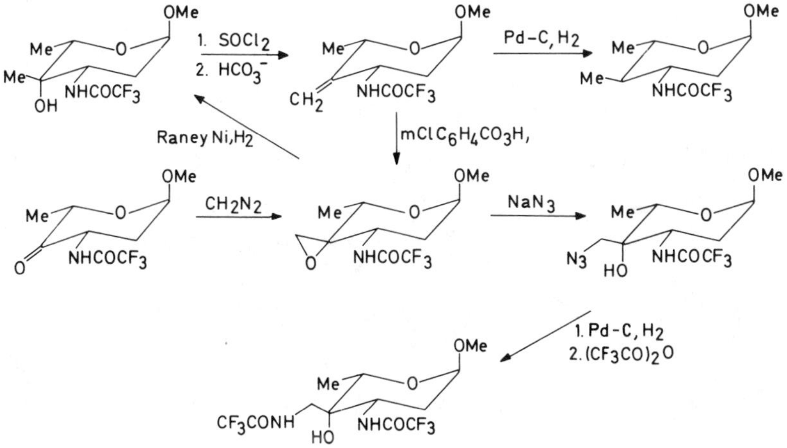

thyl 4-C-methyl-N-trifluoroacetyl- ∝-daunosaminide is easily
converted into the corresponding 4-methylene derivative, which
in turn can be transformed *via* a stereoselective reduction in
the 4-C-methyl-4-deoxy analogue and *via* a stereoselective epoxidation followed by azidolysis in the 4-C-aminomethyldaunosa̲
mine derivative (6).

Concomitantly, a new addition to the series of the 4'-0-me̲
thyl analogues (7) is provided by the synthesis of 3',4'-diepi̲
-4'-0-methyl-daunorubicin and doxorubicin (L-*ribo* configuration)
by the standard procedure indicated in Scheme 3 (8).

A different series of potentially useful compounds is that
of the furanoside analogues of the antitumor anthracyclines.

The example reported in Scheme 4 is concerned with the syn̲
thesis of 7-0-(3-amino-2,3,6-trideoxy-∝ -L-*ribo*-hexofurano̲
syl)-daunomycinone, a new isomer of daunorubicin, from 5-0-p-
-nitrobenzoyl-2,3,6- t r i d e o x y-3-trifluoroacetamido-L-*ribo*-hexo̲
furanosyl chloride in turn obtained from the equilibrium mixtu̲
re of furanosyl glycosides derived from N-trifluoroacetylristo̲
samine (9).

SCHEME 3 . Synthesis of 3',4'-diepi-4'-0 - methyl-
doxorubicin

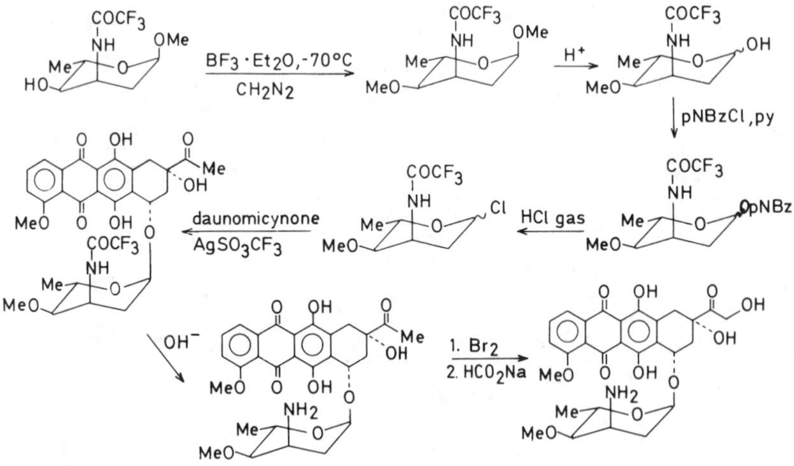

SCHEME 4. Synthesis of 7-0-(3-amino-2,3,6-trideoxy-α-
-L-ribo-hexofuranosyl)-daunomicynone

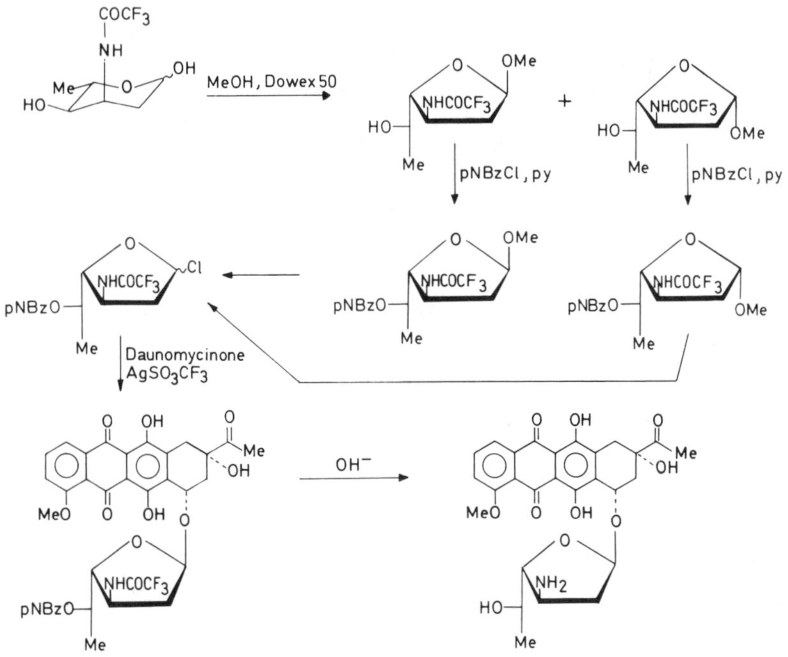

III. CHEMICAL MODIFICATION OF THE BIOSYNTHETIC GLYCOSIDES

As it was reported in previous presentations (10-12) or published in reviews covering also the patent literature (1, 13-15), chemical reactions of daunorubicin and its derivatives have been explored in our laboratory both as a source of new analogues and for the establishment of structure-activity relationship. The new compounds obtained along this line were: (a) compounds bearing modifications at the C-9 side chain by way of carbonyl reactions, nucleophilic substitutions on 14--bromodaunorubicin, or side chain oxidative degradation; (b) compounds modified at C-9 and C-10 obtained via an intermediate 9,10-anhydro derivative and also 9,10-epoxide; (c) compounds possessing two sugar residues prepared by glycosidation at C-4' of N-trifluoroacetyldaunorubicin. Recent investigations in this area have been concerned inter alia with the direct modification of daunorubicin at C-4' in order to obtain the pharmacologically important 4'-epi and 4'-deoxydoxorubicin without splitting of the biosynthetically available glycoside.

The first synthesis of 4'-epidoxorubicin (4) involved the
coupling of N,O-ditrifluoroacetylacosaminyl chloride with a
protected adriamycinone derivative according to a modified
Koenigs-Knorr reaction to give a 50% yield of the protected
α-glycoside along with a 7% of the corresponding β-glycosi-
de. Chromatographic separation followed by hydrolysis of the
protecting groups afforded 4'-epidoxorubicin (III).

III   IV

Further improvement was achieved by the use of the already
mentioned triflate procedure in the coupling of daunomycinone
with N,O-trifluoroacetylacosaminyl chloride, which gave stereo
selectively 4'-epi-N-trifluoroacetyldaunorubicin in high yield
(80%). The corresponding doxorubicin analogue was subsequently
obtained by a standard procedure (16).

More recently inversion of the configuration at C-4' in
the biosynthetic product, daunorubicin, has been carried out
upon oxidation of N-trifluoroacetyldaunorubicin with a modified Moffat reagent to give the 4'-ketone IV, whose reduction
with sodium borohydride afforded 4'-epi-N-trifluoroacetyldauno
rubicin in high yield (17). The reaction sequence was further
extended to afford the semisynthetic 4'-deoxydaunorubicin and
4'-deoxydoxorubicin as indicated in Scheme 5 (17).

It should be noted here that when the preparation of a 4'-
-O-triflate starting from daunorubicin N-trifluoroacetate was
attempted, the derivative could not be isolated, but a rearrangement product was obtained instead (Scheme 6). On the
other hand the configuration at C-3' of the key-intermediate IV
can be easily inverted by treatment with buffered silicagel
(phosphate buffer, pH 7), to give, after reduction, the analogues having the L-*ribo* and L-*xylo* configuration of the sugar
moiety.

SCHEME 5. Partial Synthesis of 4'-Deoxydoxorubicin from Daunorubicin

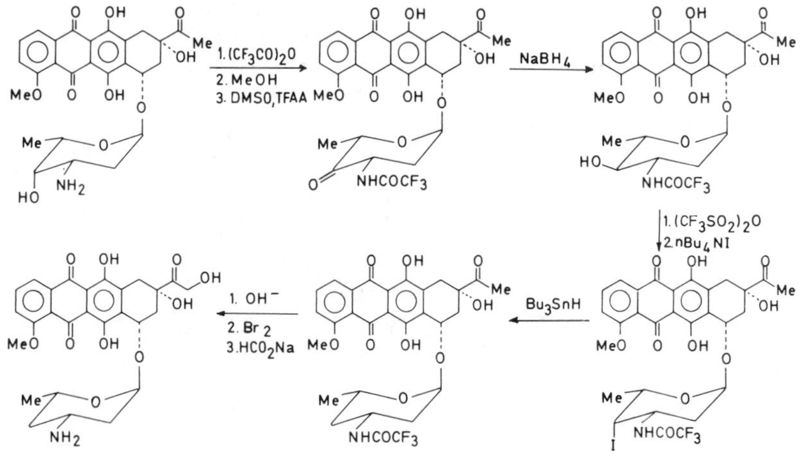

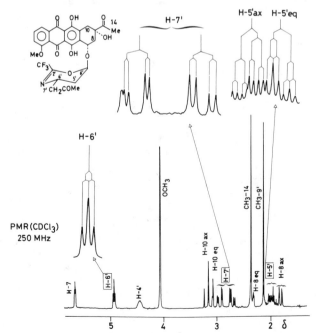

SCHEME 6. Structure and PMR Spectrum of the Rearrangement Product

Taking account of the pharmacological importance of the 4'-
-O-methyl derivatives (1,14), experiments   aimed to the direct
methylation of the N-trifluoroacetyl glycosides were also performed. The results (Scheme 7) indicated the higher reactivity
of the 11-hydroxyl in N-trifluoroacetyldaunorubicin, whereas in
the corresponding 11-deoxy analogue the methylation of the 4'-
-hydroxyl was nearly complete although accompanied in part by
methylation of the phenolic group at C-6 (18).

Treatment of daunorubicin and doxorubicin with sodium nitri
te and aqueous acetic has opened the way to a new group of C-
-branched furanosyl glycosides. As it is shown in Scheme 8, the
product of the reaction was an aldehyde that underwent the conversion to the more stable L-*erythro* form under the action of
silicagel. The analysis of the ^{13}C-NMR (acetone-d$_6$) of the epimeric 3'-C-formyl-2',3',5'-trideoxy-pentofuranosyldaunomycino-
nes allowed identification of the same because of the upfield
shifts (due to steric interactions) shown in the L-*threo* (CHO,
191.7 ; 4-CH$_3$, 16.6) in comparison to the L-*erythro* compound
(CHO, 201.5 ; 4-CH$_3$, 20.4). The aldehyde group was also sub
jected to further transformations as indicated in Scheme 8 (19).

SCHEME 7. Methylation of N-trifluoroacetylglycosides

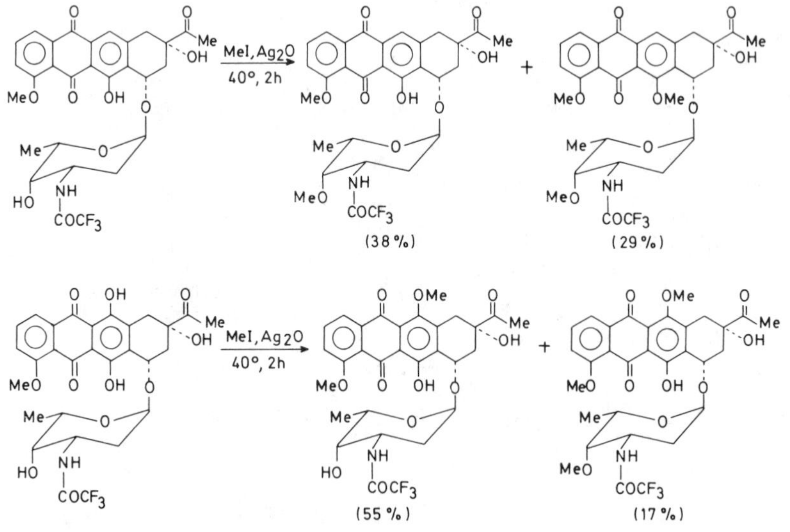

SCHEME 8. Nitrosation of Daunorubicin and Doxorubicin

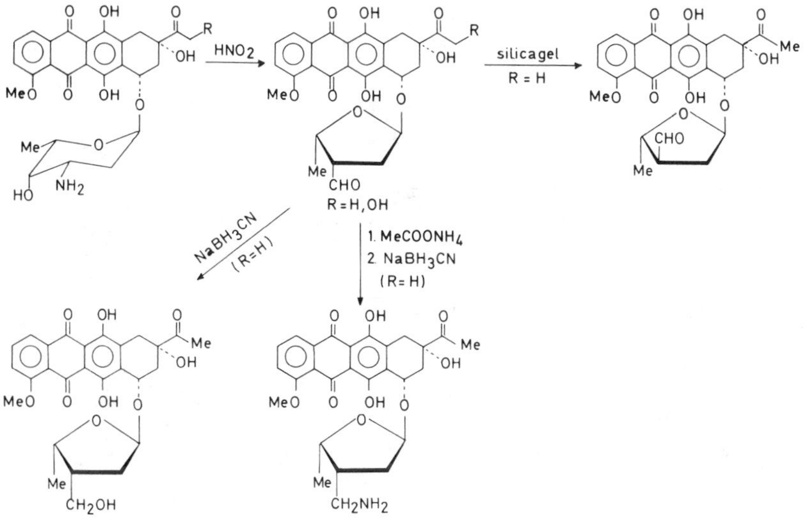

IV. SEMISYNTHESIS FROM DAUNOMYCINONE

The synthesis of the 6-and 11-methyl ethers of 4-0-demethyl daunorubicin, two structural isomers of daunorubicin, has already been reported (20). Biological testing performed under the auspices of NCI had shown that antitumor activity in the P 388 test was retained by the two analogues, especially in the former, possessing both quinone carbonyls in a chelated form. An alternative synthesis of 4-0-demethyl-6-0-methyldaunorubicin and the conversion of the latter to the corresponding doxorubicin analogue has been carried out as shown in Scheme 9. The synthetic scheme was based on the shift of the acetyl group from 6 to the 7 position occurring concomitantly to the acid catalyzed opening of the oxirane ring in 4,6,11-triacetylcarminomycinone-9,10-isopropylidene ketal. Along this line 6-0-methyl- and 6,9-di-0-methyldaunorubicins were prepared as indicated in scheme 10 whereas the synthesis of 9-0-methyldaunorubicin (Scheme 11) was also carried out in order to complete this series and derive information relevant to the consequences of 0-methylation on biological activity (21, 22).

SCHEME 9 . *Alternative Synthesis of 4-0-demethyl-*
            -6-0-Methyldoxorubicin

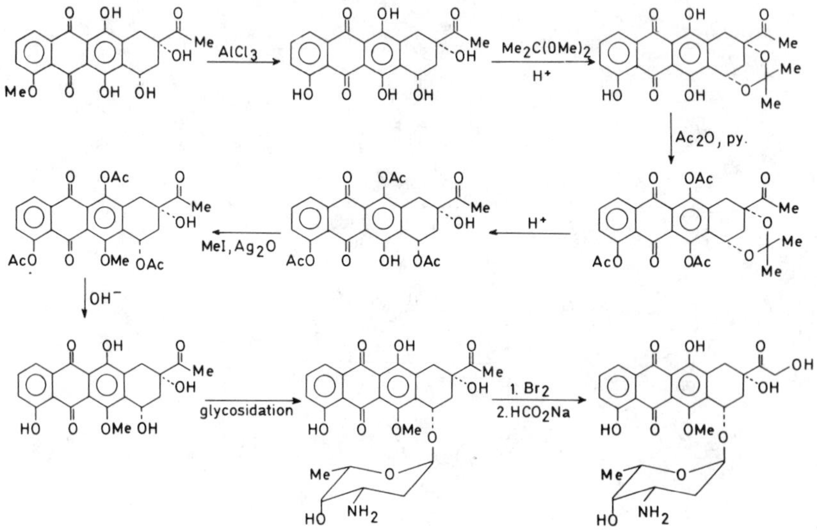

SCHEME 10. *Synthesis of 6-0-Methyl and 6,9-di-0-*
            -Methyldaunorubicins

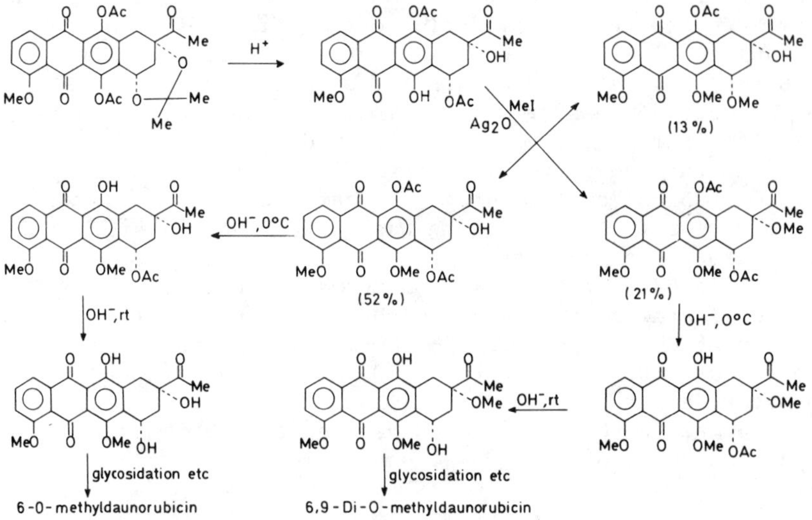

SCHEME 11. Synthesis of 9-O-Methyldaunorubicin

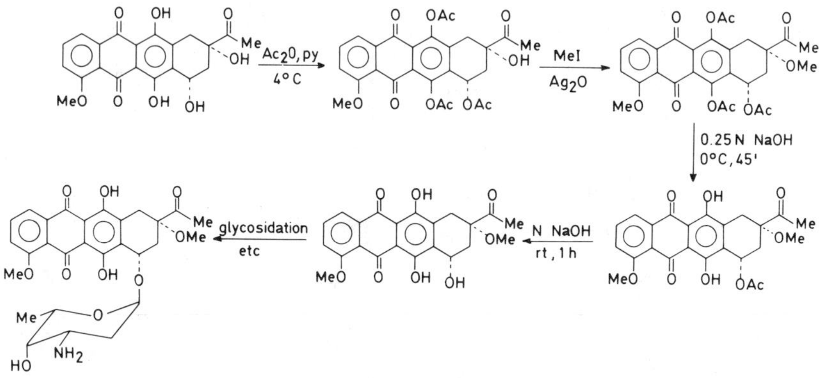

V. BIOSYNTHETIC ANALOGUES

Investigations aimed to isolate and identify new doxorubicin related compounds produced by mutant strains derived from the original daunorubicin producer, *Streptomyces peucetius*, are currently pursued in our laboratory. Different new analogues have been obtained, namely 13-dihydrocarminomycin (Va) (23), the 11-deoxy compounds in the daunorubicin-doxorubicin series (VIa-d) (24), in the carminomycin series (VIIa-b) (25) and 13-deoxycarminomycin (Vb) (26). Scheme 12 shows the reaction that allowed the chemical correlation of the different 11-deoxyanthracyclines.

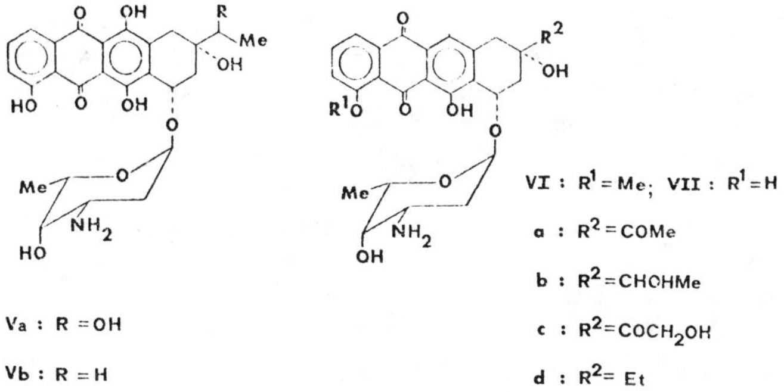

VI : R^1 = Me; VII : R^1 = H

a : R^2 = COMe

b : R^2 = CHOHMe

c : R^2 = COCH$_2$OH

d : R^2 = Et

Va : R = OH

Vb : R = H

SCHEME   12.   *Semisynthetic Correlations of 11-Deoxy
Anthracyclines derived from S.peucetius
Mutant Strains (R = H, Me)*

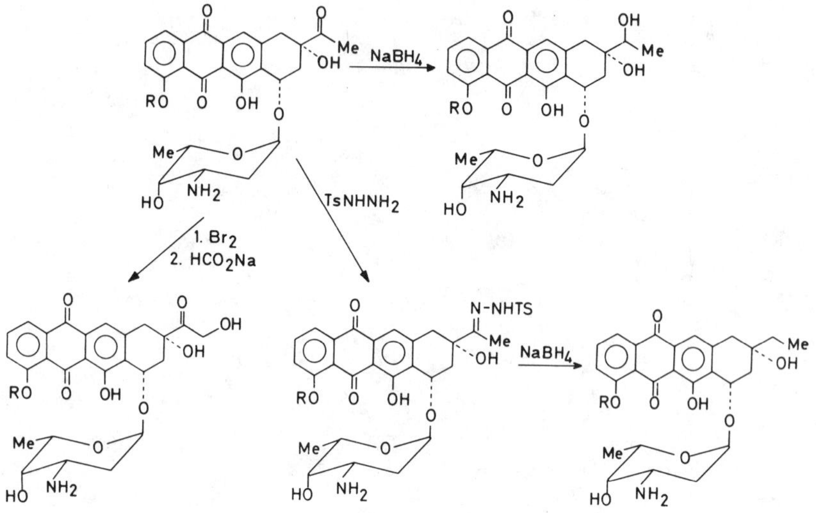

VI.   ENANTIO-4-DEMETHOXYDAUNORUBICIN

The synthesis of the enantiomeric form of natural bioactive compounds is often an attractive goal for the medicinal
chemists, because of the additional information then available on the configurational requirements for activity and of
the possible use of the unnatural form for the saturation of
non specific receptors (27). The availability of (-)-4-deme-
thoxydaunomycinone, prepared from (+)-2-acetyl-1,4-dimethoxy
tetralin according to the procedure already developed for
the synthesis of 4-demethoxydaunomycinone (1,28), prompted
us to obtain the enantio form of the strongly bioactive 4-de-
methoxydaunorubicin.

The necessary aminosugar, D-daunosamine, was obtained
starting from the already mentioned furanose form of methyl
N-trifluoroacetylristosaminide that was converted, *via* the
5-ketone, to a mixture of the starting compound and of its D-
-*lyxo* epimer (Scheme 13). Hydrolysis afforded N-trifluoroace-
tyl-D-daunosamine that was coupled with (-)-demethoxydaunomy-
cinone (29).

SCHEME 13 . *Synthesis of enantio 4-Demethoxydauno-rubicin*

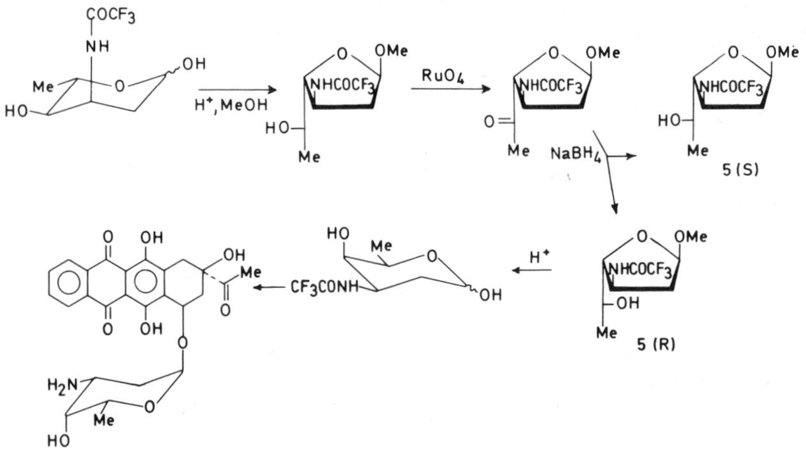

VII. BIOLOGICAL ACTIVITY

The new glycosides whose synthesis has been reported here were tested for antitumor activity in the P 388 murine lympho-cytic leukemia system by Prof. A. Di Marco, Dr. Annamaria Ca-sazza and their coworkers at Istituto Nazionale Tumori (Milan, Italy) and at Farmitalia Carlo Erba Laboratory (Nerviano, Mi-lan, Italy). All compounds were administered intraperitoneally on day 1 after tumor inoculation. Results are expressed as me-dian survival time of treated animals expressed as percent of tumor bearing untreated controls (T/C%), the optimal non toxic dose (OD $\leq$ LD$_{10}$) being indicated in parenthesis as mg/Kg body weight.

All 4'-C-methyl analogues, both in the L-*lyxo* and L-*arabino* series, were found to retain substantially the efficacy of the parent compounds as the following T/C % values were recorded: (a) daunorubicin 175 (2.9); -,4'-C-methyl 155 (20.0); -,4'--epi-4'-C-methyl 163 (0.44); doxorubicin 193 (6.6); -,4'-C--methyl 172 (7.7); -,4'-epi-4'-C-methyl 156 (2.0); (b) dauno-rubicin 163 (2.9); -,4'-C-methyl-4'-O-methyl 160 (33.7); -,4'--epi-4-C-methyl-4'-O-methyl 150 (22.5); doxorubicin 201 (6.6); -,4'-C-methyl-4'-O-methyl 172 (6.6); -,4'-epi-4'-C-methyl-4'--O-methyl 205 (10.0). Similarly behaved 3',4'-diepi-4'-O-me-thyl-doxorubicin which showed T/C % = 180 (1.9) whereas the corresponding values of doxorubicin in the same experiment were 233 (6.6). In the 4'-O-methyl series, however, the $\underline{L}$-*lyxo* compound 4'-O-methyldoxorubicin remains the most effective (1,5).

An interesting result with consequences on our general views of molecular requirements for bioactivity is the finding that the furanose analogue of 3',4'-diepidaunorubicin exhibits T/C % = 175 (66), whereas the corresponding pyranose compound gave T/C % = 181 (40). Also, the concentration inhibiting by 50% the viability of cultured HeLa cells was similar for both analogues (140 and 145 ng/ml respectively). Also, significant antitumor activity was shown by the $\underline{L}$-*threo* aldehydes reported in Scheme 8 with T/C % = 168 (50, R = H) and T/C % = 190 (100, R = OH).

Methylation of the 6- and 11-OH resulted instead in practi cally complete loss of bioactivity and of affinity for DNA as shown in a recently published paper (22). Similarly, as expected, no cytotoxic activity was shown by the enantio-4-demethoxydaunorubicin in cultured HeLa cells in vitro.

REFERENCES

1. Arcamone, F., "Doxorubicin", in Medicinal Chemistry Series Vol. 17, Academic Press, New York, (1981).
2. Casazza, A.M., paper presented at the International Symposium on Anthracycline Antibiotics in Cancer Therapy, New York, Sept. 16-18 (1981).
3. Arcamone, F., Penco, S., Redaelli, S., and Hanessian, S., *J. Med. Chem. 19*, 1424 (1976).
4. Arcamone, F., Penco, S., Vigevani, A., Redaelli, S., Fran chi, G., Di Marco, A., Casazza, A.M., Dasdia, T., Formelli, F., Necco, A., and Soranzo, C., *J. Med. Chem. 18*, 703 (1975).
5. Bargiotti, A., Cassinelli, G., Penco, S., Vigevani, A., and Arcamone, F., *Carbohydr. Res.*, in press.
6. Bargiotti, A., Casazza, A.M., Cassinelli, G., Di Marco, A., Penco, S., Pratesi, G., Supino, R., Zaccara, A., Zunino, F., and Arcamone, F., to be published.
7. Cassinelli, G., Ruggieri, D., and Arcamone, F., *J. Med. Chem. 22*, 121 (1979).
8. Cassinelli, G., Ruggieri, D., Arcamone, F., and Di Marco, A., U.S. Patent N. 4.276.289 (1981, June 30).
9. Ruggieri, D., Cassinelli, G., and Ballabio, M., Abstracts XII Convegno Nazionale Chimica Organica, Ancona, Italy. September 1980, pp 79-80.
10. Penco, S., Angelucci, F., Gozzi, F., Franchi, G., Gioia, B., Vigevani, A., and Arcamone, F., Abstracts 11th IUPAC

Symposium on the Chemistry of Natural Products, Golden
Sands, Bulgaria, September 1978, Vol. 4, pp 448-463.

11. Penco, S., Angelucci, F., Vigevani, A., Arlandini, E.,
and Arcamone, F., J. *Antibiotics* 30,764 (1977).

12. Penco, S., Vicario, G.P., Angelucci, F., and Arcamone,
F., J. *Antibiotics* 30, 773 (1977).

13. Arcamone, F., "Daunomycin and Related Antibiotics" *in*
Antibiotic Chemistry, Ed. Sammers, P., Vol. 2, pp 99-
239, Ellis Horwood Chichester (1978).

14. Arcamone, F., Medicinal Chemistry Series, Vol. 16,
Eds. Cassady, J.M., and Douros, J.D., Academic Press,
New York, pp 1-41 (1980).

15. Arcamone, F., "Doxorubicin and its Analogs" *in* Topics on
Cancer Chemotherapy, Eds. Wu Huanxing, Shen Jaxiang, and
Nicolis, F.B., China Academic Publishers, Peking, China,
p. 13 (1981).

16. Arcamone, F., Franceschi, G., and Penco, S., U.S. Patent
3,803,124 (1974, April 9).

17. Suarato, A., Penco, S., Vigevani, A., and Arcamone, F.,
Carbohydr. Res., in press.

18. Cassinelli, G., Forenza, S., Ripamonti, M.C., and Ruggieri, D., European Patent Application DE-EP 22515A (1981,
August 13).

19. Cassinelli, G., Arcamone, F., and Di Marco, A., U.S. Patent 4,254,110 (1981, March 3).

20. Masi, P., Suarato, A., Giardino, P., Iraci, G., Bernardi,
L., and Arcamone, F., *Il Farmaco Ed. Sci.* 35, 347 (1980).

21. Cassinelli, G., Forenza, S., Ripamonti, M.C., and Arcamone, F., Belg. Patent 883,759 (1980, June 30).

22. Zunino, F., Casazza, A.M., Pratesi, G., Formelli, F., and
Di Marco, A., *Biochem. Pharmacol.* 30, 1856 (1981).

23. Cassinelli, G., Grein, A., Masi, P., Suarato, A., Bernardi, L., Arcamone, F., Di Marco, A., Casazza, A.M., Pratesi, G., and Soranzo, C., J. *Antibiotics* 31,178 (1978).

24. Arcamone, F., Cassinelli, G., Di Matteo, F., Forenza, S.,
Ripamonti, M.C., Rivola, G.,Vigevani, A., Clardy, J., and
McCabe, T., J. Am. Chem. Soc. 102, 1462 (1980).

25. Cassinelli, G., Rivola, G., Ruggieri, D., Arcamone, F.,
Merli, S., Spalla, C., Casazza, A.M., Di Marco, A., and
Pratesi, G., to be published.

26. Rivola, G., Forenza, S., Cassinelli, G., Grein, A., and
Merli, S., British Patent Application 2.048.245 (1980,
December 10).

27. Brossi, A., *Pure & Appl. Chem.* 51, 681 (1979).

28. Arcamone, F., Bernardi, L., Patelli, B., Giardino, P., Di
Marco, A., Casazza, A.M., Soranzo, C., and Pratesi, G.,
Experientia 34, 1255 (1978)

29. Franchi, G., Ruggieri, D., Penco, S., and Cassinelli, G., to be
published.

MICROBIAL TRANSFORMATION OF ANTHRACYCLINE ANTIBIOTICS AND DEVELOPMENT OF NEW ANTHRACYCLINES

*Toshikazu Oki**

Central Research Laboratories
Sanraku-Ocean Co., Ltd.
Fujisawa, Japan

INTRODUCTION

The outstanding cancer chemotherapeutic efficacy of adriamycin has stimulated research in the area of anthracycline antibiotics. The search for drugs that would not exhibit its severe and cumulative dose-dependent cardiotoxicity, has led to our isolation of a new potent anthracycline, aclacinomycin A. This antibiotic produces favorable responses in patients with acute leukemia refractory to daunomycin and adriamycin, malignant lymphoma, lung, breast, ovarian, stomach and urinary bladder cancers when administered by intravenous infusion or bladder instillation. Aclacinomcin A is marketed in Japan[1] under the generic name aclarubicin. Our work leading to the development of aclarubicin has now been extended to include the preparation of new derivatives with modified aglycones or sugar moieties, in order to reduce the toxicity and/or improve biological activity of the drugs.

In this paper, I will review the biosynthesis and structure-antitumor activity relationships of some new oligosaccharide anthracycline glycosides *in vitro* and *in vivo*.

*Present address: Nagoya Biochemistry Laboratory, Pfizer-Taito Co., Ltd., Taketoyo, Japan and School of Pharmaceutical Sciences, Kobe-Gakuin University, Kobe, Japan.

I.   ANTHRACYCLINE METABOLITES PRODUCED BY MICROORGANISMS.

Since 1973, we have isolated about one hundred different anthracyclines from the culture broth of various *streptomycetes*, by microbial glycosidation of various aglycones using blocked mutants, as well as by chemical glycosidation and modification. Among the streptomycetes we studied, *S. galilaeus* and *S. coeruleorubidus* produced a number of anthracycline glycosides in the culture broth, which were shown by acid hydrolysis, methanolysis and hydrogenolysis to contain the saccharides shown in Table 1. The occurrence of daunosamine was restricted to the daunorubicin group of metabolites, whereas its *N,N*-dimethyl derivative, rhodosamine, was found in rhodomycin and the aclacinomycin group of metabolites.

A new α,β-unsaturated hexulose, named aculose, was produced by *S. galilaeus*,[2] and a unique sugar moiety was found in *S. coeruleorubidus*,[3,4] it resembled a hexose cleaved between C-3 and C-4 positions.

Table 1. Saccharides found in S. galilaeus and S. coeruleorubidus

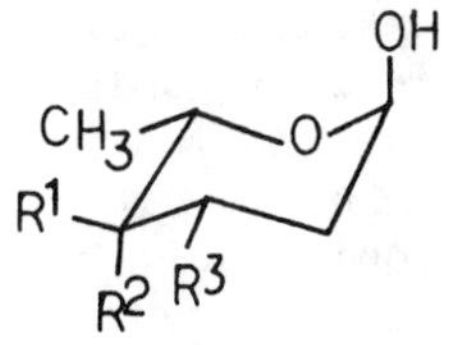

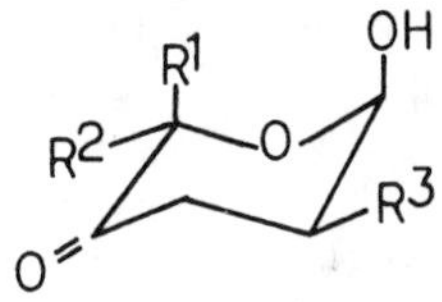

	R^1	R^2	R^3
L-Amicetose (Am)	OH	H	H
L-Rhodinose (R)	H	OH	H
2-Deoxy-L-fucose (dF)	H	OH	OH
L-Daunosamine (D)	H	OH	NH_2
N-Monomethyl D (mD)	H	OH	$NHCH_3$
L-Rhodosamine (RN)	H	OH	$N(CH_3)_2$
L-Cinerulose A (C)	H	CH_3	H
D-Cinerulose A (DC)	CH_3	H	H
L-Cinerulose B (CB)	H	CH_3	OH

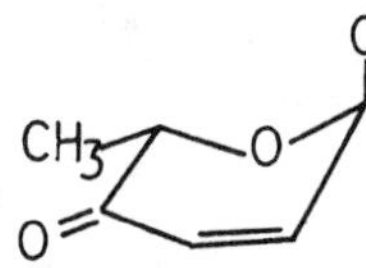

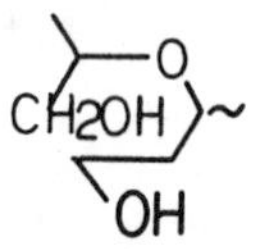

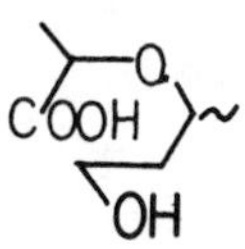

A.   Metabolites from *S. Galilaeus* MA144-M1 and its Mutant
      Strains.

      Aclacinomycins A and B, the two major antibiotics belong-
ing to a new aklavinone glycoside complex, as well as a host
of their analogues, were isolated from cultured broth of
S. galilaeus MA144-M1. They were purified by a combination
of chelation with copper and silicic acid chromatography,[5-11]
(see Table 2). Among the aglycone-type of metabolites
MA144-E1, 7,7'-bis-(7-deoxy aklavinone) was produced when
aklavinone or aklavinone glycosides were reduced at the C-7
position by microbial enzyme under anerobic conditions, rat
hepatic cytochrome P-450-reductase, xanthine oxidase, NADH
dehydrogenase and soluble DT diaphorase.[12-14] An additional
yellow minor component, named 13-methylaclacinomycin A, which
has 13-methylaklavinone as the aglycone was isolated by HPLC
in the course of the large scale production of aclacinomycin A. Several of its derivatives were prepared chemically
by reduction and hydrolysis.[11]

      During the genetic studies aimed at obtaining high-yield
variants of aclacinomycin-producing strains, a variety of
blocked mutants were isolated from *S. galilaeus* MA144-M1 by
UV irradiation of NTG treatment. Several new aklavinone
glycosides devoid of amino sugar, and designated as MA144-U5,
U6, U7, U8 and U9 were isolated from various mutant strains.
Furthermore, new aglycones, such as 2-hydroxyaklavinone, and
its non-esterified analogue were produced by a blocked mutant
ANR-58.[9-10]

B.   Daunomycin Analogues from *S. coeruleorubidus* ME130-A4,
      its Mutant Strains and *Actinomadura* sp. D326.

      New daunomycin analogues, such as the baumycins which
have a unique residue attached to the 4' position, were
isolated from the culture broth of *S. coeruleorubidus*
ME130-A4 in association with known daunomycin-related compounds, such as daunomycin, N-acetyl daunomycin, their
aglycones and ε-rhodomycinone.[3,4] Baumycins A and B were
only isolated when purification was carried out under neutral
conditions (without acidic treatment). Other daunomycin
analogues having different side chains at the C-9 position,
were produced by a mutant 4N-140 of *S. coeruleorubidus*
ME130-A4, and named feudomycins. They accompanied six
daunomycinone-related aglycones in the mycelium,[15] as shown
in Table 3.

Table 2. Metabolites from $\underline{S}$. $\underline{galilaeus}$ MA144-M1 and its mutants

Producers	Metabolites	R^1	R^2	R^3	R^4
MA144-M1	Aclacinomycin A	H	H	RN-dF-C	CH_2CH_3
(Original	" B	"	"	RN-dF-CB	"
strain)	" Y	"	"	RN-dF-Ac	"
	MA144 M1	"	"	RN-dF-Am	"
	" N1	"	"	RN-dF-R	"
	" G1	"	"	RN-dF-DC	"
	" S1	"	"	RN-dF	"
	Aklavin	"	"	RN	"
	N-Monomethyl ACM	"	"	mD-dF-C	"
	N,N-Dimethyl ACM	"	"	D-dF-C	"
	MA144 A2(Cinerubin A)	OH	"	RN-dF-C	"
	" B2(" B)	"	"	RN-dF=CB	"
	" M2	"	"	RN-dF-Am	"
	" N2	"	"	RN-dF-R	"
	" S2	"	"	RN-dF	"
	" T2(Pyrromycin)	"	"	RN	"
	Aklavinone(AKN)	H	"	OH	"
	7-Deoxy AKN	"	"	H	"
	*Bisanhydro AKN	"	"	"	"
	MA144 E1(7,7'-bis(7-deoxy AKN))	"	"	Dimer	"
	ε-Pyrromycinone(ε-PMN)	OH	"	OH	"
	7-Deoxy PMN(ζ-PMN)	"	"	H	"
	** 13-Methyl ACM-A	H	"	RN-dF-C	$CH(CH_3)_2$
	" -M	"	"	RN-dF-Am	"
	" -N	"	"	RN-dF-R	"
	" -S	"	"	RN-dF	"
	" -T	"	"	RN	"
	13-Methyl AKN	"	"	OH	"
	7-Deoxy-13-methyl AKN	"	"	H	"
Mutant 7U-491	Glycoside U1	"	"	RN-dF-dF	CH_2CH_3
"	" U2	"	"	RN-dF	"
9U-653	" U5	"	"	dF-dF-C	"
"	" U6	"	"	dF-R-R	"
"	" U7	"	"	dF-dF-Am	"
"	" U8	"	"	dF-R	"
7N-1881	" U9	"	"	dF-dF	"
ANR-58	*** 58G	"	-	-	
"	2-Hydroxy AKN(58D)	"	OH	OH	"
"	2-Hydroxy-7-deoxy AKN(58C)	"	"	H	"

** 13-Methylaclacinomycins M and N were derived by reduction and S, T, 13-methyl-aklavinone and 7-deoxy-13-methyl AKN by acid hydrolysis of 13-methylaclacinomycin A, respectively.

A new *Actinomadura* sp. D326 isolated from a soil sample produced new carminomycin-analogues. These were the 4-hydroxybaumycins which have the same residue at the 4' position of carminomycin I as in baumycins.[16]

Table 3. Daunomycin analogues from S. coeruleorubidus ME130-A4, its mutants and Actinomadura sp. D326

Producers	Products	R^1	R^2	R^3	R^4
S. coeruleorubidus	Baumycin A1	OCH_3	D-X1	$COCH_3$	H
ME130-A4(Original)	" A2	"	"	"	"
	" B1	"	D-X2	"	"
	" B2	"	"	"	"
	" C1				
	(N-Formyl DM)	"	N-Formyl-D	"	"
	" C2				
	(N-Formyl DDM)	"	"	$CH(OH)CH_3$	"
	N-Acetyl DM	"	N-Acetyl-D	$COCH_3$	"
	" DDM	"	"	$CH(OH)CH_3$	"
	Daunomycin(DM)	"	D	$COCH_3$	
	ε-Rhodomycinone	OH	OH	CH_2CH_3	$COOCH_3$
	7-Deoxy-13-di- hydro DMN	OCH_3	H	$CH(OH)CH_3$	H
	7-epi-13-dihydro- DMN	"	OH	"	"
Mutant 4N-140	Feudomycin A	"	D	CH_2CH_3	H
	" B	"	"	CH_2COCH_3	"
	" D	"	"	CH_3	OH
	FMN-A(13-DeoxyDMN)	"	OH	CH_2CH_3	H
	-B	"	"	CH_2COCH_3	"
	-C	"	"	CH_3	"
	-D	"	"	CH_3	OH
	13-Dihydro FMN-B	"	"	$CH_2CHOHCH_3$	H
	DMN	"	"	$COCH_3$	"
Actinomadura sp. D326	4-Hydroxybaumycin A1	OH	D-X1	"	"
	" A2(4'-epimer)	"	"	"	"
	4-Hydroxybaumycinol A1	OH	"	$CH(OH)CH_3$	"
	" A2(4'-epimer)	"	"	"	"

DMN: daunomycinone,　DDM:daunorubicinol,　FMN:feudomycinone

C. ε-Pyrromycinone and Rhodomycinone Glycosides from
    Streptomyces sp.

Seven ε-pyrromycinone glycosides, named rhodirubin, and
three aglycone-type of compounds were isolated from the
cultured broth of *Streptomyces* sp. ME505-HE1,[17] and shown
in Table 4.

Rhodomycin-producing *Streptomyces*, such as
S. purpurascens, *S. roseoviolaceus* produced new γ-rhodomycinone oligosaccharides, which we named
roseorubicin. They have 5 sugar residues at the C-10
position.[18] Four aglycones, ε-rhodomycinone, ε-isorhodo-
mycinone, β-rhodomycinone and γ-rhodomycinone were also
detected in their mycelia.

D. Microbial Glycosidation of Various Anthracyclinones by
    Blocked Mutants.

In the course of our biosynthetic study of anthracycline
antibiotics, the microbial glycosidation of biologically
inactive anthracyclinones has been attempted. This effort
aimed at preparing active anthracyclines with better therapeutic indeces. Thus, 2-hydroxy-aklavinone was microbiologically glycosidated at C-7 with cinerulosyl-2-deoxy-
fucosyl-rhodosaminide by feeding the aglycone to a culture
of an aclacinomycin-negative mutant strain KE303 derived from
S. galilaeus MA144-M1.[19] Reduction and hydrolysis of
2-hydroxyaclacinomycin A produced 2-hydroxy-aklavinone mono-,
di- and trisaccharides.[20] Also, this mutant KE303 produced
the corresponding cinerulosyl-deoxyfucosyl-rhodosaminyl
rhodomycinones by feeding the culture with various rhodomycinones.[21,22] Carminomycinone fed to the culture of
mutant KE303 was reduced at C-13 position and glycosidated
to trisarubicinol.[23]

Blocked mutant IU-222 derived from *S. coeruleorubidus*
ME130-A4 could glycosidate ε-pyrromycinone or ε-rhodomycinone
to 1-hydroxydaunorubicinol and 1-hydroxy-*N*-formyl-dauno-
rubicinol.[24]

On the other hand, since daunomycinone and adriamycinone
could not be microbiologically glycosidated, their oligosaccharide glycosides were semisynthesized by glycosidation
of daunomycinone or 14-*O*-acetyladriamycinone with $(CF_3SO_2)_2O$
followed by deprotection of 3"-acetyl group with
K_2CO_3.[25] The structures of these microbially and chemically
glycosidated products are summarized in Table 5.

Table 4. Rhodomycinone and pyrromycinone glycosides from Streptomycetes

Producers	Products	R¹	R²	R³	R⁴
S. purpurascens	Roseorubicin A	H	H	OH	RN–RN–dF–R–R
S. roseoviolaceus	" B	"	"	"	RN–RN
S. violacens	ε–RMN	"	OH	"	COOCH₃
S. violarus	ε–IsoRMN	OH	"	"	"
	β–RMN	H	"	"	OH
	α–RMN	"	H	"	"
Streptomyces sp. ME505-HE1	Rhodirubin A	OH	RN–dF–R	H	COOCH₃
	" B	"	RN–R–R	"	"
	" C (Cinerubin A)	"	RN–dF–C	"	"
	" D (Musettamycin)	"	RN–dF	"	"
	" E (Marcellomycin)	"	RN–dF–dF	"	"
	" G	"	RN–dF–DC	"	"
	Pyrromycin	"	RN		"
	ε–PMN	"	OH		"
	7-Deoxy-ε-PMN (ζ-PMN)	"	H		"
	Bisanhydro PMN (η-PMN)	"	"		"

RMN: rhodomycinone, PMN: pyrromycinone

Table 5.   Microbial glycosidation of various anthracyclinones by a blocked mutants
and chemical glycosidation

$$R^1 \quad O \quad HO \quad R^4 \quad R^3$$

$$R^5 \qquad\qquad\qquad\qquad\qquad OH$$

$$R^6 \quad O \quad R^2 \quad R^7$$

Produced by	Aglycones fed (Substrates)	Products		R^1	R^2	R^3	R^4	R^5	R^6	R^7
Mutant KE303	ε-RMN	ε-RMN-A		H	OH	CH_2CH_3	$COOCH_3$	H	OH	RN-dF-C
	ε-isoRMN	ε-isoRMN-A		OH	"	"	"	"	"	"
	β-RMN	β-RNM-A		H	"	"	OH	"	"	"
	β-isoRMN	β-isoRNM-A		OH	"	"	"	"	"	"
	α₂-RMN	α₂-RMN-A		"	H	"	"	"	"	"
	γ²RMN	γ²RNM-A		H	OH	"	RN-dF-C (C7:H)	"	"	"
	CMN/carmino-mycinol	Trisarubicinol		"	"	CH(OH)CH₃	H	"	"	"
	2-Hydroxy AKH	2-Hydroxy ACM-A		"	"	CH₂CH₃	COOCH₃	OH	"	RN-dF-C
Oxido-reductase	ACM-A	" -B		"	"	"	"	"	"	RN-dF=CB
Reduction	"	" -M		"	"	"	"	"	"	RN-dF-Am
"	"	" -N		"	"	"	"	"	"	RN-dF-R
Hydrolysis	"	" -S		"	"	"	"	"	"	RN-dF
"	"	" -T		"	"	"	"	"	"	RN
Mutant 1U-222	ε-PMN	1-Hydroxy dauno-rubicinol		OH	"	CH(OH)CH₃	H	H	"	D
	or									
	ε-RMN	1-Hydroxy-N-for-myldaunorubicinol		"	"	"	"	"	"	N-formyl D
Chemical	DMN	DMN -A		H	"	COCH₃	"	"	OCH₃	RN-dF-C
Glycosidation	"	" -S		"	"	"	"	"	"	RN-dF
"	"	" -L		"	"	"	"	"	"	mD-dF-C
"	"	" -K		"	"	"	"	"	"	D-dF-C
	AMN	3"-O-Acetyl-AMN-A		"	"	COCH₂OH	"	"	"	RN-AcdF-C

RMN; rhodomycinone, PMN; pyrromycinone, AKN; aklavinone, ACM; aclacinomycin,
AcdF; 3-O-acefyl-2-deoxyfucoside CMN; carminomycinone, DMN; daunomycinone,
AMN; adriamycinone
Blocked mutants KE303 and 1U-222 were derived from S. galilaeus MA144-M1 and
S. coeruleorubidus ME130-A4, respectively.

E.   Biosynthesis of Anthracycline Antibiotics.

^{13}C-Labeled aklavinone was obtained from the culture of
a strain, 3AR-33, which accumulated aklavinone by the genetic
loss of glycosidation ability, supplemented with various
acetates and propionate labeled at the C-1 and/or C-2 position
with carbon-13.   The incorporation of $[1-^{13}C]$ acetate resulted
in enrichment of C-2, 4, 5, 6, 7, 10a, 11a, 12a and 15, while
that of $[2-^{13}C]$ acetate enriched C-1, 3, 4a, 5a, 6a, 8, 10,
11 and 12.[26]   This indicated the consecutive incorporation of
intact acetate in the aklavinone molecule, which was further
confirmed by the fact that all resonances, except those of
C-9, 13, 14 and 16, in ^{13}C-NMR spectrum of aklavinone
enriched with $[1,2-^{13}C]$ acetate were accompanied by two
satellite signals due to the spin $^{13}C-^{13}C$ coupling. $[1-^{13}C]$
Propionate enriched aglycones showed only one signal at C-9.
It was, therefore, concluded that the ring carbon of

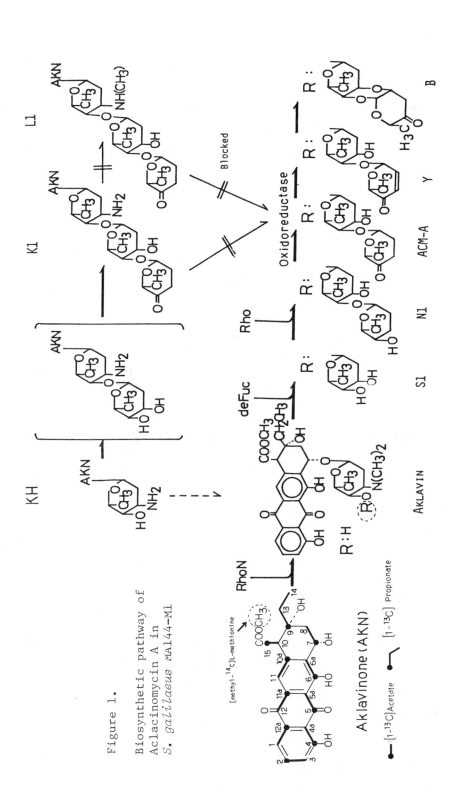

Figure 1.

Biosynthetic pathway of
Aclacinomycin A in
S. galilaeus MA144-M1

aklavinone, as well as daunomycinone, was built up from nine
acetates and one propionate residues. It was also possible
to confirm by using ^{14}C-labeled methionine that the methyl
ester at C-16 and the N,N-dimethyl group in rhodosamine
originated from methionine.

In experiments on the bioconversion of various
aklavinone glycosides, we demonstrated that MA144-N1
(rhodinosyl-deoxy-fucosylrhodosaminyl aklavinone) was biosynthesized from aklavinone by a step-wise glycosidation via
N-methylation of daunosaminylaklavinone (KH)[21] as shown in
Figure 1.

From the structural elucidation of the new natural
aglycones found in *Streptomyces* and the ^{13}C-NMR analytical
results of steffimycinone, nogalarol and daunomycinone
reported by Paulick and others,[27-29] it is clear that the
starter carbon unit in the formation of the polyketide leading to the anthracyclinones is usually an acetate or
propionate. However, in feudomycinone B, sulfurmycinone
and 13-methyl-aklavinone the isopropyl and acetonyl group
appears at C-9. This would arise from an irregularity which
utilizes isobutyrate and acetoacetate or butyrate as a
starter.

The microbial reduction of the glycosidic bond at C-7
and that of the side chain carbonyl group at C-13 in anthracycline antibiotics is well known,[12,14,30,31] but the
oxygenation of the C-14 position in DM, DDM, CM and FM has
not yet been reported. We found that the mutant 2N-267,
which was derived from *S. peucetius* subsp. *caesius* by treatment of NTG, could not produce adriamycin, but could convert
DM, DDM, CM and FM efficiently to adriamycin using the
resting mycelia treated with Mg-ion and a lytic enzyme under
aerobic condition at optimal pH of 8.5. The aglycones
themselves, such as daunomycinone, carminomycinone,
feudomycinones and even adriamycinone, were not directly
glycosidated to adriamycin.[32]

The overall biosynthetic pathway of anthracyclinones, as
illustrated in Figure 2, was examined by microbial modification and glycosidation of aklavinone, rhodomycinones and
other aglycones using various blocked mutants derived from
S. galilaeus, S. coeruleorubidus, S. purpurascens and
S. peucetius.[33] We have demonstrated that the aglycone
aklavinone is a precursor in the biosynthesis of daunomycinone, and that daunomycin is biosynthesized via glycosidation of ε-rhodomycinone followed by 10-demethoxycarbonylation

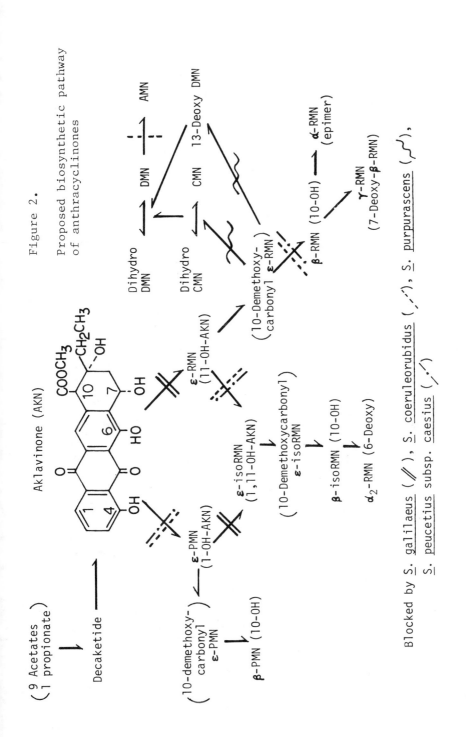

Figure 2.

Proposed biosynthetic pathway of anthracyclinones

Blocked by S. galilaeus (⫽), S. coeruleorubidus (‚‚‘), S. purpurascens (〜),
S. peucetius subsp. caesius (‚‘)

Toshikazu Oki

Table 6. Antitumor activity against L1210 leukemia and mutagenicity of various anthracycline compounds

| Compounds | IC_{50} (nM)[*1] | | | IC ratio | T/C (%)[*2] | Ames'[*3] |
	Growth	DNA Synthesis	RNA	DNA/RNA	(OD)	test
Adriamycinone	>1,000	>10,000	>10,000	—	—	±
Aklavinone	>5,000	>10,000	>10,000	—	—	-
7-con-O-methylnogarol	76	4,600	8,100	0.6	—	-
MA144 U5	>1,000	>10,000	>10,000	—	—	-
" U9	>1,000	>10,000	>10,000	—	—	-
ACM	12	370	47	7.9	203 (4)	-
N-Monodemethyl " (MA144 L1)	70	1,900	240	7.9	140 (15)	±
N,N-Didemethyl " (" K1)	280	2,600	570	4.4	105 (30)	+
MA144 S1	17	290	57	5.1	175 (5)	-
Aklavin	41	630	280	2.2	159 (20)	±
3"-O-Acetyldaunomycinone-A	4	300	20	15.0	210 (5)	-
Daunomycinone-A	4	210	21	10.0	144 (1.25)	-
" -S	10	410	58	7.1	150 (2.5)	-
" -K	120	1,500	210	7.0	162 (7.5)	-
N,N-Dimethyl DM	11	290	120	2.4	164 (0.63)	-
DM	38	800	300	2.7	191 (1.25)	+
Roseorubicin A	38	1,800	190	9.5	118 (0.25)	-
" B	88	3,100	580	5.4	159 (0.78)	-
3"-O-Acetyladriamycinone-A	5	370	14	26.4	144 (0.3)	
N,N-Dimethyl ADM	18	340	140	2.4	164 (1.25)	-
ADM	37	2,600	1,000	2.6	292 (1.25)	+
Cinerubin A	7	310	36	8.6	163 (1.5)	-
4-O-Methyl ACM	48	580	74	7.8	193 (30)	-
6-O- " "	36	1,600	110	14.4	180 (10)	-
Carminomycin I	10	390	490	0.8	—	+
4-Hydroxybaumycin A1	8	290	140	2.1	156 (0.16)	+
Baumycin A1	22	1,700	560	3.1	200 (0.04)	+
4-Demethoxy DM	10	160	280	0.6	—	
4-Demethoxy-11-deoxy "	21	460	710	0.6	—	
4-Demethoxy ADM	12	430	560	0.8	—	
Daunorubicinol	850	7,600	3,000	2.5	124 (7)	+
1-Hydroxy "	42	3,300	1,100	3.3	140 (2.5)	+
2-Hydroxy ACM	42	1,030	170	5.9	194 (6)	-
10-epi-ACM	25	3,400	1,200	2.8	—	-
10-Demethoxycarbonyl "	66	800	450	1.8	—	-
Museffamycin	7	310	59	5.3	—	-
Collinemycin (10-epi- ")	56	3,400	630	5.4	—	-

Continued

Table 6 (continued)

Compounds	IC_{50} (nM)[*1] Growth	DNA Synthesis	RNA	IC ratio DNA/RNA	T/C (%)[*2] (OD)	Ames'[*3] test
7-epi-10-Demethoxycarbonyl ACM	160	1,100	730	1.5	—	-
10-Demethoxycarbonyl MA144 S1	140	750	290	2.6	—	-
7-epi-10-Demethoxycarbonyl MA144 S1	295	1,325	750	1.8	—	-
Feudomycin D	1,500	11,000	15,000	0.8	—	+
" A	31	580	580	1.0	135 (2.5)	+
" B	1,500	2,800	1,500	1.9	—	+
Auramycin A	25	630	120	5.3	—	-
Sulfurmycin A	17	480	43	11.1	—	-
ACM-B	26	620	62	10.0	186 (1)	-
" -Y	12	190	12	15.8	114 (5)	-
MA144 M1	14	470	43	10.9	185 (4)	-
" N1	14	420	52	8.1	173 (2.5)	-
" G1	25	800	120	6.8	163 (8)	-
" U1	39	1,300	96	13.9	182 (8)	-
4'"(R)-Amino ACM	15	160	16	10.0	129 (2.5)	-
4'"(R)-N-Acetamide "	58	580	53	10.9	138 (5)	-
ACM oxime	36	820	63	13.0	177 (2.5)	-
ε-RMN-A	7	420	48	8.8	154 (1.25)	-
ε-isoRMN-A	4	730	66	11.1	—	-
β-RMN-A	6	360	97	3.7	214 (5)	-
β-isoRMN-A	22	1,530	190	8.0	—	-
α_2-RMN-A	1,100	2,200	1,100	2.0	—	-
γ-RMN-A	73	550	180	3.0	—	-
Trisarubicinol	13	470	69	6.8	216 (5)	-

Abbreviation: -A: cinerulosyl-2-deoxyfucosyl-rhodosaminide, ACM: aclacinomycin A, DM: daunomycin, ADM: adriamycin, RMN: rhodomycinone

[*1] Growth: L1210 cells (4×10^4 cells/ml) were cultured in RPMI 1640 medium containing 20% calf serum with test compound (0.01-0.5 µg/ml) at 37°C under 5% CO_2-95% air atmosphere. Cytotoxicity was expressed as IC_{50} of the control growth on day 2.
Macromolecular biosynthesis: After preincubation of L1210 cells (5×10^5 cells/ml) with test compound (0.01-2.5 µg/ml) at 37°C for 15 min, [2-^{14}C]-thymidine or -uridine was added with 0.05 µCi/ml, and incubated for 60 min at 37°C. Uptake of precursor was terminated by rapid chilling and adding 1 ml of cold 10% TCA to 1 ml of the incubation mixture. The precipitate was washed twice with 2 ml of cold 5% TCA, and dissolved in 0.25 ml of 99% formic acid. The radioactivity was counted with a Aloka LSC-653 liquid scintillation spectrometer in Bray's scintillator. IC_{50} values were estimated by Probit analysis.

[*2] In vivo antitumor activity: CDF_1 mice transplanted intraperitoneally with 10^5 L1210 leukemia cells were treated by i.p. administration of the compound daily for 10 days starting 24 hrs after implantation. Antitumor activity was evaluated in terms of the percentage increase in survival time over the control (T/C).

[*3] S. typhimurium TA98 without S9.

and further β-oxidation of ethyl group at C-9. 10-Decarbo-
methoxyaklavinone and carminomycinone exhibited positive
precursor activity for the formation of daunomycin. However,
aklavinone and rhodomycinone monosaccharides, such as
7-O-daunosaminyl aklavinone (MA144-KH), 7-O-rhodosaminyl-
aklavinone (aklavin) and 7-O-rhodosaminyl-ε-rhodomycinone
(11-hydroxyaklavin) could not be converted to daunomycin,
but 13-deoxydaunomycin (feudomycin A) was oxidized to an
intermediate in the daunomycin biosynthesis. It is clear
that the glycosidation of the precursor aglycone by
S. coeruleorubidus is strictly restricted by methylation of
hydroxyl at C-4 and by the oxidation of the ethyl group at
C-9 to an acetyl group, since daunomycinone, dihydro-
daunomycinone and adriamycinone could not be directly
glycosidated.[9,21,32,34]

F. Structure-Activity Relationships.[8,35-40]

    A study of the effect of 61 anthracyclines on growth,
macromolecular biosynthesis, in vivo antitumor activity
against L1210 leukemia cells and mutagenicity showed
(see Table 6), the following structure-activity relationships:

    1. The amino function on the aglycone or sugar moiety
is essential for in vitro and in vivo activities. Aglycones
excepting nogalarol and glycosides possessing only neutral
sugar were found to be biologically inactive.

    2. Disaccharides and trisaccharide glycosides of
anthracyclinones were more potent in vitro than the monosaccharide derivatives. However, the length of the sugar
chain did not correlate well with in vivo antitumor activity.
In all aklavinone, daunomycinone and γ-rhodomycinone glycosides, the trisaccharides were the most potent in in vitro
cytotoxicity and in inhibitory effect on RNA and DNA
synthesis. Roseorubicin A, having a pentasaccharide at the
C-10 position, was the most potent in vitro, but was found
to be less active in vivo showing only 118% T/C. The
antitumor effect was prominent in aclacinomycin A and
N,N-dimethyl daunomycin.

    3. The sugar chain length influenced the ratio of
inhibition (IC_{50}) of DNA versus RNA synthesis. The ratio of
the concentration needed to inhibit DNA synthesis to that
needed to inhibit RNA synthesis (DNA/RNA) was 1 to 4 in
monosaccharide glycosides (Group I), while in trisaccharide
glycosides (Group II) the IC_{50} ratio was 7 to 10. In
disaccharide glycosides, the ratio was 5 to 6. It, thus,

seems that trisaccharide glycosides preferentially inhibited
RNA synthesis. We have first found that aclacinomycin A and
its related oligosaccharide glycosides inhibited RNA
synthesis to a greater degree than DNA synthesis.[8] When the
concentrations required for 50% inhibition (IC_{50}) of whole
cellular RNA and DNA synthesis were plotted, the effects of
anthracyclines on the nucleic acid synthesis was classified
into two groups, as shown in Figure 3.

Group I anthracyclines, mostly monosaccharides including
DM, AM, CM aklavin, shown by dotted line, inhibited DNA and
RNA synthesis at approximately an equal concentration
(IC_{50} ratios of 1 to 4), while IC_{50} values of group II
anthracyclines, such as aclacinomycins, cinerubins and related trisaccharides, the ratio was over 7.

Preferential inhibition of RNA synthesis was also
exhibited in semisynthetic daunomycinone and adriamycinone
trisaccharides showing IC_{50} ratios of 7 to 26, while their
monosaccharides; daunomycin and adriamycin showed IC_{50}
ratio of about 2.

--------: Adriamycin-type(Group I)

————————: Aclacinomycin-type(Group II)

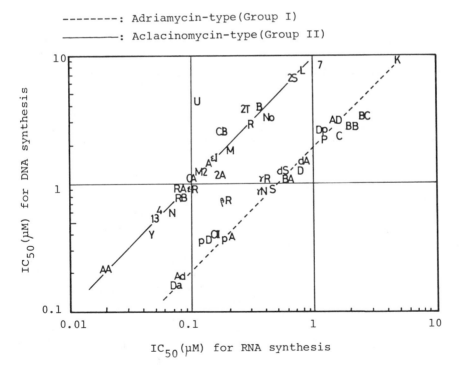

Figure 3.   Inhibitory effect of anthracyclines on DNA and RNA
            synthesis in cultured L1210 cells.

4. Anthracyclines having as N,N-dimethyl group attached
to the amino sugar were more potent *in vitro* than their
analogues having an N-methyl or a primary amino group.
N,N-Dimethyl glycosides of aklavinone and ε-pyrromycinone
were most active *in vivo*. Conversely the N,N-dimethyl derivatives of daunomycinone and adriamycinone glycosides were more
toxic and less active than the corresponding primary amino
compounds.

5. Anthracyclines having alkylamino groups at C-3' of
the amino sugar were non-mutagenic in the Ames' test, but
primary amino compounds, such as adriamycin, daunomycin and
MA144-K1 induced mutagenic activity. Thus, N-demethylation
of rhodosamine-containing anthracyclines induced the mutagenic
activity, and N-methylation of daunosamine-containing compounds suppressed mutagenicity.

6. The hydroxyls at C-1, C-2, C-4, C-6 and C-11 influenced significantly the *in vitro* and *in vivo* activity.

a) Anthracyclines lacking the hydroxyl at C-6 (α_2-rhodo-
mycinone glycosides) were lower in their cytotoxicity and
inhibitory effect on RNA and DNA synthesis than those containing the C-6 hydroxyl.

b) Anthracyclines having a methoxyl group at C-4 or
C-6, instead of a hydroxyl group, were 2-5-fold lower
in vitro and *in vivo* potency.

c) Hydrophobicity at C-4 position and *in vitro* potency
increased in parallel: Methoxyl < Hydrogen-bonded OH < Deoxy.
4-O- and 6-O-Methylaclacinomycin A, daunomycin and baumycin Al
having the methyl group at C-4 or C-6 position showed 3-fold
lower *in vitro* and *in vivo* potency than the corresponding
hydroxyl compounds.

d) The hydroxyl at C-1 and/or C-11 position enhanced
the *in vivo* and *in vitro* potency, but decreased *in vivo*
antitumor activity.

e) The hydroxyl at C-2 position decreased the *in vitro*
potency, but increased the *in vivo* antitumor activity.
Cinerubin A, ε-RNA-A, 1-hydroxyldaunorubicinol and
demethoxydaunomycin, which have the hydroxyl at C-1 and/or
C-11, were more potent *in vitro* and more toxic *in vivo* compared to the corresponding deoxy compounds at C-1 and/or C-11
position. Thus, a hydroxyl group at C-1 and/or C-11 was
effective in increasing the potency. 2-Hydroxy-aclacino-

mycin A was one-third less potent *in vitro*, but produced a
more favorable therapeutic index within a broad range of
doses against L1210 leukemia-bearing mice than
aclacinomycin A.

    7. 10-Methoxycarbonyl group in the S-configuration
decreased markedly the inhibitory effect on RNA synthesis.
The removal of this group at the C-10 position also resulted
in a marked reduction of activity.
    Also, the replacement of the 10-methoxycarbonyl group
with a hydroxyl group, i.e. β-RMN-A, lowered the inhibitory
activity on RNA synthesis to one-tenth of aclacinomycin A.
It is, therefore, suggested that the C-10 position correlates
closely with the inhibition of RNA synthesis and cytotoxicity.
    Configuration at C-7 position is also closely related to
the *in vitro* potency. 7-Epimers having R-configuration were
found to be far less potent than those with an S-configuration.

    8. The side chain at C-9 of aklavinone- and daunomyci-
none glycosides produced slight influence on cytotoxicity and
inhibitory effect on RNA and DNA synthesis. 9-Ethyl,
-isopropyl and -acetonyl derivatives had equal activities.
The methyl derivative had the least activity. There may be
an optimal length of the C-9 side chain. Reduction at C-13
of daunomycinone glycosides decreased markedly the *in vitro*
and *in vivo* activity.

G.   Prospects of New Developement of Anthracycline
    Trisaccharides.

    As mentioned above, the position of hydroxyl group on the
aromatic ring influenced the degree of cytotoxicity and
inhibitory effect on RNA and DNA synthesis, as well as
in vivo antitumor activity. Among anthracycline trisaccharides possessing the same cinerulosyl-2-deoxyfucosyl-
rhodosaminide moiety as in aclacinomycin A prepared by direct
fermentation, by microbial glycosidation using blocked
mutants and by chemical glycosidation, 2-hydroxyaclacino-
mycin A, β-rhodomycinone-A and semisynthetic daunomycinone-A
showed the increased antitumor activity against L1210
leukemia with broad effective dose range and low toxicity in
comparison with aclacinomycin A (Figure 4). Particularly,
efficacy of β-rhodomycinone-A would be superior than
adriamycin with low toxicity and comparable antitumor activity.
The most interesting property of these trisaccharides is
their oral activity. In contrast with the absence of activity

of adriamycin when administered orally, 2-hydroxy-
aclacinomycin A and β-rhodomycinone-A showed optimal on
L1210-bearing mice at an oral dose approximately 2 to 3 times
the intravenous dose.

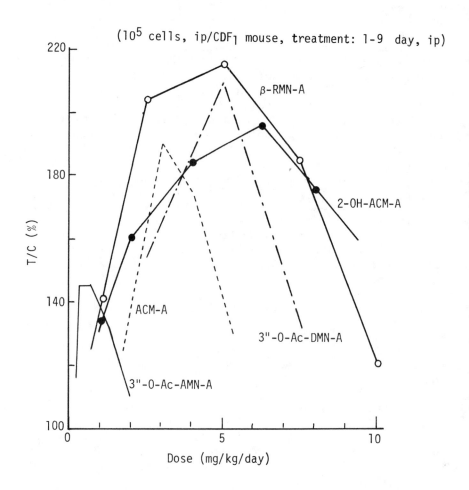

Figure 4.   Antitumor effects of anthracycline trisaccharides
            having cinerulosyl-2-deoxyfucosyl-rhodosaminide
            moiety against L1210 leukemia (10^5 cells,
            ip/CDF$_1$ mouse, treatment: 1-9 day, ip).

Finally, these promising trisaccharides must be characterized and evaluated by further studies on pharmacodynamics, particularly, susceptibility to rat hepatic cytochrome-P450 reductase or xanthine oxidase, specific tissue distribution in mice and pharmacokinetics, and on acute cardiotoxicity predicted by ECG and EM using golden hamsters and rabbits. Further important parameters to select for clinical trial seem to be the penetration into the cells, depending on pH, which would relate to pKa of the compounds, and the leakage from cells, as well as the intracellular localization of the compounds. From these results, a clinical candidate will be selected as a second generation of aclacinomycin A.

ACKNOWLEDGMENTS

I express my sincere thanks to Professor H. Umezawa and Dr. T. Takeuchi, Institute of Microbial Chemistry, Tokyo, for leading the research programs and generosity to permit this publication, and I wish to acknowledge the assistance of the many staff members at the Institute of Microbial Chemistry and Central Research Laboratories of Sanraku-Ocean Co., Ltd., who participated in these studies. I am indebted to Professor H. S. El Khadem for editing this manuscript and for his valuable assistance in the preparation of the final copy.

REFERENCES

1   T. Oki, S. Oka, T. Takeuchi and H. Umezawa, *Recent Results Cancer Res.*, *76*, 21 (1980).

2   A. Yoshimoto, T. Ogasawara, I. Kitamura, T. Oki, T. Inui, T. Takeuchi and H. Umezawa, *J. Antibiotics*, *32*, 479 (1979).

3   T. Komiyama, Y. Matsuzawa, T. Oki, T. Inui, Y. Takahashi, H. Naganawa, T. Takeuchi and H. Umezawa, *J. Antibiotics*, *30*, 619 (1977).

4   Y. Takahashi, H. Naganawa, T. Takeuchi, H. Umezawa, T. Komiyama, T. Oki and T. Inui, *J. Antibiotics*, *30*, 622 (1977).

5 T. Oki, Y. Matsuzawa, A. Yoshimoto, K. Numata,
   I. Kitamura, S. Hori, A. Takamatsu, H. Umezawa,
   M. Ishizuka, H. Naganawa, H. Suda, M. Hamada and
   T. Takeuchi, *J. Antibiotics*, *28*, 830 (1975).

6 T. Oki, I. Kitamura, A. Yoshimoto, Y. Matsuzawa,
   N. Shibamoto, T. Ogasawara, T. Inui, A. Takamatsu,
   T. Takeuchi, T. Masuda, M. Hamada, H. Suda, M. Ishizuka,
   T. Sawa and H. Umezawa, *J. Antibiotics*, *32*, 791 (1979).

7 T. Oki, I. Kitamura, Y. Matsuzawa, N. Shibamoto,
   T. Ogasawara, A. Yoshimoto, T. Inui, H. Naganawa,
   T. Takeuchi and H. Umezawa, *J. Antibiotics*, *30*, 801
   (1979).

8 T. Oki, *Jap. J. Antibiotics*, *30*, S-70 (1977).

9 A. Yoshimoto, Y. Matsuzawa, T. Oki, T. Takeuchi and
   H. Umezawa, *J. Antibiotics*, *34*, 951 (1981).

10 Y. Matsuzawa, A. Yoshimoto, N. Shibamoto, H. Tobe, T. Oki,
   H. Naganawa, T. Takeuchi and H. Umezawa, *J. Antibiotics*,
   34, 959 (1981).

11 K. Soga, H. Furusho, S. Mori and T. Oki, *J. Antibiotics*,
   34, 770 (1981).

12 T. Oki, T. Komiyama, H. Tone, T. Inui, T. Takeuchi and
   H. Umezawa, *J. Antibiotics*, *30*, 613 (1977).

13 T. Komiyama, T. Oki and T. Inui, *J. Antibiotics*, *32*,
   1219 (1979).

14 T. Komiyama, T. Oki, T. Inui, T. Takeuchi and
   H. Umezawa, *Gann*, *70*, 403 (1979).

15 T. Oki, Y. Matsuzawa, K. Kiyoshima, A. Yoshimoto,
   H. Naganawa, T. Takeuchi and H. Umezawa, *J. Antibiotics*,
   34, 783 (1981).

16 Y. Matsuzawa, A. Yoshimoto, K. Kouno and T. Oki,
   J. Antibiotics, *34*, 774 (1981).

17 I. Kitamura, N. Shibamoto, T. Oki, T. Inui, H. Naganawa,
   M. Ishizuka, T. Masuda, T. Takeuchi and H. Umezawa,
   J. Antibiotics, *30*, 616 (1977).

18 Y. Matsuzawa, A. Yoshimoto, T. Oki, T. Unui, T. Takeuchi
    and H. Umezawa, *J. Antibiotics*, *32*, 420 (1979).

19 T. Oki, A. Yoshimoto, Y. Matsuzawa, T. Takeuchi and
    H. Umezawa, *J. Antibiotics*, *34*, 1495 (1981).

20 Y. Matsuzawa and T. Oki, *J. Antibiotics*, *34*, 1495 (1981).

21 T. Oki, A. Yoshimoto, Y. Matsuzawa, T. Takeuchi and
    H. Umezawa, *J. Antibiotics*, *33*, 1331 (1980).

22 Y. Matsuzawa, A. Yoshimoto, T. Oki, H. Naganawa,
    H. Takeuchi and H. Umezawa, *J. Antibiotics*, *33*, 1341
    (1980).

23 A. Yoshimoto, Y. Matsuzawa, T. Oki, T. Takeuchi and
    H. Umezawa, *J. Antibiotics*, *34*, 1492 (1981).

24 A. Yoshimoto, Y. Matsuzawa, T. Oki, H. Naganawa,
    T. Takeuchi and H. Umezawa, *J. Antibiotics*, *33*, 1150
    (1980).

25 H. Tanaka, T. Yoshioka, Y. Shimauchi, Y. Matsushita,
    Y. Matsuzawa, T. Oki and T. Ishikura, *J. Antibiotics*,
    in press.

26 I. Kitamuro, H. Tobe, A. Yoshimoto, T. Oki, H. Naganawa,
    T. Takeuchi and H. Umezawa, *J. Antibiotics*, *34*, 1498
    (1981).

27 R. C. Paulick, M. L. Casey and H. W. Witlock, *J. Am.
    Chem. Soc.*, *98*, 3370 (1976).

28 P. F. Wiley, D. W. Elrod and V. P. Marshall, *J. Org.
    Chem.*, *43*, 3457 (1978).

29 M. L. Casey, R. C. Paulick and H. W. Witlock, *J. Org.
    Chem.*, *43*, 1627 (1978).

30 N. R. Bachur, *J. Pharmacol. Exp. Ther.*, *177*, 573 (1971).

31 R. L. Felsted, D. R. Richter, N. R. Bachur, *Biochem.
    Pharmacol.*, *26*, 1117 (1977).

32. T. Oki, Y. Takatuski, H. Tobe, A. Yoshimoto, T. Takeuchi
    and H. Umezawa, *J. Antibiotics*, *34*, 1229 (1981).

33   A. Yoshimoto, T. Oki and H. Umezawa, *J. Antibiotics*, *33*, 1199 (1980).

34   A. Yoshimoto, T. Oki, T. Takeuchi and H. Umezawa, *J. Antibiotics*, *33*, 1158 (1980).

35   Y. Matsuzawa, T. Oki, T. Takeuchi and H. Umezawa, *J. Antibiotics*, *34*, 1596 (1981).

36   T. Oki, in "Anthracyclines: Current Status and New Developments" (S. Crooke ed.), p. 323. Academic Press, New York (1980).

37   T. Oki, T. Takeuchi, S. Oka and H. Umezawa, *Recent Results in Can. Res.*, *74*, 207 (1980).

38   H. Tanaka, T. Yoshioka, Y. Shimauchi, T. Oki and T. Inui, *J. Antibiotics*, *34*, 850 (1981).

39   H. Tanaka, T. Yoshioka, Y. Shimauchi, Y. Matsuzawa, T. Oki and T. Unui, *J. Antibiotics*, *33*, 1323 (1980).

40   S. Hori, M. Shirai, S. Hirano, T. Oki, T. Unui, S. Tsukagoshi, M. Ishizuka, T. Takeuchi and H. Umezawa, *Gann*, *68*, 685 (1977).

NOGALAMYCIN CHEMISTRY AND ANALOG SYNTHESIS[1]

Paul F. Wiley

Cancer Research
The Upjohn Company
Kalamazoo, Michigan

The antibiotic nogalamycin was isolated almost 20 years ago at The Upjohn Company (2). It was highly active against Gram-positive bacteria and was active against L1210 and KB cells *in vitro*. Although nogalamycin was active against two solid tumors *in vivo*, its relatively poor activity caused cessation of testing.

The gross structure of nogalamycin (*1*), its relative stereochemistry, and the absolute stereochemistry of the neutral sugar are known. However, there is some uncertainty regarding the absolute stereochemistry of the amino sugar and absolute stereochemistry at C-7, C-9, and C-10. Proton and carbon NMR spectra established that the aminosugar has either

[1]*This work was supported in part by Contract N01-CM-77100 and previous contracts from the Division of Cancer Treatment, National Cancer Institute, National Institutes of Health, Education and Welfare.*

1

the α-L- or α-D-glucopyranose configuration (3). The neutral
sugar, nogalose, was shown to have the α-L-rhamnose configuration. On the basis of CD studies and X-ray crystallography
(4,5) structure _1_ in which C-7 is S, C-9 is S, C-10 is R, and
the aminosugar has the α-L-glucopyranose configuration was
assigned. In this assignment the absolute configuration is
based on CD with the relative configuration in ring A and in
the sugar based on X-ray crystallography. Since such a
structure would necessitate that C-9 have a configuration
opposite to that in other anthracyclines, it is felt that the
mirror image of that portion of _1_ exclusive of nogalose cannot
be totally ruled out as the structure until further results
from X-ray crystallography can be obtained.

        Because of the slight uncertainty as to absolute stereo-
chemistry in nogalamycin and its analogs, the prefixes dis and
con are used to designate, respectively, those compounds in
which the oxygen atoms at C-7 and C-9 are _trans_ and _cis_.
Nogalamycin itself has the dis structure.

About sixty analogs of nogalamycin have been prepared.
These can almost all be included in two series: the nogalarol
series and the nogarol series. The difference between the two
is the presence of the carbomethoxy group at C-10 in the nogalarol series and its absence in the nogarol series. Only
two compounds fall outside these two classes. These compounds
have the carboxyl group at C-10. As indicated in Scheme 1,
nogalamycin is readily hydrolyzed to its corresponding acid,
nogalamycinic acid (2). This occurs in 0.5 N KOH at room temperature. The unionized form of 2 is indicated, but it exists

Scheme 1

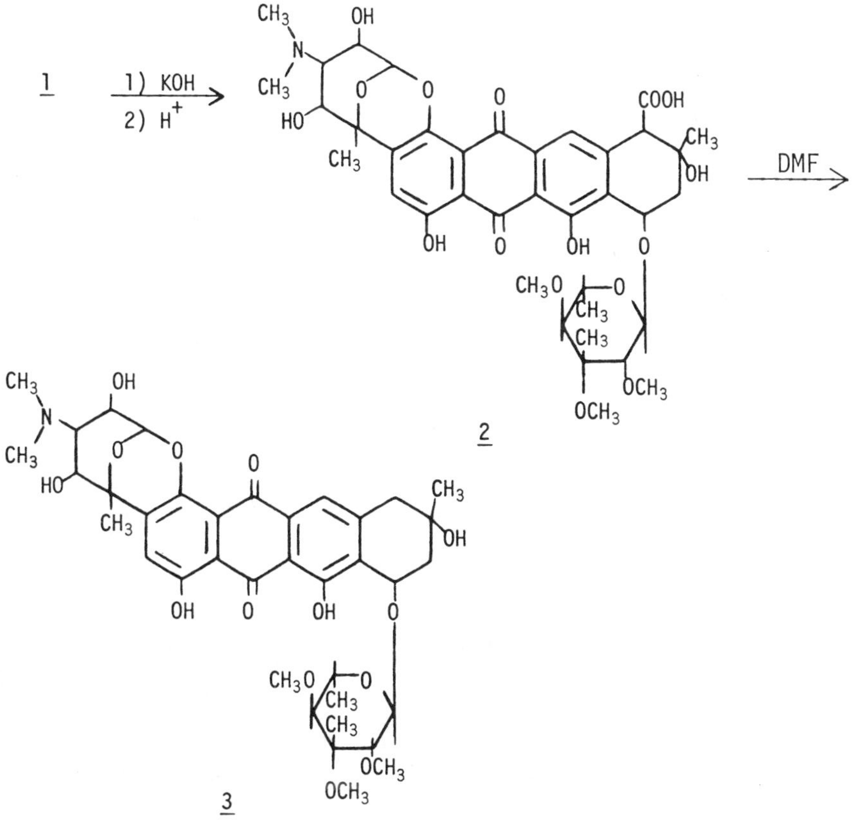

as the zwitterion. The acid *2* readily decarboxylates upon
solution in DMF to give disnogamycin (*3*). The latter compound
was more active in the L1210 *in vitro* cytotoxicity assay than
was nogalamycin.

During early structural investigations on nogalamycin, it
was found that acidic methanolysis (Scheme 2) replaced nogalose with a methoxy group (*4*). In the original work the dis
isomer was isolated, but subsequently the con isomer (*5*) was
also obtained. 7-Dis-O-methylnogalarol was found to be
superior to nogalamycin as an antitumor compound. When disnogamycin was obtained, it was treated with acidic methanol to
obtain 7-con- and 7-dis-O-methylnogarol (*6*,*7*). These pairs of
compounds (*4-5* and *6-7*) differed only in stereochemistry at
C-7. 7-Con-O-methylnogarol was found to be the most active of
the nogalamycin analogs, and it will be discussed in more
detail subsequently. The ratio of compounds *6* and *7* formed in
the reaction was about 4:6. Purification was quite difficult
as aromatization of ring A occurred readily to form nogarene
(*9*), solubility was a problem, and removal of solvents was
quite difficult.

It was found that analogous 7-O-alkyl pairs in the nogalarol and nogarol series could be obtained using ethanol and
n-propanol. The two compounds in each pair exhibit characteristic differences. In the nogarol series, the chemical shift
for C-6 in the ^{13}C NMR spectra in the dis isomers (*trans*) is
about δ 1.5 downfield from that of the con isomer (*cis*) while
the C-10 signal is about δ 1 upfield. The nogalarol pairs
show similar differences. In all cases the dis isomer was
less mobile than the con isomer in tlc using silica gel plates
and a chloroform-methanol-water (78:20:2) system. Circular
dichroism curves were quite characteristic for each isomer of

Scheme 2

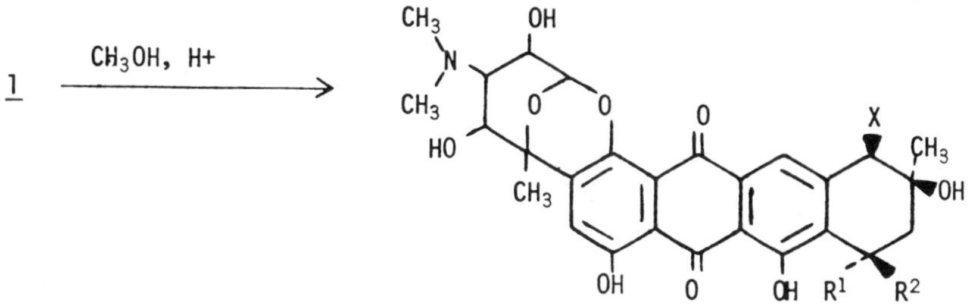

(**4**) 7-Dis-O-methylnogalarol: X = COOCH$_3$, R^1 = CH$_3$O, R^2 = H

(**5**) 7-Con-O-methylnogalarol: X = COOCH$_3$, R^1 = H, R^2 = CH$_3$O

(**6**) 7-Dis-O-methylnogarol: X = H, R^1 = CH$_3$O, R^2 = H

(**7**) 7-Con-O-methylnogarol: X = H, R^1 = H, R^2 = CH$_3$O

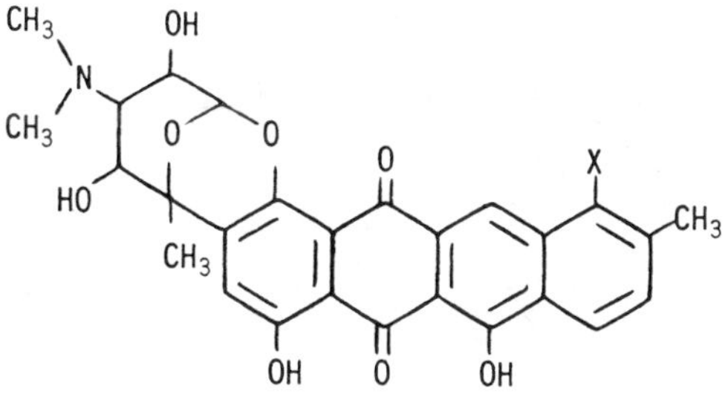

(**8**) Nogalarene: X = COOCH$_3$

(**9**) Nogarene: X = H

a pair, and all curves for con compounds were quite similar as were all dis curves.

The isomerization of various anthracyclinones at C-7 by reaction with trifluoroacetic acid followed by hydrolysis has been reported (6). Disnogamycin (*3*) was found to give a somewhat similar reaction. A solution of *3* in trifluoroacetic acid at ~15° to 25° gave a reaction product which was not completely characterized but which reacted with nucleophiles to introduce the nucleophile at C-7 with essentially complete stereospecificity. The products had the opposite chirality at C-7 to that in 3. The reaction in which the nucleophile is methoxide is indicated in Scheme 3. This reaction appears to be entirely general for nucleophiles occurring with alkoxides, mercaptides, acid anions, ammonia, primary and secondary amines, azides, and carbanions. The product in all cases was the con isomer even in one case in which the con isomer, 7-con-0-methylnogarol, was the starting material.

Scheme 3

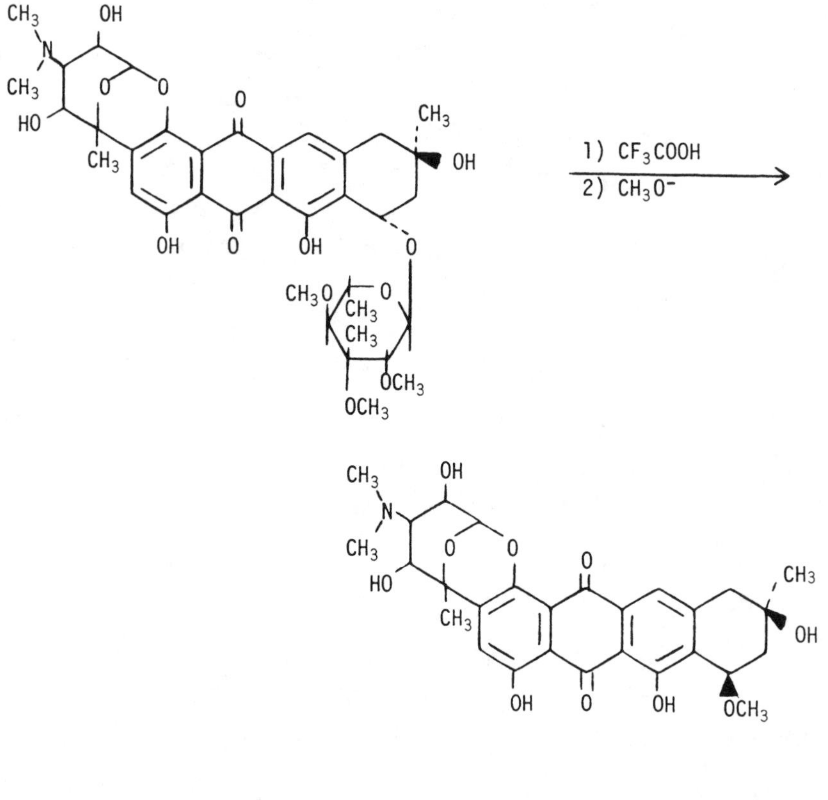

The first product after trifluoroacetic acid treatment was never obtained pure as it proved to be very difficult to purify, but it was found that the intermediate contains a tri-fluoroacetate moiety other than as a salt. It seems probable that during the course of the reaction a trifluoroacetate is formed at C-7, and this intermediate is attacked by the nucle-ophile (Scheme 4). In order to result in the observed chira-lity, the hydroxyl group at C-9 must influence the stereochem-istry of the intermediate. This may occur through an intermediate oxetane ring or its ion pair equivalent. Only ring A is indicated in Scheme 4. This procedure allowed the preparation of a large number of nogalamycin analogs although only con isomers could be obtained.

Scheme 4

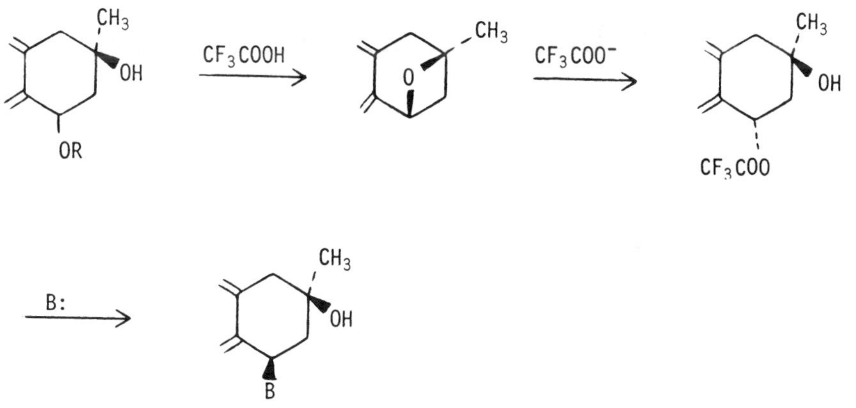

The instability to light of nogalamycin in organic sol-vents was noted very early in chemical studies on nogalamycin. It has now been found that irradiation in direct sunlight of nogalamycin and its analogs in solution in chloroform or chloroform-methanol leads to rapid conversion to two

principal products and several minor ones. Diffuse light has
the same effect, but it occurs much more slowly. The principal products are those resulting from the loss of one of the
N-methyl groups and from conversion of one N-methyl group to
N-formyl (Scheme 5). Similar photochemical N-demethylation
has been reported previously (7), but no N-formyl product was
reported. This reaction has been run with nogalamycin, disnogamycin, and 7-con-O-methylnogarol. The N-demethyl compounds were very difficult to purify and were N-acetylated for
purification and characterization.

A number of acetyl derivatives of nogalamycin and its
analogs have been prepared, but for the most part they are
relatively unstable and are mixtures which are difficult to
purify. It has now been found that acetylation occurs readily
and regiospecifically using acetic anhydride in methanol as
the acetylating agent to give good yields of 2',4'-di-O-
acetylnogalamycin and the corresponding disnogamycin derivative (*10* and *11*) Presumably a similar acetylation would occur
with all analogs retaining the dimethylamino group.

(<u>10</u>) 2',4'-Di-O-acetylnogalamycin: X = COOCH$_3$

(<u>11</u>) 2',4'-Di-O-acetyldisnogamycin: X = H

Scheme 5

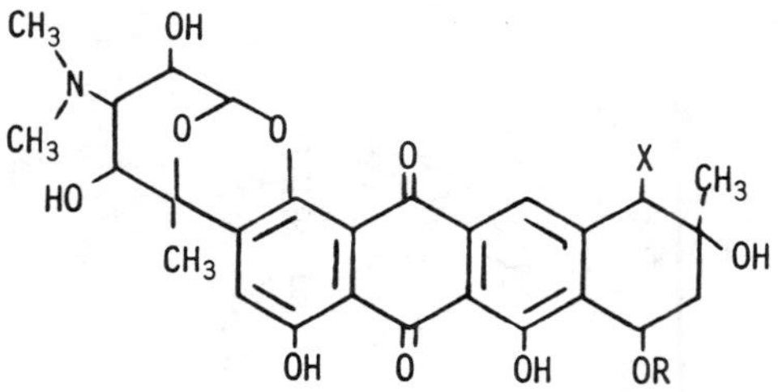

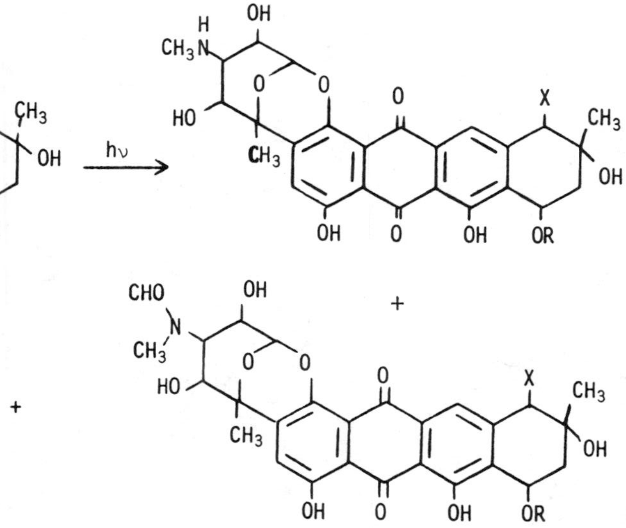

Nogalamycin: X = COOCH₃,   R = nogalosyl

Disnogamycin: X = H, R = nogalosyl

7-Con-O-methylnogarol: X = H, R = CH₃O

Those compounds having aromatized A rings (*8* and *9*) were prepared by vigorous acidic treatment of nogalamycin and disnogamycin respectively. Two further compounds having no oxygen at C-7 were prepared by catalytic reduction of *1* to give 7-deoxynogalarol (*12*) and conversion of *12* to 7-deoxynogarol (*13*) by a sequence analogous to that shown in Scheme 1.

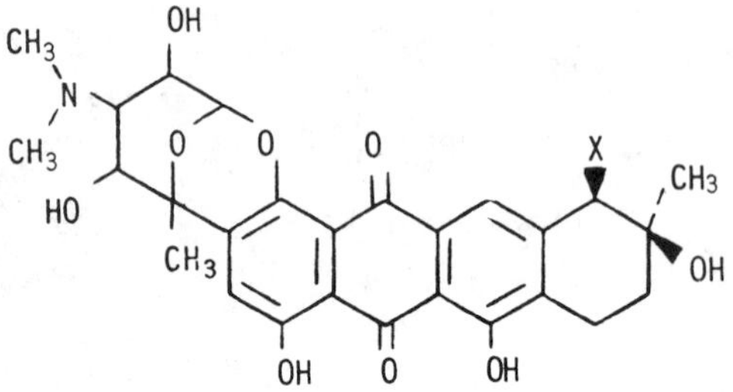

(12) 7-Deoxynogalarol: X = COOCH₃

(13) 7-Deoxynogarol: X = H

For the most part, activities of these compounds will refer to activity against L1210 cells *in vitro* or P388 which is a murine leukemia line and is an *in vivo* assay. Activity against L1210 leukemia *in vivo* and B16 melanoma *in vivo* will also be reported in some cases, and also some antibacterial activities will be mentioned.

In Table 1, a comparison of *in vitro* activities of the series going from carbomethoxy at C-10 through carboxyl to hydrogen is shown. Also, nogalamycin and disnogamycin can be compared with their analogs having a methoxy substituent at C-7 and having the same chirality as the parent compounds and with analogs lacking a C-7 substituent. These compounds

TABLE I. *Comparison of In Vitro Activity with Modification at C-7 and C-10[a]*

Compound	L1210 in vitro	
	ID_{50}	ID_{90}
Nogalamycin	0.078	0.18
Nogalamycinic acid	1.00	1.94
Disnogamycin	0.18	0.27
7-Dis-0-methylnogalarol	0.27	0.67
7-Dis-0-methylnogarol	0.41	0.91
7-Deoxynogalarol	0.58	1.51
7-Deoxynogarol	0.94	1.76

[a]*Activities against L1210 cells expressed as the μM concentration necessary to inhibit cell growth by 50% and 90%.*

TABLE II. *Comparison of In Vivo Activity with Modification at C-7 and C-10[a]*

Compound	P388 Leukemia		L1210 Leukemia	
	Dose[b]	% ILS	Dose[b]	% ILS
Nogalamycin	1	49	1	30
Nogalamycinic acid	20	56	20	18
Disnogamycin	5	93	2.5	27
7-Dis-0-methylnogalarol	25	60	50	12
7-Dis-0-methylnogarol	12.5	76	--	--
7-Deoxynogalarol	50	27	400[c]	4
7-Deoxynogarol	100	21	--	--

[a]*P388 cells were injected IP on Day 0 and drug was injected IP daily on Days 1-9 unless otherwise noted.*
[b]*mg/kg/day.*
[c]*QDx1 (2).*

exhibit no great difference in their *in vitro* activities differing by approximately an order of magnitude with nogalamycinic acid and the 7-deoxy compounds being least active.
However, the *in vivo* activities against P388 and L1210
leukemias in mice (Table II) exhibit a rather different pic-
ture. In this assay, disnogamycin is substantially more
active than the other compounds against P388 but is no more
active than nogalamycin against L1210. Nogalamycinic acid is
less potent but just as active as nogalamycin while the 7-
deoxy compounds show only marginal activity. However, the
7-O-methyl compounds are both quite active in the P388 leukemia assay.

The most extensive series prepared was one in which lower
alkoxy groups were substituted at C-7 in the series having
carbomethoxy at C-10 and in the series lacking this substituent. As these compounds were prepared by acidic alcoholysis,
two isomers differing in chirality at C-7 were obtained in
each instance. A total of twelve compounds of this type were
prepared. As indicated in Table III, the difference in activities of these compounds against L1210 *in vitro* did not differ
greatly showing at the maximum only a seven-fold difference.
However, in general the con isomers were more active than the
dis. The 7-methoxy compounds in the con series were both
quite active with 7-con-O-methylnogarol being the most active
of the group.

In the 7-alkoxy analogs of nogalamycin many were not
tested *in vivo*. Table IV shows results against P388 murine
leukemia of those compounds tested. The indication of the
in vitro test that 7-con-O-methylnogarol is the most active is
confirmed by these *in vivo* results although potency is substantially less than with either nogalamycin or disnogamycin.
In the con nogarol group, which is the only one completely

TABLE III. Activities of 7-Alkoxynogalarols and 7-Alkoxynogarols against L1210 In Vitro[a]

C-7 Substituent	Nogalarols				Nogarols			
	Dis		Con		Dis		Con	
	ID_{50}	ID_{90}	ID_{50}	ID_{90}	ID_{50}	ID_{90}	ID_{50}	ID_{90}
CH_3O	0.27	0.67	0.13	0.30	0.41	0.91	0.061	0.13
C_2H_5O	0.16	0.36	0.15	0.34	0.43	1.42	0.16	0.32
$n\text{-}C_3H_7O$	0.16	0.39	0.33	0.73	0.33	1.02	0.10	0.30

[a]Activities against L1210 cells are expressed as the μM concentration necessary to inhibit cell growth by 50% and 90%.

TABLE IV. Activities of 7-Alkoxynogalarols and 7-Alkoxynogarols against Murine P388 Leukemia[a]

Substituent	Nogalarols				Nogarols			
	Dis		Con		Dis		Con	
	Dose[b]	% ILS	Dose[b]	% ILS	Dose[b]	% ILS	Dose[b]	% ILS
CH_3O	25	60	25	98	12.5	76	12.5	197
C_2H_5O	--	--	12.5	70	--	--	6.5	63
$n\text{-}C_3H_2O$	3.13	50	10	34	3.1	50	6.3	34

[a] P388 leukemic cells were injected IP on Day 0 and drug was injected IP on Days 1-9.

[b] mg/kg/day.

tested, the activity decreases with increasing length of the alkyl group on oxygen at C-7. This is also indicated in the con nogalarol and the dis nogarol series although only two compounds can be compared in each case. A comparison of the four 7-methoxy compounds shows that nogarols are more active than nogalarols and con isomers more active than dis.

As already mentioned, various nucleophiles can be readily substituted at C-7 in disnogamycin for nogalose. It is of interest that most of these show substantial activity both *in vitro* and *in vivo*. The activities of five representative compounds of this group, all in the con series, are shown in Table V. The *in vitro* activities did not differ greatly except for the dimethylamino one. The amino compounds and the acetoxy compound show substantial *in vivo* activity on the order of nogalamycin. Even an azido substituent at C-7 gives a compound having some activity.

Table VI shows *in vitro* and *in vivo* activities of compounds derived from irradiation of nogalamycin, disnogamycin, and 7-con-O-methylnogarol. It might be expected that the N-demethyl compounds would have considerable activity, and this was the case for N-demethylnogalamycin and 7-con-O-methyl-N-demethylnogarol. The latter was not only quite active but had a potency rivaling that of nogalamycin. Somewhat surprisingly N-demethyl-disnogamycin was only marginally, if at all, active. Those compounds in which an N-methyl was replaced by N-formyl were totally inactive.

2',4'-Di-O-acetylnogalamycin and 2',4'-di-O-acetyldisnoga-mycin were quite difficult to test as they hydrolyzed readily in aqueous systems to the parent compounds. As indicated in Table VII, both showed considerable Gram-positive antibacteri-al activity and good L1210 *in vitro* activity, but these results may be due to hydrolysis. The P388 murine leukemia

TABLE V. *Activities of Acetoxy, Mercapto, Amino, and Azido Analogs*[a]

Substituent at C-7	L1210 *in vitro*		P388 leukemia *in vivo*	
	ID_{50}	ID_{90}	Dose[c]	% ILS
CH_3COO	0.51	1.43	10	87
CH_3S	0.13	0.34	8	37
CH_3NH	0.50	1.63	25	58
$(CH_3)_2N$	1.58	3.12	50	54
N_3	0.83	1.76	5	33

[a]*Activities against L1210 cells expressed as the μM concentration necessary to inhibit cell growth by 50% and 90%.*

[b]*P388 leukemic cells were injected IP on Day 0 and drug was injected IP on Days 1-9.*

[c]*mg/kg/day.*

assays were run by preparing fresh solutions immediately prior to injection. At higher levels 2',4'-di-O-acetyl-nogalamycin was toxic, and this may have precluded the finding of *in vivo* activity.

Those compounds having ring A aromatized (nogalarene and nogarene) are still active against L1210 *in vitro* having ID_{50} 0.24 and 0.23 respectively. Nogalarene was approximately as active against P388 murine leukemia as was nogalamycin although about seventy times as much drug was required.

TABLE VI. *Analogs from Irradiation*[a,b]

Compound	L1210 *in vitro*		P388 *in vivo*	
	ID_{50}	ID_{90}	Dose[c]	% ILS
N-Demethylnogalamycin	0.36	0.90	25	59
N-Formyl-N-demethylnogalamycin	>1	>1	25	12
N-Demethyldisnogamycin	0.88	>1	33	24
N-Formyl-N-demethyldisnogamycin	>1	>1	50	0
7-Con-O-methyl-N-demethyl-nogarol	0.038	0.11	1.25	73
7-Con-O-methyl-N-formyl-N-demethylnogarol	4.3	5	--	--

[a]*P388 leukemic cells were injected IP on Day 0 and drug was injected IP on Days 1, 4, and 9.*

[b]*Activities against L1210 cells expressed as the µM concentration necessary to inhibit cell growth by 50% and 90%.*

[c]*mg/kg/dose.*

As mentioned earlier, 7-con-O-methylnogarol was by far the most active against murine P388 leukemia of any of the nogala-mycin analogs tested. It was tested further against murine L1210 leukemia and murine B16 melanoma. In both tests it was highly active. As Adriamycin[tm] is the most effective anti-tumor agent used at present, 7-con-O-methylnogarol was com-pared directly with this compound (8). As can be seen in Table VIII, 7-con-O-methylnogarol is at least as active as Adriamycin against P388 *in vivo*, somewhat more active against L1210 murine leukemia *in vivo*, but less active against B16 melanoma. However, 7-con-O-methylnogarol has only about one-tenth the potency of Adriamycin. 7-Con-O-methylnogarol was

TABLE VII.   Activities of 2',4'-di-O-acetyl Derivatives[a,b]

Test	2',4'-di-O-acetyl-nogalamycin	2',4'-di-O-acetyl-disnogamycin
L1210 in vitro	ID_{50} 0.060 mcg/ml	ID_{50} 0.062 mcg/ml
P388 in vivo	3 (6.25 mg/kg/dose)	41 (50 mg/kg/dose)
Bacillus subtilis	29	24
Bacillus cereus	23	15
Sarcinea lutea	25	20
Streptococcus pyogenes	32	28
Mycobacterium avium	26	22

[a]P388 leukemia cells were injected IP on Day 0 and drug was injected IP on Days 2, 4, and 9. Results are expressed as % ILS.

[b]Antibacterial assays are expressed in zone sizes in mm.

just as active when injected IP against IV-injected cells as against IP-injected tumor cells. This indicated that its activity was not due to contact toxicity. Adriamycin was essentially inactive when tested in this way. Also, 7-con-0-methylnogarol is as active when administered orally as when injected although about twice as much drug was required.

In view of the activity of 7-con-0-methylnogarol, it was tested further at the National Cancer Institute in a panel of seven tumors. Three of these tumors were the same as those shown in Table VIII, and results were much the same. In four additional solid tumors (Table IX), 7-con-0-methylnogarol was

TABLE VIII. *Comparative Antitumor Activity of 7-Con-O-Methylnogarol and Adriamycin[a]*

Tumor	7-Con-O-Methylnogarol		Adriamycin	
	Dose[b]	% ILS	Dose[b]	% ILS
P388	12.5	168	1	158
L1210	12.5	104	2	40
B16	10	114	1	166

[a]*Tumor cells were injected IP on Day 0 and drug was injected IP on Days 1-9.*

[b]*mg/kg/day.*

TABLE IX. *Antitumor Activity of 7-Con-O-methylnogarol in Various Murine Tumors[a]*

System	Site[b]	Schedule[c]	Dose (mg/kg/dose)	% ILS (cures)
Colon 26	IP	Q4Dx2(1)	25	106 (4)
Lewis Lung	IP	Q1Dx9(1)	12.5	38
				T/C (cures)
Colon 38	SC	Q7Dx2(2)	25	21 (3)
CD8F1 Mammary	SC	Q7Dx5(1)	25	1

[a]*Tests done at the National Cancer Institute.*

[b]*Site of tumor inoculation.*

[c]*Q4Dx2(1) means drug was given every fourth day for two injections starting on Day 1.*

[d]*Ratio of median tumor size of treated and control animals x 100.*

active in two colon tumors and a mammary tumor but not in
Lewis lung. These results are such that this compound is
being extensively investigated as an antitumor agent.

In summary, it can be said that substantial modification
of nogalamycin at three positions—C-7, C-10, and the
dimethylamino group—has given a number of compounds having
activity as good as or better than the parent compound. It
also has led to an analog, 7-con-O-methylnogarol, having outstanding antitumor properties.

ACKNOWLEDGMENTS

I wish to thank Mrs. Jian Johnson, Mr. David W. Elrod, and
Mr. David J. Houser for most of the chemical work discussed.
I also wish to express my appreciation for the use of biological data developed by Dr. L. H. Li, Dr. J. Patrick McGovren,
and Dr. Gary L. Neil and their associates. My thanks are
extended to Dr. William Krueger who did the circular dichroism
studies. A portion of the biological results was furnished by
the National Cancer Institute.

REFERENCES

1. Wiley, P. F., *J. Nat. Prod. 42*, 569 (1979).
2. Wiley, P. F., MacKellar, F. A., Caron, E. L., and Kelly,
   R. B., *Tetrahedron Lett.* 663 (1968).
3. Wiley, P. F., Kelly, R. B., Caron, E. L., Wiley, V. H.,
   Johnson, J. H., MacKellar, F. A., and Mizsak, S. A., *J.
   Am. Chem. Soc. 99*, 4030 (1979).
4. Eckle, E., Stezowski, J. J., and Wiley, P. F., *Tetrahedron
   Lett. 21*, 507 (1980).

5. Wiley, P. F., Elrod, D. W., Houser, D. J., Johnson, J. L.,
   Moscowitz, A., Pschigoda, L. M., and Krueger, W. C., *J.
   Org. Chem. 44*, 4030 (1979).

6. Brockmann, H., and Niemeyer, J., *Chem. Ber. 100*, 3578
   (1967).

7. Stenberg, V. I., Singh, S. P., Narain, N. K., and Parmar,
   S. K., *J. Chem. Soc. Chem. Commun.*, 262 (1976).

8. Neil, G. L., Kuentzel, S. L., and McGovren, J. P., *Cancer
   Treat. Rep. 63*, 1971 (1979).

APPROACHES TO MORE EFFECTIVE ANTHRACYCLINES
BY ANALOG SYNTHESIS AND EVALUATION[1]

Edward M. Acton
Carol W. Mosher
John M. Gruber[2]

Life Sciences Division
SRI International
Menlo Park, California

I. INTRODUCTION

Present efforts to develop new anticancer agents derived
from anthracyclines can take advantage of an excellent back-
ground of knowledge and experience. This includes an aware-
ness of the clinical applications and limitations of doxorubicin and several analogs, wider knowledge of structure-
activity relationships than ever before, and a better under-
standing of proposed biochemical mechanisms of action. The
need for new anthracyclines was recently defined (1) in terms
of four factors, involving not only diminished toxicity but
improved activity. The practical approach is still the derivatization of natural anthracyclines, as in general the
total synthesis of these complex molecules is not yet feasible for the amounts needed in drug development. Doxorubicin (2), because of its unique clinical importance, would
seem to be a logical starting material for semisynthetic analogs, but daunorubicin (1) is the more feasible because it
is more readily and less expensively obtainable by

[1]*Supported by Cancer Research Emphasis Grant CA 25711 from the
National Cancer Institute, DHHS.*

[2]*Present address: Zoecon Corp., Palo Alto, California*

fermentation. Daunorubicin is also more stable and more soluble than doxorubicin and therefore easier to use in synthetic reactions. Anthracycline activity can be altered by such small differences in structure as the 14-OH that distinguishes 2 from 1, but is also consistent with such wide changes in structure as between 2 and aclacinomycin A.

Our current interests focus on two sites in the anthracycline structure, the quinone and the sugar amine. The quinone is a key site of biochemical action involving quinone redox properties that are relevant to proposed mechanisms of biological activity (2,3). The amine function readily undergoes reductive alkylation in one step with a variety of aldehydes and ketones, and this can be used to introduce a wide variety of structural changes while amine basicity is retained (4,5).

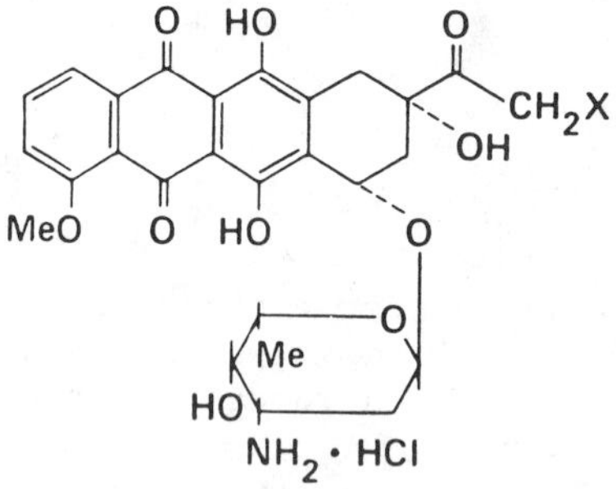

1, X = H, daunorubicin,

2, X = OH, doxorubicin (Adriamycin)

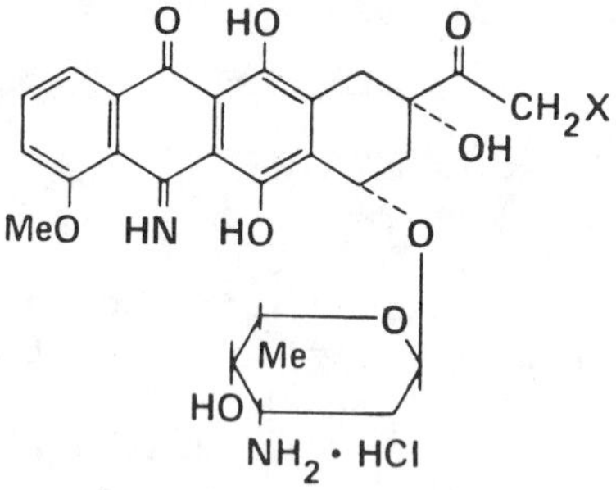

3, X = H, 5-iminodaunorubicin

4, X = OH, 5-iminodoxorubicin

II. IMINO DERIVATIVES

So far, the only type of change at the quinone in the entire series of anthracyclines has been the conversion to the 5-imine (6,7). Treatment of daunorubicin with cold methanolic ammonia gave exclusively the 5-imine 3, uniquely stabilized by H-bonding with both peri substituents--in a complementary sense the NH is an H-bond donor to the 4-OMe and an H-bond receptor from the 6-OH (6). No appreciable amination was observed at the 12-position where only one H-bond would be possible. The chemical stability of the 5-imine was demonstrated under both hydrolytic and reductive conditions (unpublished results). Prolonged treatment of <u>3</u> with dilute acid at room temperature produced selective cleavage of the sugar moiety, without loss of the imine from the resultant aglycone <u>5</u>. Reductive cleavage of the sugar with sodium dithionite produced the 7-deoxy aglycone <u>6</u>, also without loss of the imine, and sodium cyanoborohydride at pH 4.5 selectively produced the 13-dihydro derivative <u>7</u> of <u>3</u>.

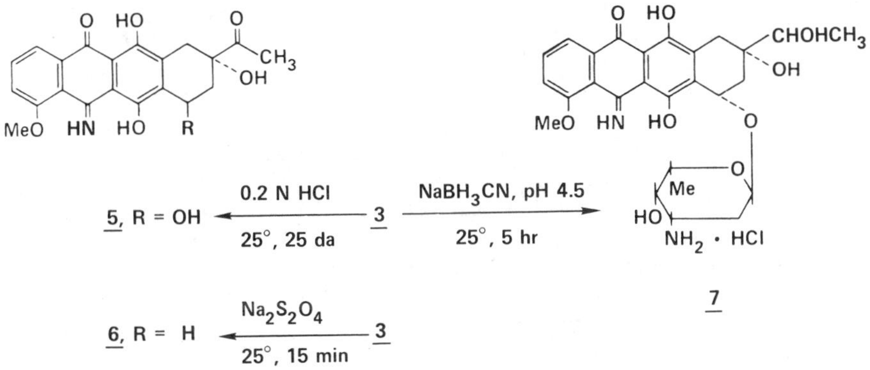

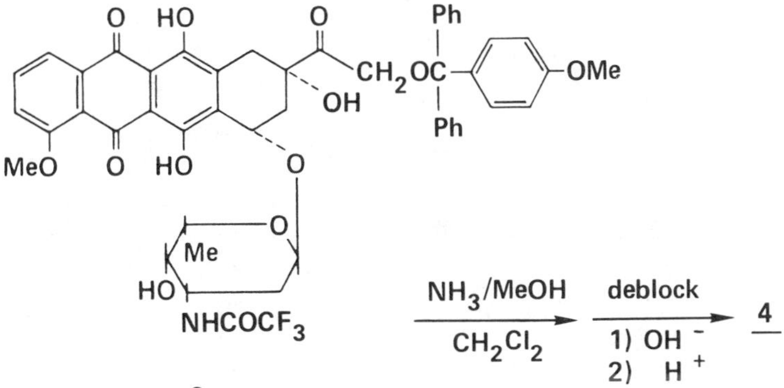

Doxorubicin, on the other hand, upon treatment with methanolic ammonia produced little of the 5-imine <u>4</u>. Instead there was extensive decomposition, no doubt brought about by base lability of the hydroxyketone side chain. Successful synthesis of 5-iminodoxorubicin (<u>4</u>) required prior blocking of the 14-OH (7). Conversion to the p-anisyldiphenylmethyl ether was the method of choice, but this in turn required initial N-trifluoroacetylation, in order to avoid alkylation of the amine as well as the 14-OH with p-anisyldiphenylmethyl chloride. Ammonolysis of the resultant N-trifluoroacetyl 14-O-p-anisyldiphenylmethyl ether (8) occurred with minimal decomposition. After removal of the blocking groups, 4 was obtained in 21% yield overall from 2, in five steps requiring chromatographic purification at two points.

Biological test results for the imino compounds 3 and 4 are summarized in Table I, in comparison with the parent anthracyclines 1 and 2 (6,7). The results include antitumor screening data against leukemia P388 in mice, obtained under auspices of the National Cancer Institute. Antitumor efficacy (% T/C) is measured by the survival time of mice treated at the optimum dose, which measures the potency of the drug, compared to the survival time of tumor-bearing controls. The dose schedule used, with the implanted tumor allowed to progress for four days and become systemic before treatment on days 5, 9, and 13, produces a deliberately stringent test (i.e., T/C = 130% for the clinically useful 1 is little more than the T/C of 125% defined as the minimum for significant

Table I   Comparison of Biological Properties of the 5-Imino Derivatives[a]

| Compound | Activity versus mouse leukemia P388 | | Leukemia L1210 cells inhibn of synth ED_{50}, μM | | ΔT_m of isolated helical DNA in solution | Microsomal O_2 consumption, stimulation relative to 2 |
	Efficacy % T/C	Optimum dose q4d 5,9,13 mg/kg	DNA	RNA	°C	%
3	130	3	1.6	1.3	6.2	8.2
4	217	100 (highest dose)	2.0	2.1	6.9	7.5
1	130	8	1.0	0.3	11.2	82, 109
2	160	8	1.5	0.7	13.4	100
	NCI		D.L. Taylor, SRI			J.H. Peters, G.R. Gordon SRI

[a]The data are from ref. 7, except for the data on 4 versus P388, which are new and at a higher dose.

activity). Conversion to the quinonimine was unexpectedly different in its effect on the antitumor properties of 1 and 2. With 5-iminodaunorubicin (3), for example, there was no change in antitumor efficacy. The lower optimum dose suggested an increase in potency, but this was not observed in other dose schedules against leukemia P388 or in tests against other mouse tumors, and the overall impression was that neither efficacy nor potency was significantly changed. This is surprising if the quinone is a mechanistically important site of action. On the other hand, with 5-iminodoxorubicin (4) there was a dramatic increase in antitumor efficacy (T/C = 217%) and a twelve-fold decrease in potency. Except for two recent examples (described below), reproducible T/C values of 217% are unsurpassed by anthracyclines against leukemia P388 in the q4d 5,9,13 schedule. (This value at 100 mg/kg supersedes the result previously reported in ref. 7 at 50 mg/kg; still higher doses need to be tested before the optimum dose and peak efficacy is established at 100 mg/kg.) The analogs 3 and 4 provide another example of the inexplicable difference in biological properties introduced by the 14-OH of doxorubicin.

The in vitro tests in Table I were chosen for relevance to the two major proposed mechanisms of anthracycline activity. DNA interactive properties are measured by the doses (ED$_{50}$) required for 50% inhibition of nucleic acid synthesis, and by the increase (ΔT_m) in thermal denaturation temperature of helical DNA upon complexation with the drug in solution. The data indicate a moderate decrease in DNA interactions for both 3 and 4. (Also indicative of this was the loss of mutagenicity by 3 against S. typhimurium tester strain TA 98.) Much more striking is the weak effect of both 3 and 4 on the consumption of oxygen by liver microsomes (7,8). The imino compounds produced less than 10% of the stimulatory effect produced by 1 or 2 (the reference standard). When 2 is added to liver microsomes with NADPH cofactor, the dramatic increase in O_2 consumption over the endogenous level apparently reflects an increased production of free radicals (2,3). This may be a generally cytotoxic effect, but much current thinking associates radical formation with anthracycline cardiotoxicity. The diminished radical production by 3 and 4, also evidenced in other studies on the altered redox properties of the imino quinone function of 3 (9), may well indicate diminished cardiotoxicity, especially since no other change of in vivo property has been observed so far upon going from quinone to imino quinone.

There is, in fact, evidence for diminished cardiotoxicity of 3, judging from the diminished electrocardiographic changes after chronic treatment in the rat (Table II). The method developed by Zbinden serially measured prolongation of the QRS complex in the electrocardiogram (10). He found that

Table II. Cardiotoxic Potency in Rats: Total Dose to Cause Electrocardiographic Changes

Compound	15% Prolongation of QRS mg/kg	10% Prolongation of QRS mg/kg	of QαT mg/kg
2	10-12	8[a]	4[a]
3	64	48[b]	36[b]
	G. Zbinden et al., ref. 10	R.A. Jensen, SRI, 1981	

[a]*After multiple doses of 1, 2, or 4 mg/kg. The cumulative dose for 10% prolongation was thus independent of regimen.* [b]*After multiple doses of 4 mg/kg. After multiple doses of 10 or 16 mg/kg, higher cumulative doses (up to 80 mg/kg) were required for 10% prolongation, suggesting an even greater decrease in cardiotoxic potency. This variability with regimen has been observed only with 3 so far. Until it can be explained, we assume the low-dose results are more reliable and less subject to questions such as bioavailability.*

the lowest cumulative dose of 3 required to produce a presumably irreversible 15% prolongation was five or six times the lowest required dose of doxorubicin (2). A 5- to 10-fold decrease in cardiotoxic potency of 3 is being confirmed in further studies at SRI of electrocardiographic changes as an assay for cardiotoxicity (11). These studies include measurement of QαT prolongation and use computer averaging and recording of the ECG waves for improved sensitivity. Preliminary results, after doses of 3 at 4 mg/kg in the rat, are shown in Table II. Further attempts are being made to investigate the possible correlation of cardiotoxic effects with radical generating capacity among anthracycline analogs.

III. N-BENZYL DERIVATIVES

Reductive N-alkylation of the anthracyclines with various aldehydes and ketones in the presence of sodium cyanoborohydride has proven to be a versatile, one-step method for adding structural changes that can modify chemical, physical and biological properties (6,7). With excess formaldehyde the reductive alkylation goes rapidly through two stages to produce the N,N-dimethyl derivatives of 1 and 2, with no apparent formation of the mono N-methyl derivatives as isolable intermediates. With higher aldehydes, however, the reaction is slower, and either mono- or dialkyl derivatives can be obtained as the major products, depending on reaction time and stoichiometry. Ketones, even acetone, produce only monoakylation. Because the N-alkylation is a reductive method, the by-products of 13-ketone reduction are usually obtained also, in smaller amounts. When isolated by chromatography, these 13-dihydro derivatives are often useful as the expected first metabolite of the various N-alkyl analogs. Most of the N-alkyl analogs have shown activity against mouse leukemia P388 but were not greatly different from the parent anthracyclines 1 or 2. Exceptions were the lipophilic N-decyl derivatives, which were inactive, and the also lipophilic N-benzyl derivatives (Table III), some of which showed notably superior antitumor activity. With mono- and dialkylation and with ketone reduction at each stage, 1 and 2 each produced a series of four N-benzyl derivatives, 9-12 and 13-16 respectively, listed in Table III with the antitumor test results. (Only for N,N-dibenzyldoxorubicin (15) was the amount produced so small as to prevent completion of the antileukemic screen, because in the extended reaction time for dibenzylation the reactive keto group of the doxorubicin molecule was almost entirely reduced to produce 16; this could perhaps be prevented by a bulky blocking group on the 14-OH.) In each series, there is a trend toward increased efficacy and decreased potency, in going from parent, to mono, to dibenzyl. In fact, the T/C values of 209% for N,N-dibenzyldaunorubicin (11) and 210% for N,N-dibenzyl-13-dihydrodoxorubicin (16) are among the highest observed (along with T/C = 217% for 4) in this antitumor screen. Such values are reproducibly surpassed only by two examples new in 1981 (described below). For further investigation, dibenzyl-daunorubicin (11) with an optimum dose of 38 mg/kg was obviously to be favored over the equally efficacious 16 but less potent at an optimum dose of 100 mg/kg. Tests against a number of other tumors in mice under the auspices of NCI (unpublished data) showed that 11 was also superior to 2 against a mouse (CD8F1) mammary tumor, and was active against a mouse colon tumor (colon 38) to which 2 was inactive. For these reasons, 11 was selected for studies in the initial steps (NCI Decision Network 2A) leading to preclinical development at NCI.

N,N-Dibenzyldaunorubicin (11) has also been tested for cardiotoxic potency in rats by the serial measurement of ECG

Table III. Antitumor Properties of N–Benzylation Products[a]

N–Benzyl derivatives	Activity versus mouse leukemia P388	
	Efficacy % T/C	Optimum dose q4d 5,9,13 mg/kg
1, R = $COCH_3$, X = NH_2	132	8
9, R = $COCH_3$, X = $NHCH_2Ph$	184	19
10, R = $CHOH-CH_3$, X = $NHCH_2Ph$	168	19
11, R = $COCH_3$, X = $N(CH_2Ph)_2$	209	38
12, R = $CHOH-CH_3$, X = $N(CH_2Ph)_2$	184	25
2, R = $COCH_2OH$, X = NH_2	160	8
13, R = $COCH_2OH$, X = $NHCH_2Ph$	190	19
14, R = $CHOH-CH_2OH$, X = $NHCH_2Ph$	135	38
15, R = $COCH_2OH$, X = $N(CH_2Ph)_2$	active, incomplete test	
16, R = $CHOH-CH_2OH$, X = $N(CH_2Ph)_2$	210	100
	NCI	

[a]*Data from ref. 4.*

changes with multiple dosing (11). The results in comparison with those for 2 are shown in Table IV. Table IV also compares the antitumor potencies for 11 and for 2, so that a preliminary estimation of the therapeutic advantage of 11 can be made. The table shows that cardiotoxic potency decreased over a range of 30- to 45-fold in going from 2 to 11 (the factor of 30 was calculated from 240/8, and 45 = 180/4). On the other hand, antitumor potency decreased only 4.8-fold (38/8 = 4.8). Hence, 11 may have an approximately 8-fold advantage over 2, based on a separation of the antitumor and cardiotoxic effects (the factor of 8 was derived by dividing 4.8 into the range 30-45). The separation of effects is probably even greater than this calculation shows, because as noted in Table IV the ECG changes observed with 11 were found

Table IV. Comparison of Potencies of Effects

	In mice	In rats	
	Antitumor potency[a]	Cardiotoxic potency[b]	
		In electrocardiogram, total dose to cause 10% widening of	
	Opt dose vs P388 (q4d, 5,9,13)	QRS complex	$Q\alpha T$ complex
Compound	mg/kg	mg/kg	mg/kg
2	8	8^c (irreversible)	4^c
11	38	240-280^d (reversible)	170-180^d
Ratio (decrease in potency for 11)	$\dfrac{1}{4.8}$	$\dfrac{1}{>30\text{-}45}$	$\dfrac{1}{>42\text{-}45}$

$$\text{Therapeutic advantage for } 11 = \frac{\text{antitumor potency ratio}}{\text{cardiotoxic potency ratio}} = \frac{\dfrac{1}{4.8}}{\dfrac{1}{30\text{-}45}} \geqslant \frac{8}{1}$$

[a]NCI. [b]Ref. 11. [c]After multiple doses (intraperitoneal) of 1, 2, and 4 mg/kg. [d]After multiple doses (intravenous) of 10 and 20 mg/kg. Hence the cardiotoxic endpoint, though reversible, appeared to be independent of dose schedule.

to be reversible after dosing stopped, in contrast to the irreversible changes produced by 2.

In vitro test results for all the N-benzyl compounds are presented in Table V. It appears that the dibenzyl compounds show little or no activity in any in vitro test system that

Table V. In Vitro Tests of N-Benzyl Series

Compound	ΔT_m of isolated helical DNA in solution °C	Leukemia L1210 cells inhibn of synth ED_{50}, μM DNA	Leukemia L1210 cells inhibn of synth ED_{50}, μM RNA	Ames mutagenicity revertant/nmol	Stimulation of microsomal O_2 consumption, % rel to 2	Redox props of quinone
1	11.2	0.66	0.33	100	109, 82	active
9 (mono)	10.2	1.6	0.17	0.5	8	
10	6.2	1.7	0.32	0.5	21	
11 (di)	1.4	>100	10	0.5	2	
12	0.6	220	8	0.5	4	~inactive
2	13.4	1.5	0.58		100	active
13 (mono)	11.3	0.65	0.09			
14	7.6	1.4	0.29			
15 (di)	-1.2	110	4.8			
16	insol	160	8.0			~inactive
	D.L. Taylor, SRI			V. Simmon, SRI	ref. 12	

was tried (4,12). Except for Ames mutagenicity, which is apparently absent from all N-alkyl derivatives, the loss of activity seems to be gradual in going from parent (1 or 2), to mono, to dibenzyl. The loss of in vitro activity was opposite to the increase in antitumor efficacy (Table III) in this progression. This divergence was at first surprising, but now seems explainable by metabolism studies of 11. Our recent measurements in tissue and plasma from rats treated (intravenous) with 11 show there is stepwise debenzylation at the amino N, in addition to the usual reduction of the 13-ketone (12). The major metabolites thus include the entire series of N-benzyl derivatives (Table III) formed from 1, as well as 1 itself. N,N-Dibenzyldaunorubicin may therefore be considered a prodrug, requiring in vivo activation, for any or all of these active analogs. Presumably, this metabolic scheme is similar to that for any of the dibenzyl analogs, 16, for example. It seems possible that the debenzylation-activation process may involve some selectivity that accounts for the apparent separation of oncolytic and cardiotoxic effects in 11. In further drug design, it may also be possible to use the metabolically cleavable N-benzyl group to create new prodrugs of other active analogs.

We speculate that debenzylation can occur by means of metabolic hydroxylation at the reactive benzylic CH_2, followed by spontaneous hydrolysis of the resultant imino acetal. An isomer of 11 that lacks an N-benzyl carbon was N-(2,2-diphenylethyl)daunorubicin (17), synthesized by reductive alkylation of 1 with diphenylacetaldehyde (unpublished results, in preparation). At a neutral pH in $H_2O-CH_3OH-CH_3CN$

1, X = NH_2

Ph$_2$CHCH=O

NaBH$_3$CN

17, X = NHCH$_2$CH$\langle$ $_{Ph}^{Ph}$

9, X = NHCH$_2$Ph

HOCH$_2$CH=O

NaBH$_3$CN

18, X = NCH$_2$Ph
             |
          CH$_2$CH$_2$OH

with the commonly used 20-fold excess of aldehyde, the yield
of 17 was 35% after about 30 min and was not improved by prolonged reaction. The yield was, however, increased to about
65% simply by adding 0.5% acetic acid. Significant reduction
of the 13-ketone, expected under acidic conditions, was not
observed--probably because of the fast reaction and excess of
aldehyde used. The biological test data for the isomers 11
and 17 are compared in Table VI. The non-benzylic compound
17 was not inactive, although it required a very high dose
(200 mg/kg). Like 11, 17 showed no binding to helical DNA
and no significant stimulation of microsomal O_2 consumption,
but unlike 11 it did inhibit nucleic acid synthesis in
L1210. No doubt metabolism studies of 17 will be required to
explain this pattern of in vivo and in vitro effects.

Table VI. Biological Results on Additional N-Benzyl Analogs

Cpd	Amino substit.	Activity versus mouse leukemia P388		Leukemia L1210 cells inhibn of synth ED_{50}, μM		ΔT_m of isolated helical DNA in solution	Microsomal O_2 consumption, stimulation relative to 2
		Efficacy % T/C	Optimum dose q4d 5,9,13 mg/kg	DNA	RNA	°C	%
11	N(CH$_2$Ph)$_2$	209	38	>100 (susp)	10	1.4	2
17	NHCH$_2$CHPh$_2$	147	200	3.5	3.8	0.1	6
9	NHCH$_2$Ph	184	19	1.6	0.17	10.2	8
18	NCH$_2$Ph | CH$_2$CH$_2$OH	240	128	6.0	2.2	5.0	10

N-Benzyldaunorubicin (9) was converted to the N-benzyl-N-
(2-hydroxyethyl) derivative 18 initially to produce a more
soluble member of the N-benzyl series, but because both the
N-benzyl and hydroxyethyl groups of 18 might be altered by
metabolic processes (debenzylation and O-conjugation, for
example), 18 could also be an interesting prodrug. The synthesis of 18 illustrated the usefulness of reductive alkylation as a general method and the advantages of acidic conditions in some cases. Attempts at N-hydroxyethylation of 9
with ethylene oxide in acetic acid solution at 25° produced

no acid degradation of the anthracycline but no alkylation
either.   Treatment of 9 with a 30-fold excess of glycol-
aldehyde in H_2O-CH_3CN acidified with 0.5% acetic acid produced after 40 minutes a 76% yield of 18.   Again, there was
little reduction of the 13-ketone.   Table VI shows that 18
was the most active anthracycline analog we have seen in
terms of antitumor efficacy.   The T/C value of 240% is markedly superior to the values of 210-215% which previously
appeared to be the highest attainable by anthracyclines
against leukemia P388 with the q4d 5,9,13 schedule.   (Another
synthetic anthracycline, the 3',4'-di-0-acetyl derivative of
3'-deamino-3'-hydroxydoxorubicin was recently reported to
show an average T/C = 244% at 128 mg/kg, ref 13).   Combining
different types of N-alkyl groups has been little tried so
far but may be a highly effective approach to new analogs.

IV. PIPERIDINO AND MORPHOLINO ANALOGS

    A distinct class of N-alkyl analogs has been generated by
reductive alkylation with dialdehydes.   For example, both
aldehyde functions of glutaraldehyde (19) gave reductive alkylation successively at the NH_2 of 1 or 2 to construct a new
6-membered ring that incorporated the amino N with the five
C's of glutaraldehyde (4,5).   The resultant piperidine com-
pounds--the 3'-deamino-3'-(1-piperidinyl) derivatives (26 and
28) of 1 and 2 and corresponding 13-dihydro derivatives (27
and 29)--all showed good antitumor activity (Table VII).
What was more unusual was that inhibition of RNA synthesis in
L1210 cells occurred at very low doses (ED_{50} = 0.04-0.05 μM
for 26-28), and was considerably more potent (factors up to
18-fold) than inhibition of DNA synthesis.   Most anthracyclines like 1 and 2 are only two or three times more potent
against RNA synthesis.   The results with 26-29 recalled the
suggestion that increased potency against RNA synthesis
denotes a Class II of anthracyclines (14).   This designation
was based on inhibition of nucleolar RNA synthesis, where
very striking increases in potency can be observed, so it is
uncertain how relevant to this are the results in Table VII
for the whole cell.   Structurally, with the piperidino
derivatives, the addition of a new ring to the sugar may have
some relevance to the fact that the Class II anthracyclines
so far have all been disaccharides or trisaccharides.
Clearly, reductive alkylation with dialdehydes and the
attachment of additional rings appeared to be an area of
further interest.

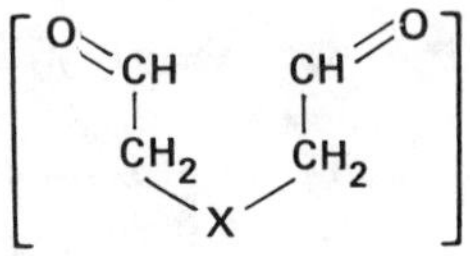

$$\left[\begin{array}{c} O{=}CH \qquad CH{=}O \\ | \qquad\qquad | \\ CH_2 \qquad CH_2 \\ {\diagdown}\,X\,{\diagup} \end{array} \right]$$

<u>19</u>, X = CH$_2$

<u>20</u>, X = CHOMe

<u>21</u>, X = CHCH$_2$OMe

<u>22</u>, X = C(CH$_2$OMe)$_2$

<u>23</u>, X = O

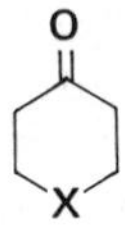

<u>24</u>, X = CH$_2$

<u>25</u>, X = O

1 or 2,
NaBH$_3$CN

1
NaBH$_3$CN

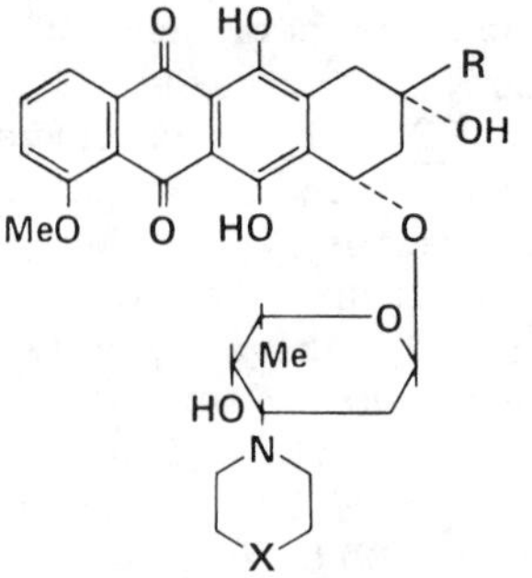

<u>26</u>, R = COCH$_3$, X = CH$_2$

<u>27</u>, R = CHOH–CH$_3$, X = CH$_2$

<u>28</u>, R = COCH$_2$OH, X = CH$_2$

<u>29</u>, R = CHOH–CH$_2$OH, X = CH$_2$

<u>30</u>, R = COCH$_3$, X = CHOMe

<u>31</u>, R = CHOH–CH$_3$, X = CHOMe

<u>32</u>, R = COCH$_3$, X = CHCH$_2$OMe

<u>33</u>, R = COCH$_3$, X = C(CH$_2$OMe)$_2$

<u>34</u>, R = COCH$_3$, X = O

<u>35</u>, R = CHOH–CH$_3$, X = O

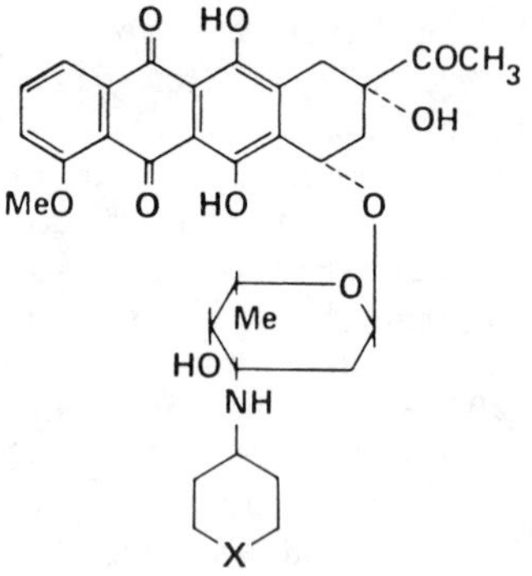

<u>36</u>, X = CH$_2$

<u>37</u>, X = O

Table VII. Biological Results of Piperidino Analogs

Compound	Amino substit.	Efficacy % T/C	Optimum dose q4d 5,9,13 mg/kg	Leukemia L1210 cells inhibn of synth[a] ED$_{50}$, μM DNA	Leukemia L1210 cells inhibn of synth[a] ED$_{50}$, μM RNA	ΔT_m of isolated helical DNA in solution[a] °C	Microsomal O$_2$ consumption, stimulation relative to 2[b] %
	Activity versus mouse leukemia P388[a]						
1	NH$_2$	130	8	0.66	0.33	11.2	82, 109
2	NH$_2$	160	8	1.5	0.58	13.4	100
26		177	6.2	0.50	0.05	16.8	87
27		162	5	0.62	0.04	12.9	
28		158	9.4	0.70	0.04	15.4	
29		136	18	0.72	0.10	12.5	
	NCI			D.L. Taylor, SRI			J.H. Peters, G.R. Gordon, SRI

[a]Data from ref. 4. [b]Data from ref. 8.

Two types of changes in the piperidino structure were first explored, with the analogs in Table VIII (15). Introduction of a ring O was provided by the morpholino analog 37, synthesized by reductive alkylation of 1 with 2,2'-oxybis-acetaldehyde (23). The N was moved out of the piperidino ring by use of cyclohexanone (24) to give N-cyclohexyl-daunorubicin 36.

Both changes were combined in the N-(tetrahydro-4-pyranyl) derivative 37, synthesized from tetrahydro-4-pyranone. In Table VIII it is immediately apparent that 34 (T/C = 166%) retained the antitumor efficacy of 2 (T/C = 160%) against mouse leukemia P388, but exhibited the activity at a greatly decreased dose--0.2 mg/kg compared to 8 mg/kg for 2 (q4d 5,9,13). This 40-fold increase in potency is the greatest reported for any anthracycline so far. It seems to be confirmed by a 20-fold increase in potency for the 13-dihydro derivative 35, and by a 20-fold potency increase of 34 against B16 melanoma (qd1; unpublished data from NCI). What this potency increase implies about the therapeutic potential of 34 has yet to be investigated in further tests, but it

Edward M. Acton *et al.*

Table VIII. Biological Comparison of Piperidino, Morpholino, and Cyclohexyl Analogs

| Compound | Amino substit. | Activity versus mouse leukemia P388 | | Leukemia L1210 cells inhibn of synth ED_{50}, μM | | ΔT_m of isolated helical DNA in solution | Microsomal O_2 consumption, stimulation relative to 2 |
		Efficacy % T/C	Optimum dose q4d 5,9,13 mg/kg	DNA	RNA	°C	%
2	NH_2	160	8	1.5	0.58	13.4	100
26		177	6.2	0.50	0.05	16.8	88
34		166	0.2	0.76	0.10	6.1	25
35		153	0.4	2.2	0.53	4.1	29
36		≤108 (inact)	≤200	64	16	0.6	57
37		136	100	2.0	0.61	4.0	68

NCI   D.L. Taylor, SRI   Refs. 12,15

seems possible that undesirable side effects may not be mag-
nified in potency to the same degree and may be missing at
the doses needed for cancer treatment with 34. Almost as
striking and even more unexpected is the complete absence of
activity for the N-cyclohexyl compound 36 up to very high
doses. The only apparent difference in structure between 26
and 36 is an increase in conformational flexibility of the N-
cyclohexyl ring relative to the piperidino ring. This seems
hardly sufficient to account for a deletion in activity, although structural rigidity often favors a specific inter-
action at a receptor site. Going from N-cyclohexyl to N-
(tetrahydropyranyl) (36 to 37) again shows the favorable
effect of the ether oxygen at the 4-position. Moderate
activity (T/C = 136%) against leukemia P388 was restored, but
a very high dose (100 mg/kg) was required. Apparently the
effect of starting with the cyclohexyl type of structure
could not be overcome. We concluded at this stage that antitumor activity in this type of structure is optimized when
the amino N is incorporated within the new ring, and when an
ether O is present at or near the 4-position of the new
ring. Presumably this ether O is at an interactive site not
previously encountered with anthracycline activity.

Activity observed with additional substituted piperidino analogs is shown in Table IX (15, and additional unpublished results). The important ether oxygen at the 4-position of the added ring was successfully moved into the side chain by use of 3-methoxyglutaraldehyde 20 in the reductive alkylation. The improved antitumor efficacy (T/C = 199%) of both the resultant 4-methoxy-1-piperidinyl analog 30 and its 13-dihydro derivative 31 suggested further elaboration of the methoxy-bearing 4-substituent on the piperidino ring. Logical extensions were the 4-methoxymethyl and 4-bis(methoxymethyl) analogs (32 and 33, respectively), which were synthesized after the correspondingly substituted glutaraldehydes (21 and 22) were synthesized. Only the bis(methoxymethyl) compound 33 has been tested so far, but the further improvement in T/C (212%) is obvious.

Table IX.   Extension of the Piperidino 4-Substituent

Compound	Amino substit.	Efficacy % T/C	Optimum dose q4d 5,9,13 mg/kg	Leukemia L1210 cells inhibn of synth ED$_{50}$, μM DNA	Leukemia L1210 cells inhibn of synth ED$_{50}$, μM RNA	ΔT_m of isolated helical DNA in solution °C	Microsomal O$_2$ consumption, stimulation relative to 2 %
		Activity versus mouse leukemia P388					
2	NH$_2$	160	8	1.5	0.58	13.4	100
26	[N-piperidine]	177	6.2	0.50	0.05	16.8	88
30	[N-piperidine, OMe]	199	6.2	0.63	0.12	13.3	82
31	OMe	199	12.5	0.58	0.08	9.5	
32	[N-piperidine] CH$_2$OMe			0.61	0.08	16.3	84
33	[N-piperidine] MeOCH$_2$ CH$_2$OMe	212	12.5	1.3	0.05	9.2	50
	NCI			D.L. Taylor, SRI		J.H. Peters, G.R. Gordon SRI	

Both 33 and 34 merit further study of their potential as antitumor drugs, as well as providing leads for the design of additional analogs. Significant increases in antitumor efficacy have been attained in the piperidino series, but so far

none of the methoxy-substituted piperidino analogs has produced a potency increase such as was provided by the morpholino structure. A new derivative that combined the increased
potency of the morpholino structure with the efficacy
increase of the methoxy-substituted morpholino structure
would be of great interest. Clearly, it is important to
continue exploring structural changes within this class of
derivatives.

The synthetic approach to the construction of the various
piperidino and morpholino rings (of 26-35; unpublished results) using dialdehydes apparently needs to be no different
from the general reductive alkylation with monoaldehydes.
Generally, aldehydes are used in large (20-fold) excess, but
initially with the dialdehydes (19, 20, and 23 in particular)
excesses were avoided in attempts to favor cyclization with
one mole of dialdehyde and minimize any open-chain dialkylation. This proved to be unnecessary. The yields of the
corresponding 1-piperidinyl (26-29), 4-methoxy-1-piperidinyl
(30, 31) and 4-morpholinyl compounds were quite low, partly
because extensive chromatographic purification was required,
involving separation of the 13-keto and 13-dihydro analogs
(15-20% and 5-10% isolated yields, respectively). Considerable by-product formation was encountered especially in the
reductive alkylation with 2,2'-oxybisacetaldehyde (23),
probably because isomerization of the intermediate aldimine
to a reactive enamine may be favored by the ether O in the β-
position. The yield of morpholino compound 34 benefited

23

when the 20-fold excess of 23 was restored, because at least
the production of 13-dihydro compound 35 was suppressed.
Other current studies indicate that the other by-products can
be minimized also and higher yields of 34 are obtainable. In
the later syntheses of the methoxymethyl and bis(methoxymethyl) compounds (32 and 33), we found that 5-fold excesses

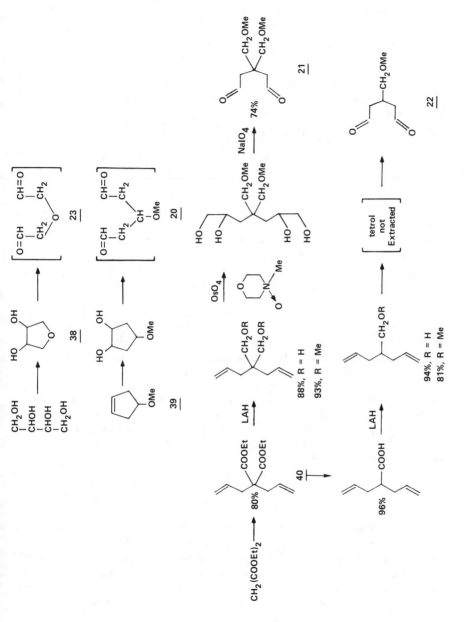

of dialdehydes 21 and 22 were sufficient. Ironically, the inactive and weakly active cyclohexyl type of compounds (36 and 37) were easily obtained in good yields (50-60%) from the ketones 24 and 25 plus cyanoborohydride.

Of the dialdehydes, only glutaraldehyde was commercially available. 2,2'-Oxybisacetaldehyde (23) was synthesized (15) from 1,4-anhydroerythritol by periodate cleavage and was used without isolation. A similar synthesis of 3-methoxyglutaraldehyde was devised from 4-methoxycycopentene (39). Both the methoxymethyl and bis(methoxymethyl) dialdehydes (21 and 22) were synthesized from the diallylation product 40 of malonic ester. These dialdehydes were conveniently isolated by extraction but apparently as mixtures of hydrated forms.

V   CONCLUSIONS

It is clear from the foregoing examples that anthracycline structure can be modified in various ways to produce active new analogs. If productive structure changes are identified (e.g., amination of the quinone, N-benzylation, or attachment of morpholinyl rings to the sugar), and if useful biological criteria can be established (e.g., diminished radical generation, slow release from prodrug forms, or large increases in antitumor potency), progress in analog development can be made toward defined objectives. More remains to be done toward optimizing each of the structural types that has been discussed. Very little has been done to combine the different types of structural changes. Eventually, combining optimized structures from different classes should produce still higher degrees of optimization. The possibilities for developing truly superior anthracycline are now probably better than ever before.

ACKNOWLEDGMENTS

The authors are indebted to Dr. R. A. Jensen for results on electrocardiographic measurement of cardiotoxic effects and to Dr. J. H. Peters and coworkers for results on metabolism and disposition studies on anthracycline analogs in advance of publication.

REFERENCES

1. Carter, S. K., *Cancer Chemother. Pharmacol.* *4*, 5 (1980).

2. Bachur, N. R., Gordon, S. L., and Gee, M. V., *Cancer Res.* *38*, 1745 (1978).

3. Bachur, N. R., Gordon, S. L., Gee, M. V., and Kon, H., *Proc. Natl. Acad. Sci. USA 76*, 954 (1979).

4. Tong, G. L., Wu, H. Y., Smith, T. H., and Henry, D. W., *J. Med. Chem. 22*, 912 (1979).

5. Acton, E. M., in "Anthracyclines: Current Status and New Developments" (Crooke, S. T., Reich, S. D., eds.) p. 15. Academic Press, New York (1980).

6. Tong, G. L., Henry, D. W., and Acton, E. M., *J. Med. Chem. 22*, 36 (1979).

7. Acton, E. M. and Tong, G. L., *J. Med. Chem. 24*, 669 (1981).

8. Gordon, G. R., Peters, J. H., and Acton, E. M., 2nd Chem. Congress, No. Amer. Continent, Amer. Chem. Soc., 25-28 Aug. 1980. BIOL 136.

9. Lown, J. W., Chen, H., Plambeck, J. A., and Acton, E. M., *Biochem. Pharmacol. 28*, 2563 (1979); Lown, J. W., Chen, H., Plambeck, J. A., and Acton, E. M., *Biochem. Pharmacol. 31*, 000 (1982).

10. Zbinden, G., Bachmann, E., Holderegger, C., *Antibiot. Chemother. 23*, 255 (1978).

11. Jensen, R. A., *Proc. Amer. Assn. Cancer Res. 22*, 269 (1981), and additional unpublished results.

12. Peters, J. H., Kashiwase, D., Gordon, G. R., Hunt, C. A., and Acton, E. M. *Proc. Amer. Assn. Cancer Res. 22*, 256 (1981).

13. Horton, D., Priebe, W., and Turner, W. R., *Carbohyd. Res. 94*, 11 (1981).

14. Crooke, S. T., Duvernay, V. H., Galvan, L., and Prestayko, A. W., *Mol. Pharmacol. 14*, 290 (1978).

15. Mosher, C. W., Wu, H. Y., Fujiwara, A. N., and Acton, E. M., *J. Med. Chem. 25*, in press (Jan. 1982).

STEREOSPECIFIC TOTAL SYNTHESIS OF
11-DEOXYANTHRACYCLINONES

Andrew S. Kende
James P. Rizzi
Margaret Logan King

Department of Chemistry
University of Rochester
Rochester, New York

I. INTRODUCTION

The "first generation" anthracycline antitumor agents adriamycin (*1a*, doxorubicin), daunomycin (*2a*, daunorubicin) and
carminomycin (*3a*) have developed over the last decade into major
chemotherapeutic agents for the treatment of neoplastic disease
in man.(1) Their broad range of antitumor activity, limited to
some degree by dose-dependent cardiotoxicity, has led to vigorous competition by organic chemists to achieve enhanced therapeutic indices for this series of naturally-occurring antibiotics.
Several hundred semisynthetic modifications of the natural anthracyclines have been carried out by the Farmitalia group
(Milan), at Stanford Research Laboratories (Palo Alto) and at
many other industrial and academic laboratories.(2) At the same
time, several groups have undertaken the more elaborate chal-
lenge of achieving the total synthesis of these and related anthracycline antibiotics.

ANTHRACYCLINE ANTIBIOTICS

141

FIGURE 1

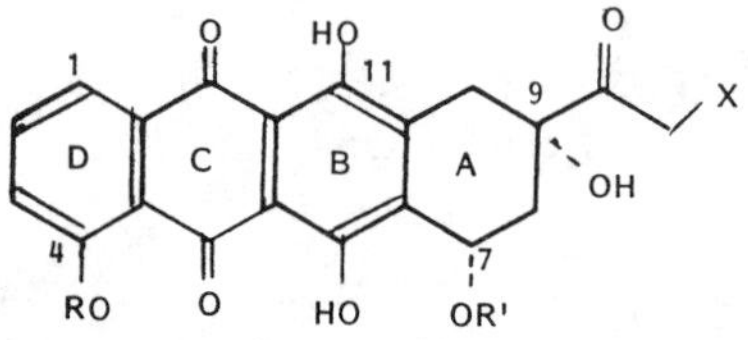

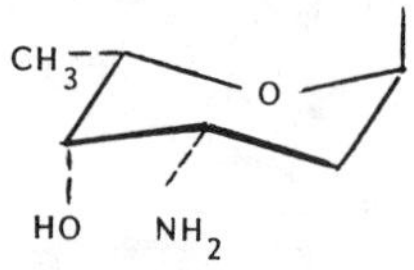

<u>1a</u> R = CH$_3$, R' = $\underline{4}$, X = OH

<u>1b</u> R = CH$_3$, R' = H, X = OH

<u>2a</u> R = CH$_3$, R' = $\underline{4}$, X = H

<u>2b</u> R = CH$_3$, R' = X = H

<u>3a</u> R = X = H, R' = $\underline{4}$

$\underline{4}$
(L-daunosamine)

As noted by T. R. Kelly in his excellent 1979 review, (3) the synthesis of anthracyclines may be divided into three tasks 1) construction of the aglycone, known as an anthracyclinone (eg *1b* , *2b*), 2) synthesis of L-daunosamine (4), and 3) coupling of the two units, preferably with each in the natural optically active form.   The first total synthesis of the anthracyclinone (±)- daunomycinone (*2b*) was achieved by Wong (Winnipeg) in 1973, (4) and the first "practical" synthesis of *2b* was carried out using a Diels-Alder sequence by the Rochester group in 1976. (5) By the latter date, the requisite aminosugar L-daunosamine (4) had been synthesized, (6) and efficient procedures to couple this sugar to the aglycone had been developed in several laboratories. (7) With the subsequent *tour de force* by Kelly (Boston) which gave the aglycone *2b* in 36% yield over 10 steps from napthazarin, (8) and striking improvements in the chiral synthesis of L-dauno samine (4) by the Roche group (Nutley), (9) one could conclude that by 1980 the total synthesis of the "first generation" anthracycline antibiotics was essentially a closed chapter in organic synthesis.

As is frequently the case in such matters, a new series of naturally-occurring anthracycline antitumor agents having attractive therapeutic properties came to light at about this time. These "second generation" anthracyclines had as a common structural feature an 11-deoxy B-ring, thus differing in that respect from the anthracyclines previous discussed. Among the new agents were 11-deoxydaunomycin (*5a*, 11-deoxydaunorubicin), 11-deoxyadriamycin (*6a*, 11-deoxydoxorubicin) and 11-deoxycarminomycin (*7*), by the Arcamone group at Farmitalia, (10) and the aclacinomycins, represented by aclacinomycin A (*8a*), isolated by the Oki and Umezawa groups in Japan.(11)

FIGURE 2

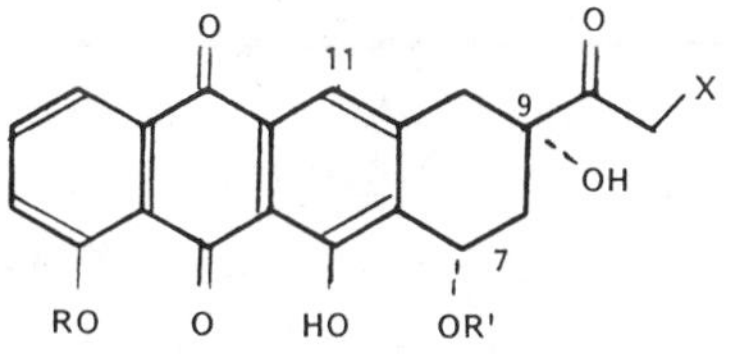

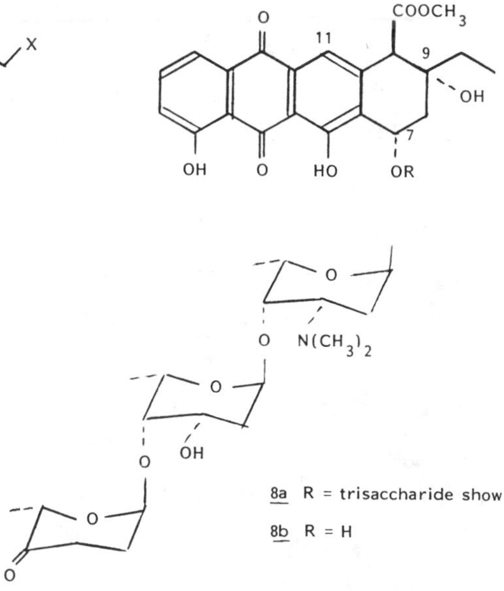

5a R = CH$_3$, R' = 4, X = H
5b R = CH$_3$, R' = X = H
6a R = CH$_3$, R' = 4, X = OH
6b R = CH$_3$, R' = H, X = OH
7   R = X = H, R' = 4

8a R = trisaccharide shown
8b R = H

Reports of good antitumor properties and reduced cardiotoxicities for some of these new agents, as well as the nonmuta-
genicity and good clinical activity exhibited by aclacinomycin A,
(12) once again attracted the scrutiny of synthetic chemists.
Their interest was further stimulated by the recent report from
the Japanese groups that extremely efficient bioconversion of
aklavinone (*8b*) and its congeners to intact aclacinomycins
could be achieved by mutant strains of *Streptomyces galilaeus*.
(13) This opened the possibility that new, synthetic aglycones
closely resembling aklavinone could be transformed in practical
yields to novel, non-natural aclacinomycin antitumor agents.

In this article we describe selected results from our laboratories during the period 1979–1981 that have led to several efficient total syntheses of certain 11-deoxyanthracyclinones. We
describe the strategic considerations that directed our approaches
the synthetic routes, and a comparison of our results with other
work in this highly competitive field.

II. GENERAL STRATEGY

At the outset of these studies it had been demonstrated that
a variety of synthetic strategies, including but not limited to
Diels–Alder routes, could achieve both regiochemical and stereochemical control in the synthesis of daunomycinone (*2b*) and its
congeners. The presence of hydroxyl groups at both the C-6
and C-11 positions in these compounds permitted the imaginative
exploitation of various Diels–Alder strategies based on B-ring
quinone intermediates, as discussed by Kelly.(3) Moreover,
these hydroxyl groups served to deactivate the two anthraquinone carbonyl groups toward attack by organometallic reagents, permitting reasonably efficient introduction of the C-9
side chain as illustrated in Figure 3 for the conversion *9 → 10*.
(14)

FIGURE 3

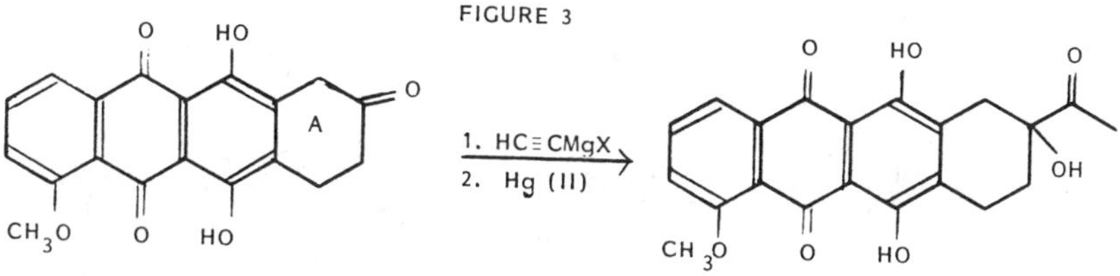

1. HC≡CMgX
2. Hg (II)

9

10

Un fortunately, the 11-deoxyanthracyclinones possess neither the local symmetry nor the chemospecific stabilization noted above. As a result, Diels-Alder strategies could not be readily employed,(15) and chemoselective transformations such as the one illustrated for the 11-deoxy analogs of ketone 9 proceeded poorly. Therefore a new strategy had to be adopted to achieve our synthetic objectives. The basic strategy we selected for our present work could be summarized by the convergent scheme depicted in Figure 4.

In this strategy, an AB bicyclic synthon designed to contain the maximum substituent pattern compatible with the proposed chemistry will be linked (arrow 1) to a nucleophilic D-ring synthon as shown. Subsequently, the C-ring will be generated by cycloacylation of the B-ring as implied (arrow 2). The chemistry proposed here has as its origin the known syntheses of simple anthraquinones described in 1978 by Baldwin, by Raphael and by Snieckus.(16) For example (Figure 5), heteroatom-directed o-lithiation of 3-methoxybenzanilide by

FIGURE 4

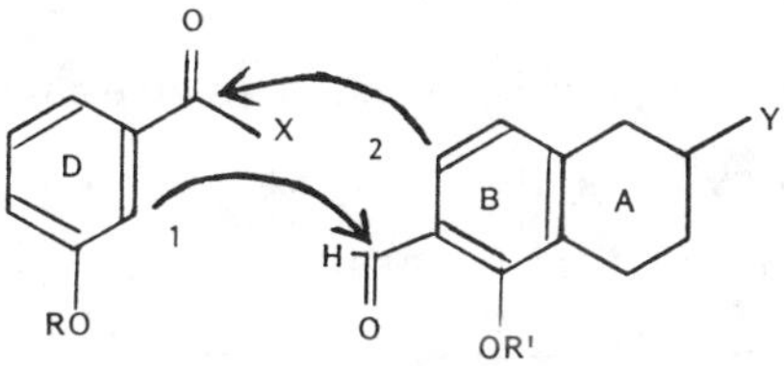

FIGURE 5

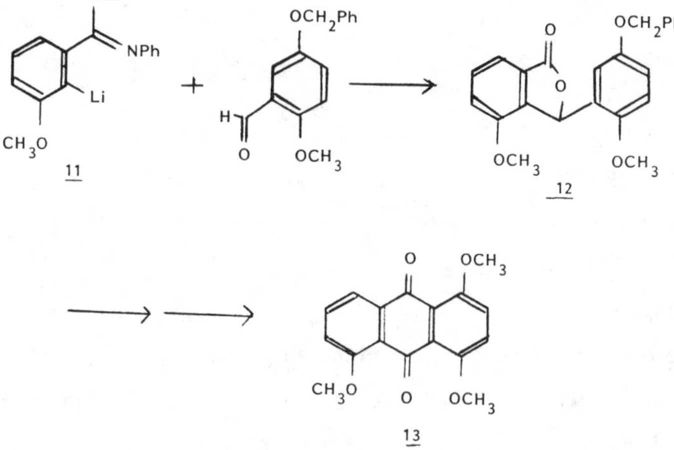

n-butyllithium gives rise to the dilithio derivative *11*, which reacts with a benzaldehyde to give a phthalide (*12*) on acidic work-
up. Reductive cleavage of the phthalide (*12*) to an o-benzylbenzoic acid, followed by cyclodehydration, gives the corresponding anthrone which can be oxidized to the anthraquinone
13. (16a)

We selected the above strategy because it was expected to
be 100% regiospecific (o-benzylbenzoic acids cyclize without
Hayashi rearrangement) and because it offered the possibility
of maximum convergence provided the AB synthon were properly
designed. Applications of this strategy to the synthesis of our
target aglycones are discussed in the following sections.

III. TOTAL SYNTHESIS OF CHIRAL AKLAVINONE

Early attempts in our laboratories to prepare aklavinone
(*8b*) from the tetracyclic ketone *14* by way of the unsaturated
nitrile *15* (Figure 6) proved to be unattractive because of the
difficulty in converting CN to $COOCH_3$ and also introducing the
requisite 9α hydroxyl group. (17)

FIGURE 6

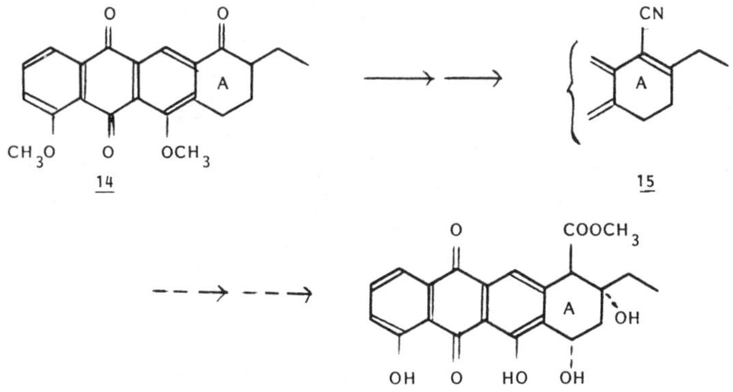

In order to overcome this problem, and to provide a more convergent synthesis of aklavinone, we designed a synthesis based on our central strategy in which the C-10 exocyclic carbon was introduced early in our synthetic sequence. This was achieved at the AB synthon stage by the sequence shown in Figure 7. Commercially available 5-methoxy-1-tetralone was selectively monoethylated by the Rathke procedure (18) involving the boronate derived from the lithium enolate; other alkylation methods gave severe mixtures of starting ketone, mono-alkyl and dialkyl derivatives. Conversion of the 2-ethyl ketone to the "trisylhydrazone" 16 followed by reaction of the latter with 2 equivalents of n-butyllithium according to the protocol of Chamberlin, Stemke and Bond (19) gave the vinyl anion 17. This could be trapped directly with paraformaldehyde to yield 45% of carbinol 18, mp 87-89°C, after chromatography. Alternatively, vinyl anion 17 could be reacted with dimethylformamide, followed by $NaBH_4$ reduction of the intermediate unsaturated aldehyde, to give the same carbinol (18) in 54% overall yield. The selective introduction of a formyl group ortho to the B-ring methoxyl (to provide a suitable AB aldehyde synthon) required a bit of ingenuity. In particular, there was concern

FIGURE 7

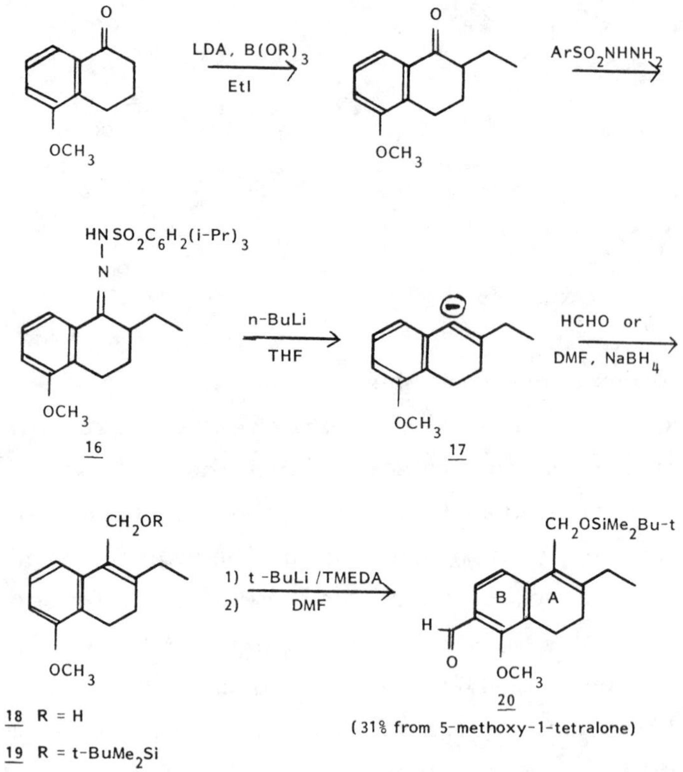

18 R = H   (31% from 5-methoxy-1-tetralone)

19 R = t-BuMe$_2$Si

that heteroatom-directed lithiation of *18* or a protected derivative could result in metalation *para* rather than *ortho* to the
methoxy group. Indeed, the lithiation of the methyl ether of
carbinol *18* followed by quenching with dimethylformamide led to
mixtures containing predominantly the undesired 8-formyl compound. To avoid the observed coordination of lithium cation
with the carbinol oxygen, a bulky blocking group had to be employed. Thus, treatment of carbinol *18* with t-butyldimethyl-
silyl chloride and imidazole in dimethylformamide gave quantita-
tively the silyl ether *19*, which with one equivalent of t-butyl-

lithium-TMEDA complex in hexanes at 0°C, followed by addition to dimethylformamide in tetrahydrofuran gave the key AB aldehyde 20, mp 50-51°C, in 80% yield.

Generation of the nucleophilic dilithium derivative 21 of 3-methoxybenzanilide was carried out by addition of 2.0 equiv. of n-butyllithium-TMEDA complex in THF, then stirring at -20°C for five hours. In subsequent studies we have found that replacement of THF by dry 1,2-dimethoxyethane leads to more reproducible results, since the latter solvent is not attacked by organolithium reagents. Addition of aldehyde 20 to the solution of 21, followed after 16 hours by workup with cold aqueous oxalic acid led directly to the phthalide 22, mp 111-113°C. Use of oxalic acid rather than mineral acids led to complete retention of the silyl ether group. As pictured in Figure 8, conversion of this phthalide to the tetracyclic anthraquinone 24 followed relatively standard chemistry. The only difficult step was the benzylic oxidation of the labile anthrone 23. It was found that immediate air oxidation of this anthrone by adding it slowly to a stirred solution of Triton B in methanol gave the best yields of the stable, crystalline yellow anthraquinone 24, mp 233-234°C.

At this stage of the synthesis, major difficulties were encountered in O-demethylation of 24 to the dihydroxyanthraquinone system, a step which we wished to carry out prior to conducting the delicate A-ring chemistry leading to the sensitive 9α-hydroxylated aklavinone system. Lewis acid reagents ($AlCl_3$, BBr_3) on quinone 24 or the corresponding benzoate or acetate ester, led to immediate decomposition. Nucleophilic demethylation procedures with such nucleophiles as thioethoxide, cyanide or $PhNNaCH_3$ only gave A-ring aromatization. After considerable experimentation, selective O-demethylation was achieved using lithium iodide in the presence of benzoic acid in 1:1 pyridine-collidine at 145°C for 90 minutes.(20) Under these exact

FIGURE 8

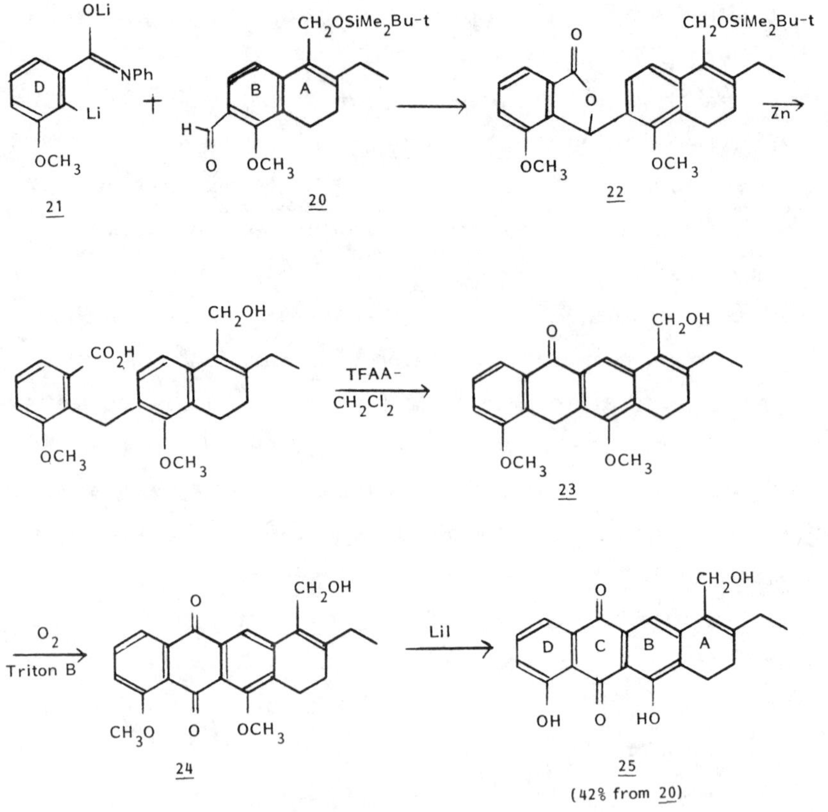

conditions, the anthraquinone *24* was reproducibly converted to triol *25*, mp 199–201°C, in 92% yield, accompanied by about 3% of the A-ring aromatized congener. Since separation of this impurity from *25* was difficult, the two products were carried through together for two more steps, where purification proved easier.

Completion of the synthesis of (±)-aklavinone from the triol *25* is depicted in Figure 9. Epoxidation of this triol with m-chloroperbenzoic acid in aqueous dichloromethane containing sodium bicarbonate buffer gave 90% of the epoxide *26*, mp 185–187°C. Oxidation of the alcohol using pyridinium chlorochromate gave 79% of the epoxy aldehyde *27*, which was easily separated from aromatic impurities by preparative thin-layer chromatography. Sodium chlorite oxidation of aldehyde *27* by the extremely useful procedure of Lindgren and Nilsson (21) gave, after diazomethane treatment, the epoxy ester *28*, mp 221–224°C, in 98% yield.

At this point we had to face the task of stereospecific epoxide hydrogenolysis. Previous experience in our laboratories as well as the 1965 work of Brockmann (22) had shown that Pd over $BaSO_4$ in a solvent mixture of ethanol-triethanolamine could be employed for the efficient and selective catalytic hydrogenolysis of a benzylic C–O bond in the anthracyclinone series. When these conditions (Pd–$BaSO_4$, 1:1 EtOH–triethanolamine, H_2, 1 atm., room temperature, 2.5 hours) were applied to the epoxy ester *28*, there was formed a single β-hydroxy ester, mp 220–222°C, in 76% yield. The chemical identity of this compound with 7-deoxyaklavinone (*29*), itself a natural product known as galirubinone D, (23) was confirmed by comparison of its nmr spectrum with that of an authentic sample (by C-7 hydrogenolysis of aklavinone)from the laboratories of Dr. P. Confalone at Hoffmann-La Roche in Nutley. From independent studies at Roche, Dr. Confalone has noted that the presence of triethanolamine is essential for this epoxide hydrogenolysis to proceed cleanly.(17) Since the liquid-phase Pd-catalyzed hydrogenolysis of cyclohexene epoxides is not typically stereospecific,(24) direct C–O hydrogenolysis in our system is regarded as unlikely. We suggest that the observed stereospecificity might arise from initial reduction of epoxy ester *28* to the C-ring hydroquinone, followed by elimination to give a quinone methide, followed by stereospecific capture of a C-10 hydrogen (proton) from the pseudoequatorial α-side.

FIGURE 9

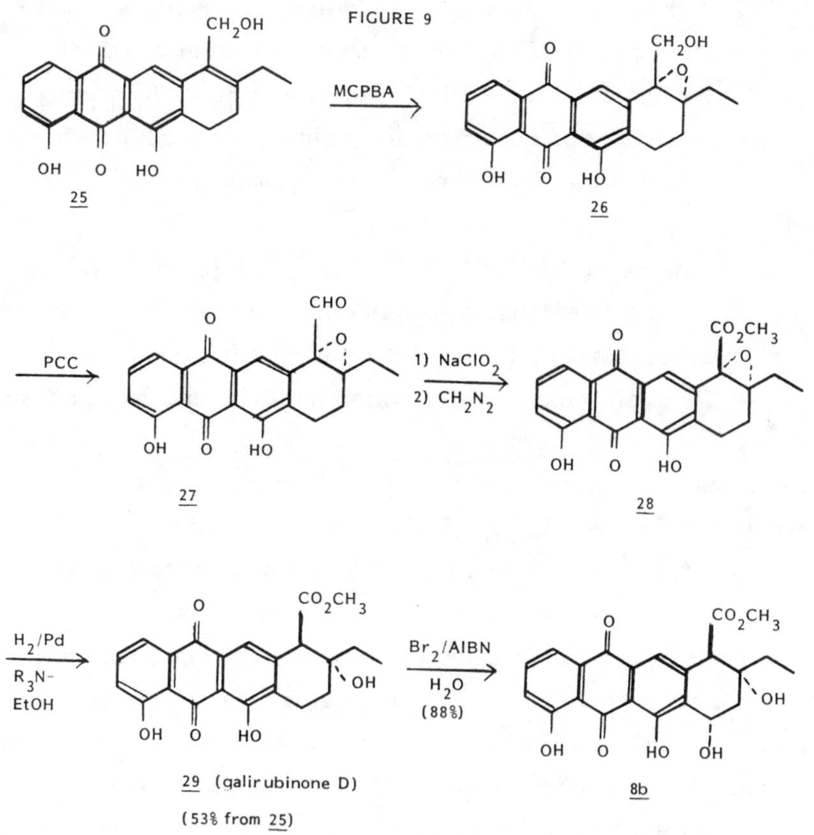

25

MCPBA →

26

PCC →

27

1) NaClO$_2$
2) CH$_2$N$_2$ →

28

H$_2$/Pd
R$_3$N–
EtOH →

29 (galirubinone D)

(53% from 25)

Br$_2$/AIBN
H$_2$O
(88%) →

8b

    To introduce the requisite C-7 oxygen, 7-deoxyaklavinone
(*29*) was subjected to homolytic bromination (2.0 equivalents
Br$_2$, AIBN, CCl$_4$, reflux, 1 hour) followed by solvolysis of
the crude 7-bromo derivative in 1:1 H$_2$O–THF to give an 88%
yield of (±)-aklavinone, identical by ms, uv, tlc behavior and
400 MHz ^{1}H-nmr spectrum with natural aklavinone kindly supplied by Dr. T. Oki (Sanraku Ocean Ltd.) and Dr. Confalone.

FIGURE 10

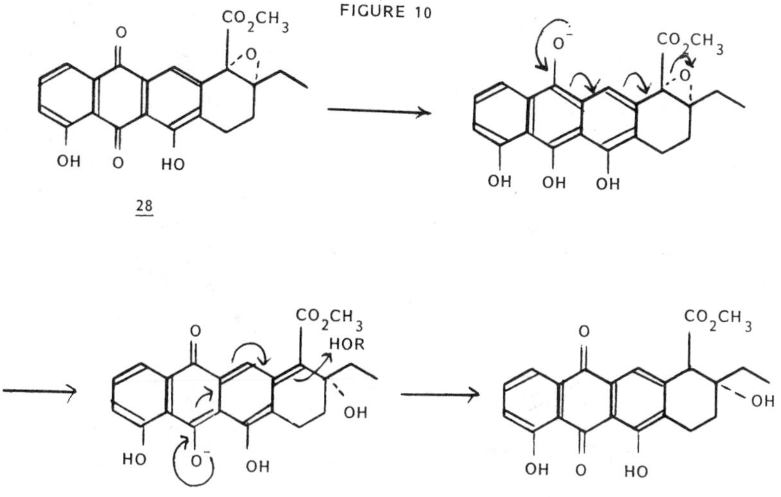

The exclusive formation of the "natural" 7 α-hydroxy epimer from the kinetic solvolysis of the 7-bromo intermediate in this last sequence was gratifying, but not without some precedent. As summarized in Figure 11, the kinetic solvolysis of 7-brominated 7-deoxyanthracyclinones gives predominantly the 7 β-hydroxy compounds when C-9 β bears an acetyl group, whereas the 7 α-hydroxy compounds are formed when the C-9 β substituent is alkyl. (An exception to this correlation is 7,11-dideoxycarminomycinone (30) which leads mainly to the kinetic 7 α-hydroxy derivative.) We would suggest the possibility that in the absence of C-13 carbonyl there is a modest stereoelectronic preference for axial approach to the sp^2-hybridized C-7 carbon (as quinone methide or carbocation), aided perhaps by hydrogen-bonding of the entering nucleophile by C-9 α hydroxyl. In the dauno-mycinone series, participation by the C-13 carbonyl could favor the 7 β-hydroxy product.

FIGURE 11

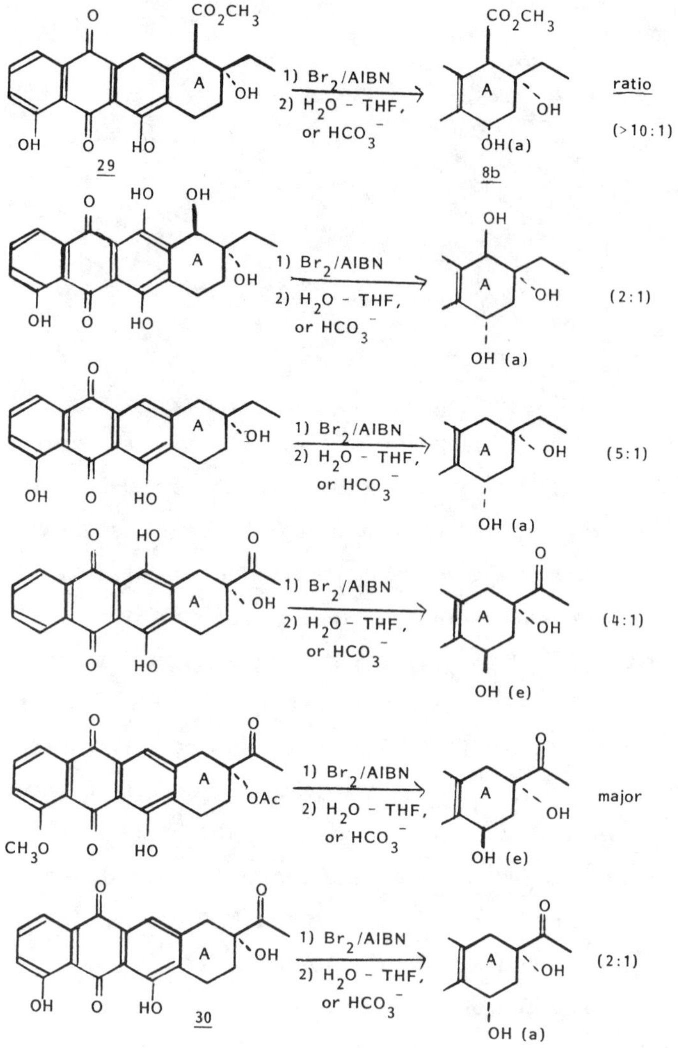

Since the key functionalization of C-10 in our synthesis involves epoxidation of an allylic alcohol (cf 25 → 26), it was
attractive to explore in this context the enantioselective epoxidation method developed by Sharpless.(25)   Treatment of alcohol
25 in CH_2Cl_2 at -10°C for 3 days with 5 equiv. of $Ti(iPrO)_4$ and
10 equiv. t-BuOOH in the presence of 5 equiv. (-)diethyl d-
tartrate gave an 85% yield of the optically active epoxy alcohol
26 (Figure 12). Based on the model of Sharpless it was predicted that the major enantiomer formed in this epoxidation
would be that of the natural series, as shown (26). In the event,
400 MHz ^{1}H-nmr analysis of the diastereomeric mixture of α-
methoxy-α-trifluoromethylphenylacetate (MTPA) (26) esters
derived from the epoxy alcohol product showed an enantiomeric
excess of 53 ± 2% of the major isomer. This value, as well as the
absolute configuration obtained, was confirmed by converting

FIGURE 12

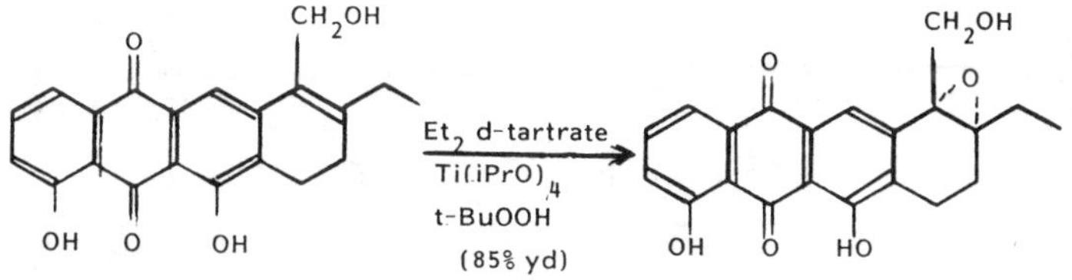

1) PCC
2) NaClO$_2$
3) CH$_2$N$_2$

4) H$_2$/Pd
5) Br$_2$,
   H$_2$O

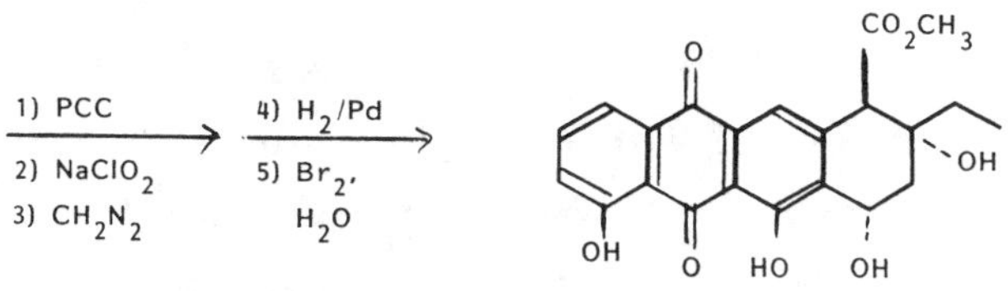

obsd $[\alpha]_D$ = +112°

lit $[\alpha]_D$ = +213°

aklavinone, 8b

the optically active epoxy alcohol *26* to aklavinone. As long as recrystallizations of intermediates or final product are avoided (due to preferential crystallization of racemates), we could show that the aklavinone thus produced has $[\alpha]_D$ = +112° (dioxane), corresponding to 53% e.e. of natural aklavinone, $[\alpha]_D$ = +213° (dioxane).

The above sequence comprises a completely stereoselective and partially enantioselective total synthesis of aklavinone in 16 steps from commercially available 5-methoxy-1-tetralone, with an overall yield of about 6.5%.

IV. TOTAL SYNTHESIS OF (±)-11-DEOXYDAUNOMYCINONE

Early in 1980 it was believed that if efficient and regiospecific access to the 11-deoxy tetracyclic ketone *31* could be devised, the introduction of a C-9 side chain by known methods would lead swiftly to a practical synthesis of 11-deoxydaunomycinone (*6b*).

Based on this premise, J.-P. Gesson and coworkers at the University of Poitiers developed an elegant and substantially regiospecific synthesis of ketone *31* by a Diels-Alder sequence involving addition of diene *33* to juglone, *32* (Figure 13).(27) At about the same time, S. D. Boettger in our laboratories synthesized *31* by a lengthier but completely regiospecific route from 5-ethoxy-2-tetralone ketal *34*. Unfortunately, access to tetracyclic ketone *31* did not lead smoothly to the target aglycone *6b*. It was found in our laboratories that the conventional ethynylation at C-9 with $HC{\equiv}CMgBr$ was exceptionally poor (22% yield), giving mainly unreacted ketone *31* under mild conditions and apparent destruction of the quinone system by C-12 attack under forcing conditions. The alternative procedure involving formation of the C-9 cyanohydrin ether followed by Grignard addition to the cyano group was likewise unsuccess-

FIGURE 13

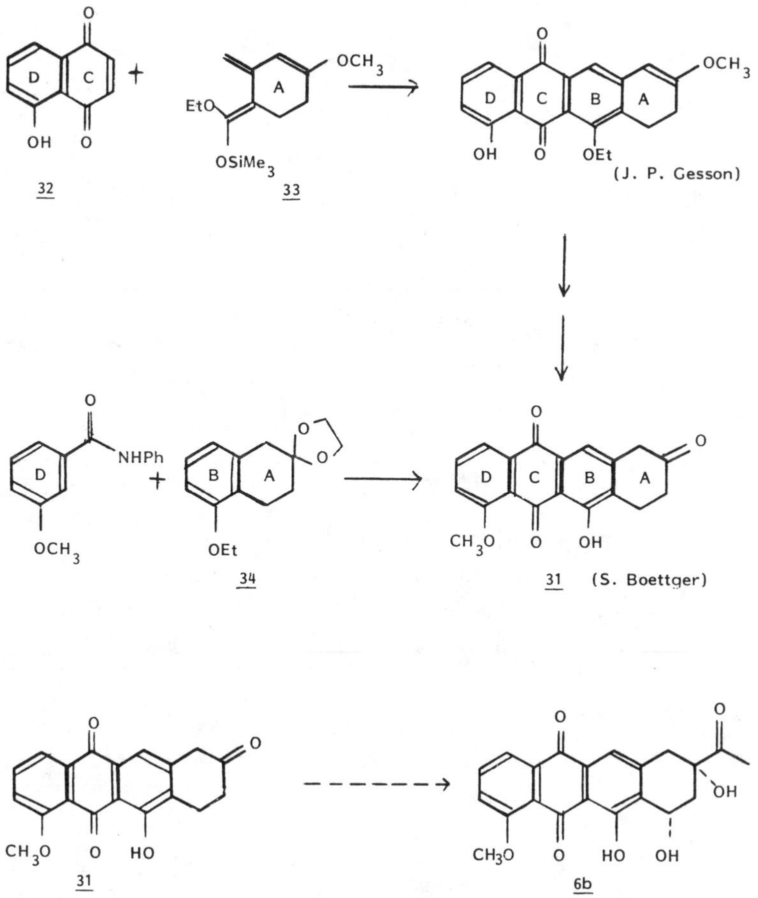

ful. (29) It soon became apparent that the chemical reactivity of ketone 31 differed significantly from that of its well-studied, 11-hydroxylated counterpart 9. Accordinqly, a new reaction sequence had to be designed to overcome this roadblock. We describe here our results toward this objective, Fias. 14-15 depict a new, efficient and reqiospecific synthesis of 11-deoxydaunomycinone from readily available bicyclic intermediates.

FIGURE 14

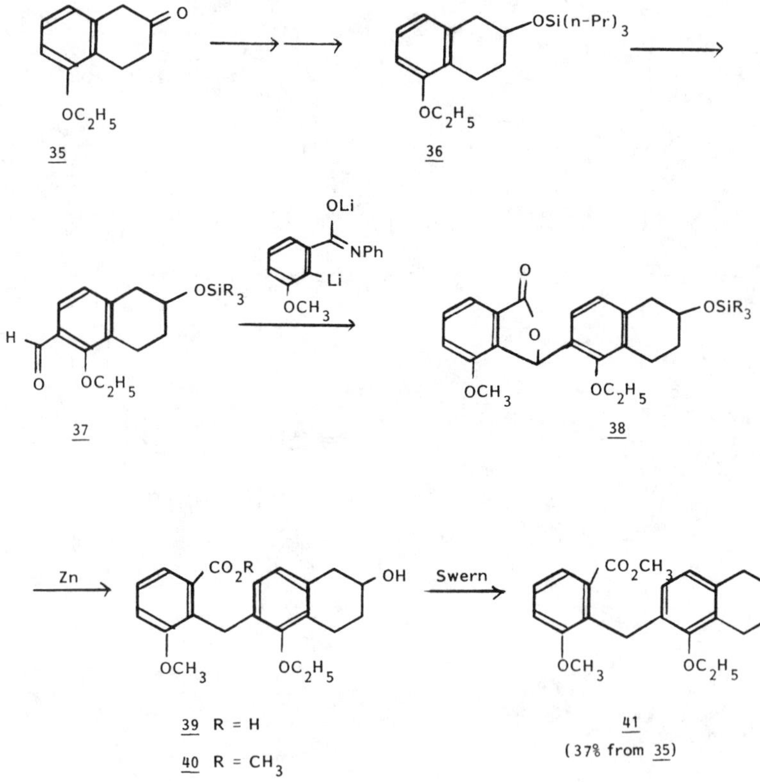

The starting material of our synthesis is 5-ethoxy-2-tetra-
lone (*35*), directly available on the kilogram scale by sodium-
ethanol reduction of 1,6-diethoxynapthalene.   Reduction of
ketone *35* with sodium borohydride followed by protection with
tri-n-propylsilyl chloride gave the silyl ether *36*.   The choice
of the (n-Pr)$_3$Si- rather than the more conventional t-BuMe$_2$Si-
blocking group was dictated by the improved yields in the following metalation step.   Reaction of silyl ether *36* with 1.5
equivalents of t-butyllithium and TMEDA in hexane at 0°C for

5 hours, followed by quenching with dimethylformamide, gave 63% of the single ethoxyaldehyde *37*. Reaction of this aldehyde with the dilithio derivative *11* of the Baldwin anilide in 1,2-dimethoxyethane (superior to tetrahydrofuran), followed by oxalic acid workup gave the phthalides *38* which were reduced with zinc powder in 10% KOH containing pyridine to the crystalline hydroxyacid *39*. The yield of acid *39* from aldehyde *37* was 61%.

The tricyclic methyl ester *40*, prepared from *39* with diazomethane, underwent smooth Swern oxidation using oxalyl chloride and dimethyl sulfoxide to give the key benzyltetralone ester *41*. Without further purification, this ketone was reacted with excess HC≡CMgBr in tetrahydrofuran to give, under the appropriate

FIGURE 15

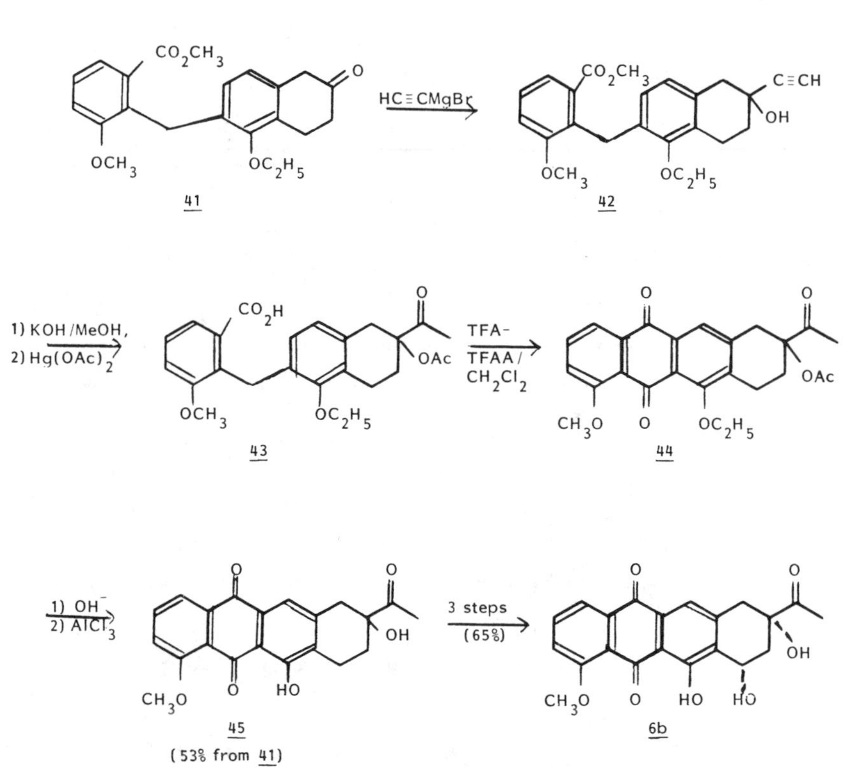

conditions, a 74% overall yield of ethynyl carbinol *42* from ester *40* (Figure 15). Saponification followed by mercuric acetate "hydration" of the side chain gave the ketoacid *43*, which was cyclized in $CF_3CO_2H-(CF_3CO)_2O$ in methylene chloride to an anthrone that was immediately oxidized by Jones reagent to the crystalline anthraquinone *44* (71% overall from carbinol *42*).

The deblocking of 9-O acetyl and of 6-O ethyl, while leaving the 4-O methyl ether intact, was expeditiously solved by brief deacetylation of *44* with 5% methanolic NaOH at room temperature, followed by treatment with 3 molar equivalents of $AlCl_3$ in nitro-benzene at 50°C for three hours, as suggested by the work of Johnson.[28] This produced a quantitative yield of (±) 7,11-di-deoxydaunomycinone (*45*), identical in [1]H-nmr and other pro-perties with those reported by Johnson, as well as with a small sample prepared earlier by S. Boettger in our laboratories from ketone *31* by a far more tedious sequence.[29]

The efficient ethynylation of benzyltetralone *41* worked out in our scheme has made possible convenient access to racemic 7,11-dideoxydaunomycinone (*45*) in 14 steps from 5-ethoxy-2-tetralone with an overall yield of 20%. The C-7 oxygenation of *45* by ketal formation, homolytic bromination and acid hydrolysis to give racemic 11-deoxydaunomycinone (*6b*) in 65% yield, as described by Johnson (28) corresponds therefore to a 17 step synthesis of this antibiotic in 13% overall yield.

V. COMPARISONS WITH OTHER ROUTES

Since the total synthesis of anthracyclinones is a very active field it is useful to place our syntheses of aklavinone and 11-deoxydaunomycinone in perspective through comparison with recent work by other investigators.

In the summer of 1981 the Kishi group (Harvard) (30) and the Confalone group (Roche) (17) reported completed syntheses of aklavinone. Figure 16 briefly summarizes these, and gives the

FIGURE 16

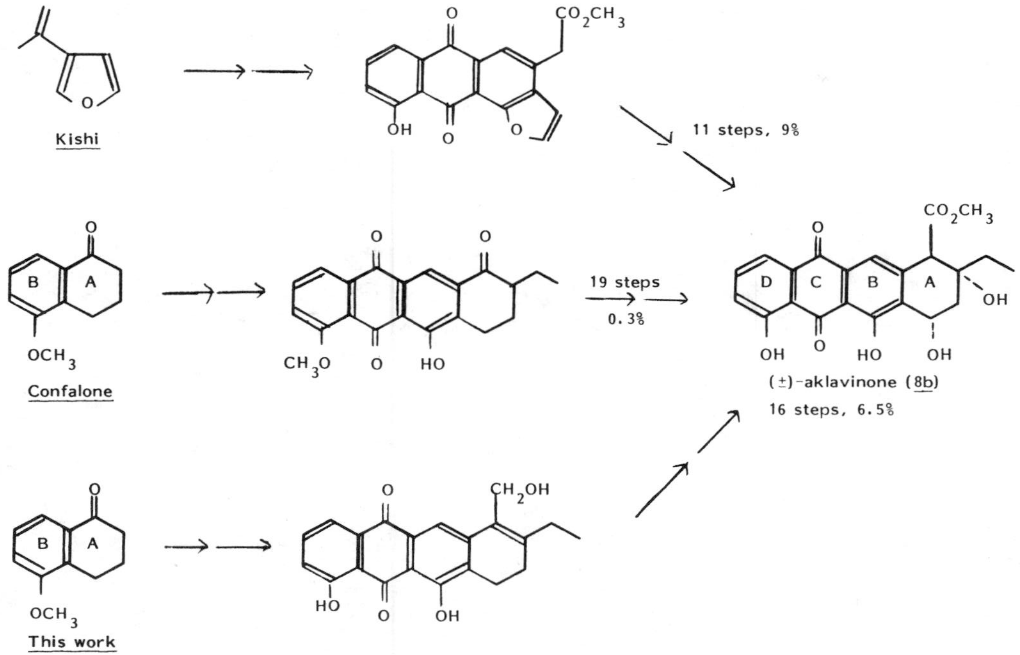

FIGURE 17

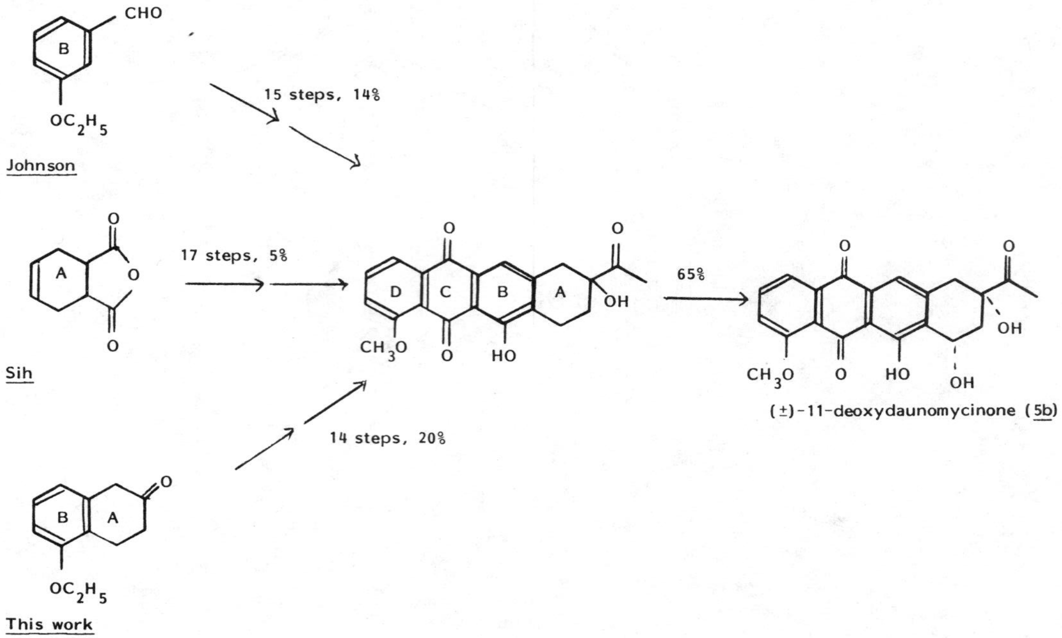

number of steps and overall yield from commercial (or equivalent) starting materials. More recently, Li and Wu at Syntex have described a novel total synthesis of aklavinone involving Michael addition-cyclization of a cyanophthalide A-ring to a bicyclic C-D enone synthon; the overall yield of the sequence however was under 2%.(31)

Figure 17 compares our synthesis of ($\pm$)-11-deoxydaunomy- cinone with that from two other laboratories. It is clear that in length and yield our sequence compares favorably with those reported to date. With the inevitable improvements in synthetic methodology anticipated, it is likely that syntheses of racemic 11-deoxyanthracyclinones in 20% yield over about a dozen steps will soon be achieved.

ACKNOWLEDGMENTS

We are grateful to Professor F. Arcamone (Farmitalia Carlo Erba), Dr. P. Confalone (Hoffman LaRoche Company), Dr. T. Oki (Sanraku Ocean Company) and Professor Y. Kishi (Harvard University) for reference samples, unpublished data and valuable discussions. Partial support of this research by grant CA-11326, awarded by the National Cancer Institute (USPHS), by a Pharmacology Training Grant T-32-GM-07141 awarded by the NIH to J. R., and by an Elon Huntington Hooker Foundation award to M. L. K. is gratefully acknowledged.

References

1. Brown, J. R. *Prog. Med. Chem.*, 1978, *15*, 125.
2. For a thorough review of this effort see Arcamone, F.,
   "Doxorubicin", Academic Press, New York, 1981.
3. Kelly, T. F. *Annu. Rep. Med. Chem.*,1979, *14*, 288.
4. Wong, C. M.; Schwenk, R.; Popien, D.; Ho, T.-L. *Can. J.
   Chem.*, 1973, *51*, 466.
5. Kende, A. S.; Tsay, Y.-G.; Mills, J. E. *J. Am. Chem. Soc.*,
   1976, *98*. 1967.
6. (a) Marsh, J. P. Jr.; Mosher, C. W.; Acton, E. M.;
   Goodman, L. *Chem. Comm.*, 1967, 973 (b) Horton, D.;
   Weckerle, W. *Carbohydr. Res.* 1975, *44*, 227.
7. See reference 3, pp 296-297.
8. Kelly, T. R.; Vaya, J.; Ananthasubramanian, L. *J. Am.
   Chem. Soc.* , 1980, *102*, 5983.
9. Grethe, G.; Witt, T.; Sereno, J.; Uskokovic, M. *Abstr.
   178th Meeting, Am. Chem. Soc.*, 1979, ORGN 126.
10. Arcamone, F.; Cassinelli, G.; Dimatteo, F.; Forenza, S.;
    Ripamonti, M. C.; Rivola, G.; Vigerani, A.; Clardy, J.
    McCabe, T. *J. Am. Chem. Soc.*, 1980, *102*, 1462.
11. Oki, T.; Kitamura, I.; Matsuzawa, Y.; Shibamoto, N.;
    Ogasawara, T.; Yoshimoto, A.; Inui, T. *J. Antibiot.*, 1979,
    32, 801, and earlier references therein.
12. Hori, S.; Shirai, M.; Shinchi, H.; Oki, T.; Inui, T.;
    Tsukagoshi, S.; Ishizuka, M.; Takeuchi, T.; Umezawa,
    H. *Gann*, 1977, *68*, 685,
13. Oki, T.; Yoshimoto, A.; Matsuzawa, Y.; Takeuchi, T.;
    Umezawa, H. *J. Antibiot.* 1980, *33*, 1331.
14. See for example ref. 5. An interesting variant of this ap-
    proach is that of Krohn, K.; Tolkien, K. *Tetrahedron Lett.*
    1978, 4023.

15. See however the work of J. P. Gesson, described in section IV.

16. (a) Baldwin, J. E.; Blair, K. W. *Tetrahedron Lett.*, 1978, 2559 (b) Forbes, I.; Pratt, R. A.; Raphael, R. A. *Ibid.*, 1978, 3965 (c) Osmund de Silva, S.; Snieckus, V. *Ibid.*, 1978, 5103.

17. Confalone, P. N.; Pizzolato, G. *J. Am. Chem. Soc.*, 1981, *103*, 4251; also Rizzi, J. P.; Kende, A. S., unpublished observations.

18. Rathke, M. W.; Lindert, A. *Synthet. Comm.*, 1978, 9.

19. Chamberlin, A. R.; Stemke, J. E.; Bond, F. T. *J. Org. Chem.*, 1978, *43*, 147.

20. Harrison, I. T. *Chem. Commun.* 1969, 616.

21. Lindgren, B. O.; Nilsson, T. *Acta. Chem. Scand.*, 1973, *27*, 888.

22. Brockmann, H.; Niemeyer, J.; Brockmann, H. Jr., Budzikiewicz, H. *Chem. Ber.*, 1965, *98*, 3785.

23. Eckardt, K. *Chem. Ber.*, 1967, *100*, 2561.

24. Accrombessi, G. C.; Geneste, P.; Olive, J.-L. *J. Org. Chem.*, 1980, *45*, 4139.

25. Sharpless, K. B.; Katsuki, T. *J. Am. Chem. Soc.*, 1980, *102*, 5974.

26. Dale, J. A.; Dull, D. L.; Mosher, H. S. *J. Org. Chem.*, 1969, *34*, 2543.

27. Gesson, J. P.; Jacquesy, J. C.; Mondon, M. *Tetrahedron Lett.*, 1980, 3351.

28. Kimball, S. D.; Watt, D. R.; Johnson, F. *J. Am. Chem. Soc.*, 1981, *103*, 1561.

29. Boettger, S. D.; Kende, A. S., unpublished observations.

30. Pearlman, B. A.; McNamara, J. M.; Hasan, I.; Hatakeyama, S.; Sekizaki, H.; Kishi, Y. *J. Am. Chem. Soc.*, 1981, *103*, 4248.

31. Li, T.-t.; Wu, Y. L. *J. Am. Chem. Soc.*, 1981, *103*, 7007.

REGIOSPECIFIC, CONVERGENT STRATEGIES FOR ANTHRACYCLINONE SYNTHESIS USING QUINONE BIS- AND MONOKETALS[1]

John S. Swenton

Department of Chemistry
The Ohio State University
Columbus, Ohio

INTRODUCTION

Anthracycline antibiotics have been of much interest in recent years due to the demonstrated therapeutic value in cancer chemotherapy (1). The intact antibiotic consists of a glycon and an aglycon portion, and most synthetic approaches would have as one of the final steps this coupling as illustrated in Scheme I for daunomycinone (2). Since daunosamine and related fraudulent sugars are available, considerable effort has concentrated on an effective synthesis of the aglycon portion of the antibiotic (3). While the majority of synthetic work has involved the rhodomycinone class of aglycons, undoubtedly new work will focus more on the other classes of anthracyclinones (Scheme II).

[1]The synthetic electrochemical equipment and the development of the electrochemical synthetic methods were generously supported by the National Science Foundation. The National Cancer Institute generously supported the application of this chemistry to synthesis of the anthracyclinones.

ANTHRACYCLINE ANTIBIOTICS

167

Scheme I. Aglycon-Glycon Coupling Route

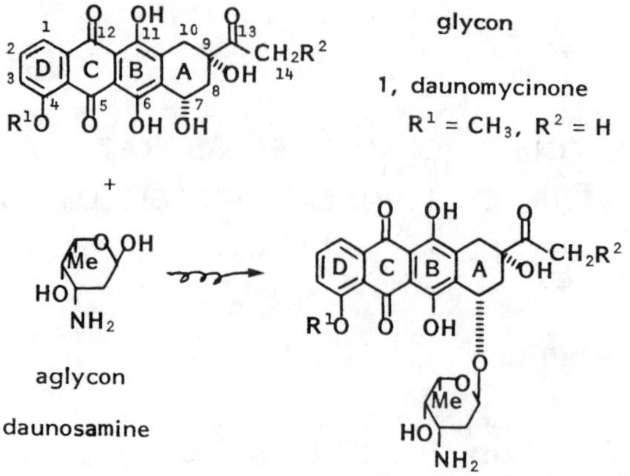

glycon

1, daunomycinone

$R^1 = CH_3$, $R^2 = H$

+

aglycon

daunosamine

daunorubicin, $R^1 = Me$, $R^2 = H$
adriamycin, $R^1 = Me$, $R^2 = OH$

*Scheme II. Representative Members of Aklavinone,
Citromycinone, and Rhodomycinone Aglycons*

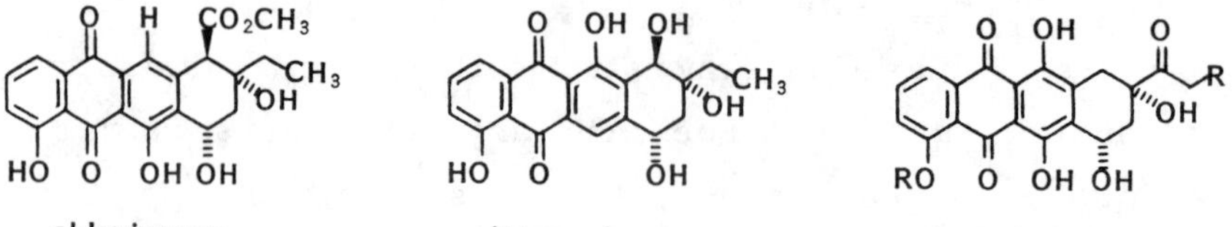

aklavinones

citromycinones

rhodomycinones

Daunomycinone, **1**, and its 4-demethoxy analogue have been the common targets of synthetic studies in the rhodomycinone area. Two especially pertinent experiments by Wong (4a) and Brockmann (5) were critical to early routes to these aglycons. Wong had shown that free radical bromination of the tetracyclic ring system followed by solvolysis of the labile bromide allowed introduction of oxygen functionality at C_7. Since Brockmann and his coworkers had demonstrated that benzylic hydroxyl groups in related systems could be equilibrated with their epimers using trifluoroacetic acid, the stereochemistry at

C_7 of the anthracyclinone was not of initial concern in the synthetic strategy. Thus, most of the early synthetic studies focused on the synthesis of the 7-deoxydaunomycinone (often without regiochemical control) or the 7-deoxy-4-demethoxy analogue followed by benzylic bromination, solvolysis of the labile C_7-bromo compound, equilibration of the C_7 stereochemistry with trifluoroacetic acid, and chromatographic separation of the C_7-epimers. We consider this particular literature sequence when applied to (±) daunomycinone itself as unacceptable if a reasonably efficient method for multigram preparation of the compound is desired.[2] As noted later, a similar sequence is even less acceptable when applied to the citromycinone aglycon. More recently we and others have developed synthetic routes to the rhodomycinone aglycons in which the C_7-oxygen function is incorporated earlier in the synthetic sequence (6,7). This method appears to have resulted in more efficient syntheses of these molecules.

Our overall objective in this area was to develop an efficient, convergent route to fully functionalized, optically active anthracyclinones. Since functionalization of 7-deoxydaunomycinone systems in an acceptable manner was not available, we chose approaches in which the C_7-oxygen function would be present when the tetracyclic ring was formed. This in turn would require mild conditions for preparation of the tetracyclic ring system of the antibiotic since A-ring precursors having the C_7- and C_9-oxygen substituents present would undoubtedly decompose under harsh reaction conditions. Furthermore, in connection with tissue distribution and

[2]*It has been stated that "The above seven-step sequence makes available ca. 3 g. of (±) daunomycinone from 100 g. of diquinone 8" (4c). However, experimental details (4f) describe the preparation of only 1.2 mg of (±) daunomycinone by this procedure!*

metabolism studies being performed by Professor L. Malspeis, a ^{14}C-ring-labeled adriamycin was required (8). We hoped that the synthesis developed here could also be adapted to the preparation of the radiolabeled system for these pharmacological studies.

THE METALLATED QUINONE BISKETAL
1,4-DIPOLE STRATEGY TO
RHODOMYCINONE AGLYCONS

Our first approach which was inspired by the general strategy outlined in Scheme III involved the reaction of a

*Scheme III. Metallated Quinone
1,4-Dipole Strategy*

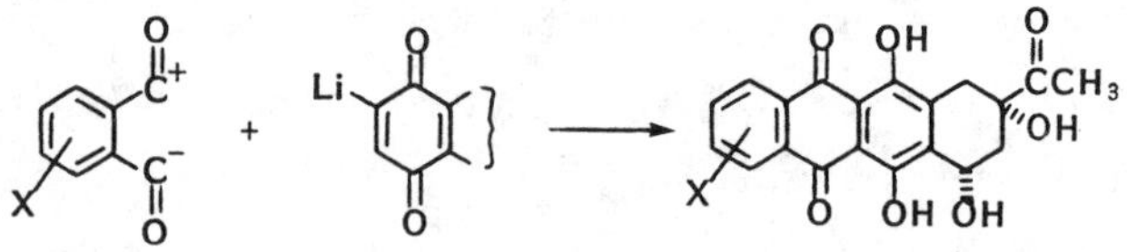

metallated quinone equivalent (9) (Scheme IV); however, a stable entity which would function as the required 1,4-dipole

*Scheme IV. A Metallated Quinone Equivalent
via an Anodic Oxidation-Metal
Halogen Exchange Sequence*

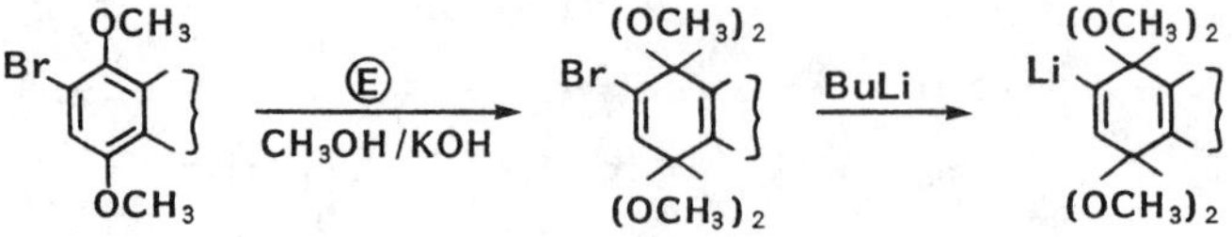

species was not apparent. After numerous attempts to implement this approach, it was found that reaction of the ethylene ketal of benzocyclobutendione (10), 2, with the lithiated quinone 3 afforded 4 in 70% yield. Hydrolysis of 4 gave the known

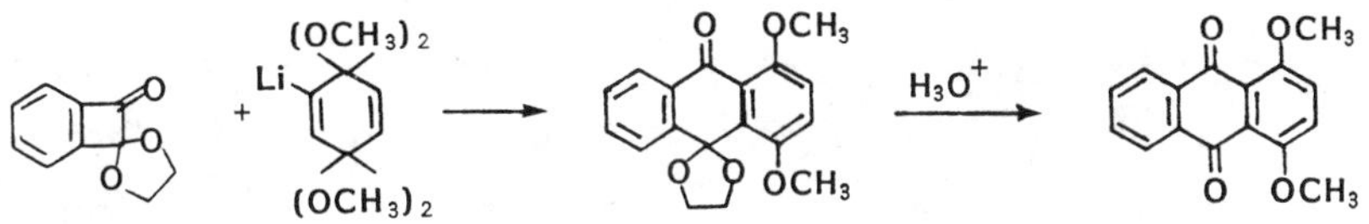

5 in quantitative yield, thus confirming the structure of 4. There are several mechanistic pathways which can be envisioned for this interesting annelation reaction (Scheme V).

Scheme V. Mechanistic Possibilities for Annelation Reaction

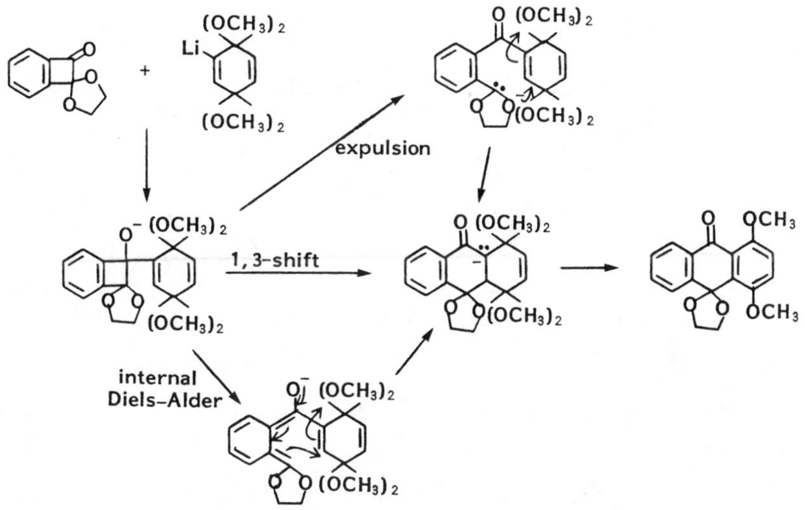

Studies are in progress to elucidate the mechanism and will be reported elsewhere.

The success of this initial study in forming a simple anthraquinone system prompted examination of the more complex AB-ring precursor 6. Aside from demonstrating the applicability of this chemistry to form a tetracyclic system, the course of the reaction of butyllithium with 6 was needed. If deprotonation of the hydroxyl group in 6 preceded metal-halogen

exchange, then the hydroxyl group in the fully functionalized
AB-ring system (vide infra) did not need to be derivitized
prior to reaction of 6 with butyllithium. However, if metal-
halogen exchange were faster than deprotonation, the hydroxyl
group would have to be protected (11). Reaction of one equivalent of n-butyllithium with 6 followed by quenching the reaction with methanol afforded recovered 6, establishing that
deprotonation was considerably faster than metal-halogen exchange in this system. Reaction of 6 with two equivalents of
n-butyllithium and then addition of 2 afforded the tetracyclic
compound 7a which was then hydrolyzed to 7b directly in an

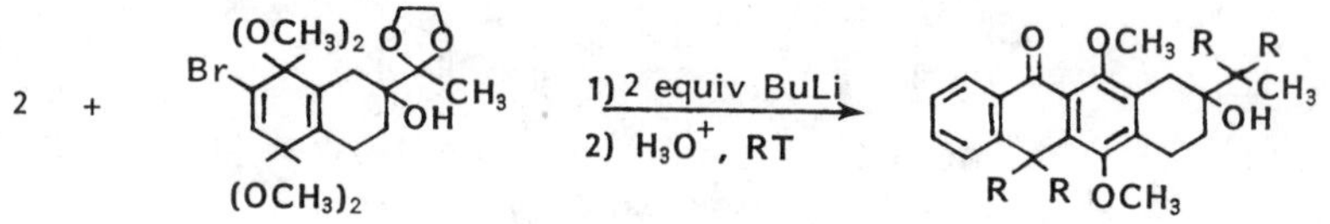

unoptimized overall yield of 47%. Having now developed the
chemistry which would in principle allow the synthesis of a
fully functionalized anthracyclinone in one step from a
benzocyclobutenone monoketal and an AB-ring precursor, the
synthesis of the fully functionalized AB-ring system was required to apply the strategy to the anthracyclinone itself.

Synthesis of the AB-Ring System

Since the penultimate step in the preparation of the required
AB-ring system for coupling with the benzocyclobutenedione
monoketal would be electrochemical bisketal formation, substituents in the A-ring must be stable to these electrolysis conditions. Thus, the oxygen at the eventual C_7 position could not

be present as a hydroxyl group since secondary benzylic hydroxyl functions complicate the electrochemical step (12). On
the other hand, aromatic compounds having benzylic methyl
ethers undergo smooth oxidation to quinone bisketals (12).
Published model studies indicated tertiary hydroxyl groups
(i.e., C_9) and ketals were stable towards electrochemical oxidation (12); thus, 8 became the synthetic objective. Based on
our previous work, 8 should afford 9 in high yield.

8a, R^1 = OCH$_3$, R^2 = H   9
 b, R^1 = H, R^2 = OCH$_3$

The eventual route to the tetralin 8 (Scheme VI) began with
11 which was available in 79% overall yield from 10. Since the
experimental details are in press, only important points of the
synthesis will be noted. Sodium borohydride reduction of 11
gave a mixture of 12a and 12b, the ratio of which depends upon
the temperature of the reaction. At -15 °C to -20 °C, primarily
the *cis*-hydroxyl acid is formed (12a/12b $\sim$ 20:80), and preparative reactions were performed at this temperature (14, 15).
Initially, the synthetic sequence was carried through with the
pure 12b obtained from lactonization of the crude reduction
mixture, extraction of the trans acid, 12a, and then hydrolysis of the crude lactone back to 12b. Thus, in our initial
studies, the sequence 12b → 12d → 13b → 14b was performed
using pure compounds. Since the oxygenation step (13 → 14)
was not stereospecific and required silica gel chromatography
to separate 14a and 14b, in scale-up work 11 was carried out

to **15** without separation of isomers and then **15a** and **15b** separated by silica gel chromatography (24–32% overall yield from
11).

The synthetic sequence **10** → **15** proceeds in a standard
fashion except that the oxygenation of the ester enolate of **13**
to give **14** was always complicated by incomplete conversion of

Scheme VI.   *Synthesis of Anthracyclinone*
AB-Ring System

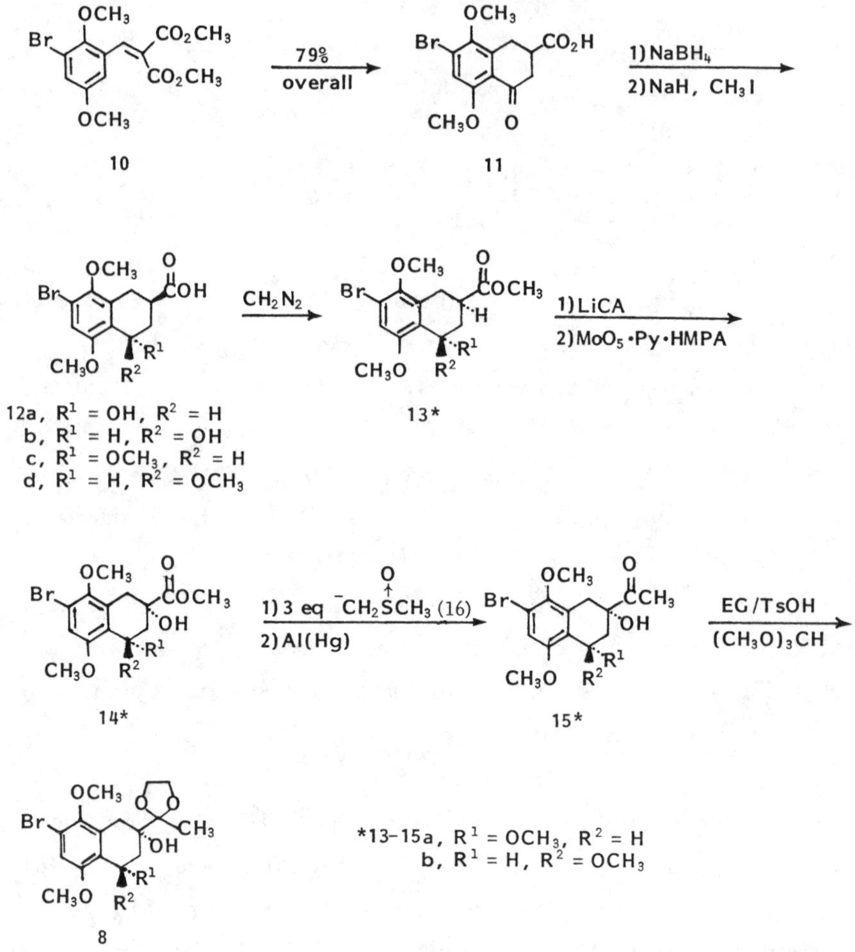

*13-15a, $R^1 = OCH_3$, $R^2 = H$
b, $R^1 = H$, $R^2 = OCH_3$

reactant. In some runs, VPC analysis indicated > 95% conversion to the hydroxyl ester **14** while under seemingly identical conditions, ca. 75:25 mixtures of **13** and **14** were observed. The most delicate step of the entire reaction is the ketalization of **15** to give **8**. There appears to be a fine balance between high-yield ketalization of **15** without side reactions and a complex reaction mixture. More than a score of ketalization procedures were attempted before reaction conditions supplied by Professor Paul Dowd led to successful execution of the reaction. Not only is the reaction time important for this particular system, but also the time is dependent upon the batch of reagent (i.e., ethylene glycol, trimethylorthoformate, toluenesulfonic acid). Thus, ketalization of **15** provided the functionalized AB-ring system for the coupling reaction.

A Regiospecific Route to Benzocyclobutendione Monoketals

The generality of the chemistry outlined in Scheme III depends on the availability of benzocyclobutendione monoketals as the CD-ring precursors. While the parent system was easily prepared via monoketalization of the Cava dione (13), routes to unsymmetrical benzocyclobutendione monoketals had not been studied. Since the D ring of many of the natural aglycons contains a methoxy or hydroxyl group in C_4, an efficient route to **20** was desired. Numerous classical routes to **20** failed; thus, a markedly different approach was explored. Pyrolysis of the acid chloride **16a** afforded the benzocyclobutenone **17a** (16) which was subsequently ketalized to give **18a**. In contrast to previous lack of success in cleanly brominating benzocyclobutenone ketals, **18a,** which has a benzylic trimethylsilyl group, rapidly undergoes free radical bromination to furnish crystalline **19a**. A similar sequence using **16b** gave

Scheme VII. Synthesis of Benzocyclobutendione
Monoketals

16a, R = H   17a (73%)   18a (90%)
    b, R = OCH₃   b (44%)   b (73%)

19a (73%)   2, R = H (85%)
    b (96%)   20, R = OCH₃ (85%)

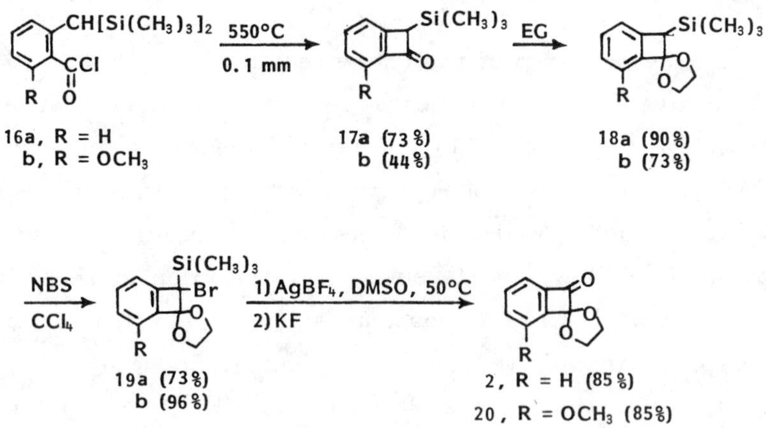

the required methoxy system **19b**. These compounds were then
transformed to the required dione monoketals by heating with
silver tetrafluoroborate (17) in dimethylsulfoxide followed by
treatment of the reaction mixture with potassium fluoride.
This latter reaction may be regarded as the silicon analogue of
the Kornblum oxidation and could proceed as illustrated below.

Scheme VIII. Proposed Mechanism for
Conversion of Bromosilane to Ketone

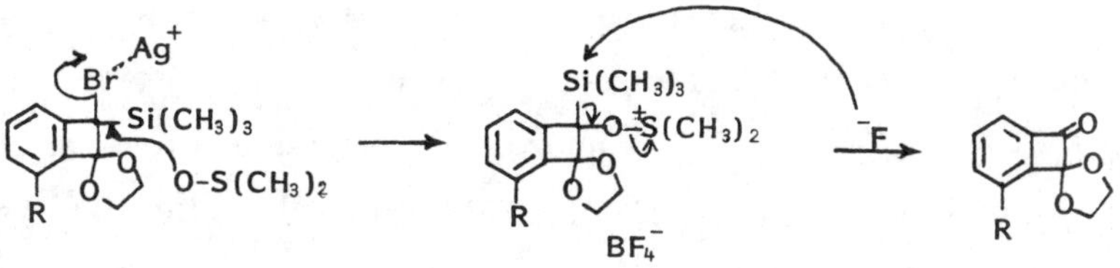

While the chemistry here has been used to prepare **2** and **20**,
it would appear to offer a general route not only to benzocyclobutendione monoketals but to the diones themselves via hydrolysis.

(±) 4-Demethoxydaunomycinone and
(±) Daunomycinone

For completion of the synthesis, there remained the anodic oxidation of **8** to its bisketal and the coupling of the lithiated bisketal to the benzocyclobutendione monoketal **2**. This chemistry was examined first with the trans (trans here will refer to the OCH_3 and OH functions) compound **8b** since this was the major isomer from our synthetic sequence (Scheme VI). As expected from model studies, anodic oxidation of **8b** gave **9b** as a crystalline solid in 81% yield. Treatment of **9b** with two equivalents of *n*-butyllithium gave the dilithio compound **21b**. When **21b** was reacted with **2** and the product hydrolyzed,

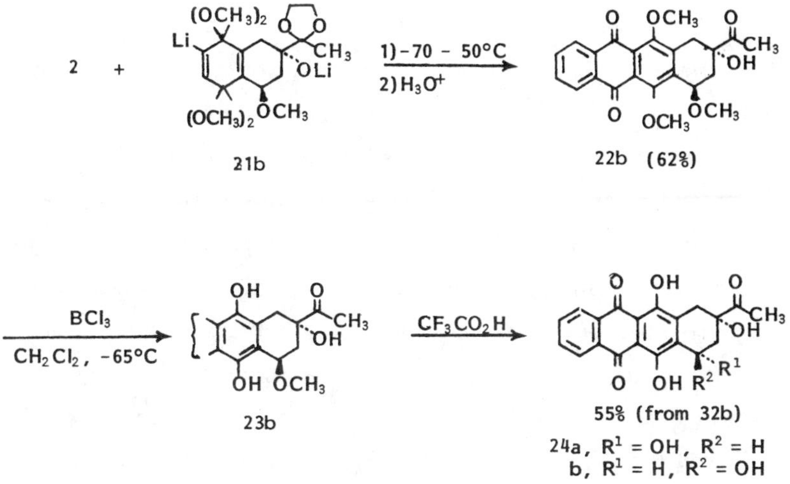

22b was isolated in 62% yield. This compound showed identical physical (TLC, mp) and spectroscopic (IR, NMR) properties with a sample of **22b** supplied by Professor Wong. While aluminum chloride (18) appears as the reagent commonly utilized in the literature for demethylation of aromatic ethers akin to **22b**, boron trichloride was more convenient and furnished **23b** in nearly quantitative yield. The subsequent solvolysis of the C_7-methoxy group initially encountered difficulties since the reaction of 23b with trifluoroacetic acid at room temperature gave poor yields of a mixture of 24a and 24b. However, if the trifluoroacetic acid was cooled to a slush and then 23b added, chromatography of the crude product afforded 4-demethoxydaunomycinone, 24a (33%), its epi-isomer, 24b (22%), and ca. 7% of aromatized material. The recovered epi-material, 24b, can be epimerized via treatment with trifluoroacetic acid to 24a (39%) with 27% of 24b recovered. Practially, two cycles of this type can be employed, raising the overall yield of the desired 4-demethoxydaunomycinone from 23b to 44%. We have utilized this chemistry to produce gram quantities of 4-demethoxydaunomycinone.

Since the solvolysis/epimerization sequence for converting 23b to 24a was less efficient than desired, we briefly explored the chemistry of 15a, the minor ketone from our synthesis. If this chemistry proceeds well, then a stereospecific synthesis of 15a and a demethylation of 21a would circumvent the solvolysis/epimerization sequence for 23b (the a series of compounds has the opposite stereochemistry at C_7 of the tetracyclic system). Unfortunately, the ketalization step 15a → 8a (56%), the electrolysis step 8a → 9a (58%), and the coupling step to form 21a (44%) all proceeded in substantially lower yield than for the compounds having the hydroxyl and the methoxyl groups trans. Thus, further work along this line was not pursued (19).

For the synthesis of the (±) daunomycinone, the organolithium compound 21b was reacted with 20 and the crude material hydrolyzed to yield 56% of 25. Since the conversion of 25 to daunomycinone is known (4a), this formally comprises a convergent, regiospecific synthesis of daunomycinones.

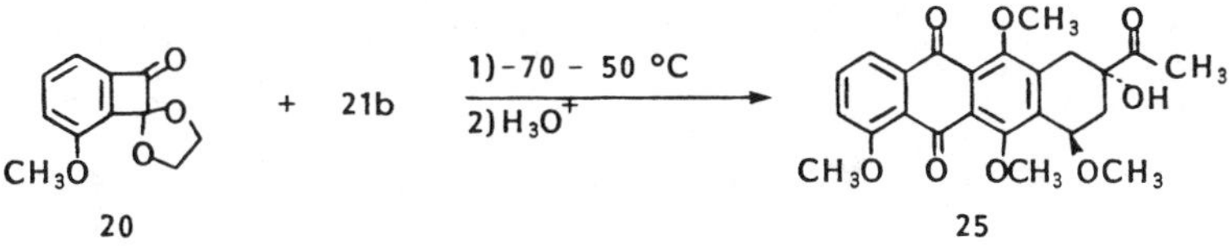

In summary, this approach provides a usable, convergent synthesis of 4-demethoxydaunomycinone and appropriate analogues but has several drawbacks for daunomycinone itself. First, the AB-ring system with the proper relative stereochemistry (*cis*-C_7,C_9-oxygen substituents) gave much lower yields in the ketalization, electrolysis, and coupling steps. Thus, if the chemistry is performed on the trans compound because of the high yield in the steps, a tedious separation of isomers will be required. However, the major unsolved problem at this state is the inefficient method (4a) for demethylation of **25** regiospecifically at the C_6- and C_{11}-methoxy group to the daunomycinone system (12% overall). While several approaches are available to circumvent this problem, the results obtained in the next section have rendered this approach to daunomycinone itself only of academic interest; thus, a better sequence for conversion of **25** to daunomycinones was not investigated.

THE QUINONE MONOKETAL 1,4-DIPOLE STRATEGY TO ANTHRACYCLINONES

The chemistry outlined in the previous section, while affording a regiospecific, convergent route to the anthracyclinone nucleus, had two drawbacks for daunomycinone/adriamycinone itself: the specific demethylation of the C_6- and C_{11}-methoxy groups in the presence of the C_4-methoxy group and the modest yields in several steps when the A-ring precursor

had the requisite cis stereochemistry between the oxygen functions of the A-ring.   These complications would be especially
troublesome in the synthesis of the ^{14}C-ring-labeled system of
high specific activity.   While our overall objective was still the
same -- a regiospecific, convergent synthesis involving the
coupling of a CD-ring precursor (^{14}C-ring-labeled) with an
AB-ring fragment (fully functionalized and optically active)--
a modified strategy was chosen.

This modified approach which essentially reverses the polar-
ity considerations of the reactants from that previously discussed is outlined in Scheme IX.   An especially attractive

*Scheme IX.   Quinone Monoketal 1,4-Dipole
Strategy to Anthracyclinones*

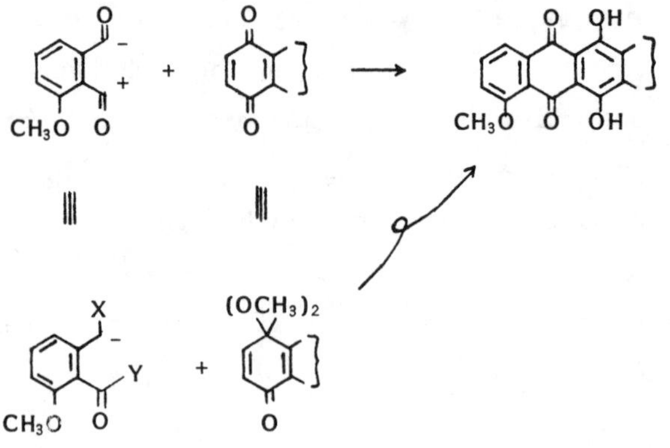

feature of this strategy was that a number of molecules (Table
1) which could serve as the 1,4-dipole equivalent were already
in the literature.   Furthermore, a quinone monoketal readily
available via an electrolysis/hydrolysis sequence from 1,4-di-
methoxy aromatic compounds (20) appeared as a viable regiospecific quinone equivalent.   While at the inception of this work
the only Michael-type addition of a carbon nucleophile to a quinone monoketal was its reaction with dimethylsulfoxonium ylid,

TABLE 1. *Potential 1,4-Dipole Equivalents*

dipole	substrate	product
CO_2CH_3 ... CO_2CH_3 **26**	CO_2CH_3	CO_2CH_3, CH_3, CO_2CH_3, OH — Schmid 1965 (21)
$SO_2\emptyset$ ... CH_3O **27**	O	OH, CH_3O OH O — Hauser 1977 (22)
28	CO_2CH_3	OH, CO_2CH_3, CH_3 — Sammes 1978 (23)
CN ... O **29**	CO_2CH_3	OH, CH_3, CO_2CH_3, OH — Kraus 1978 (24)

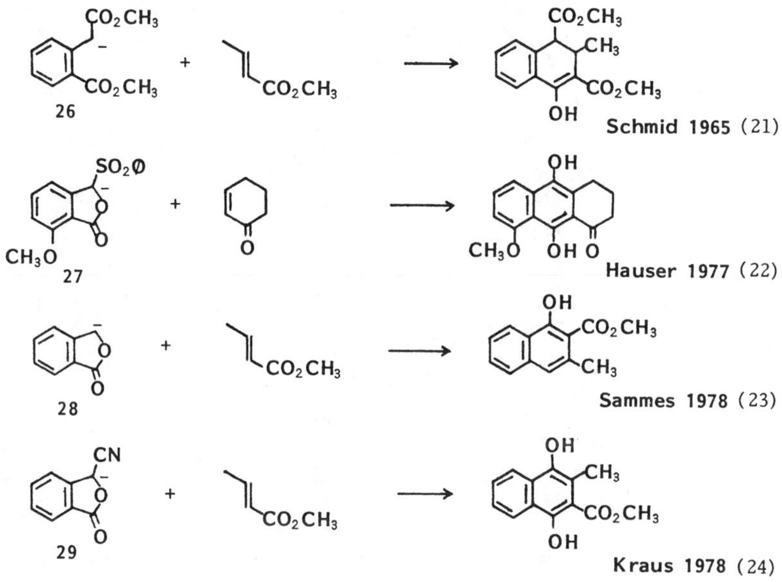

shortly after our studies were initiated, the addition of malonate anions to these protected quinone derivatives was reported (25).

To explore the feasibility of this strategy, the Schmid system was examined first. When the anion from dimethylhomophthalate, **26**, was reacted with quinone monoketals **30–34** (Table 2), there was obtained after silica gel chromatography the products **35–39** (26). These results nicely afforded the intact tetracyclic system under reaction conditions we felt would be compatible with a fully oxygenated A-ring precursor. There remained only the oxidative decarboxylation of compounds such as **38** or **39** to the anthraquinone-ring system to complete the model study. Chemistry aimed at converting **38** to **40** under

TABLE 2. *Reaction of Dimethylhomophthalate with Quinone Monoketals*

entry	monoketal	product	yield[a] (%)
1	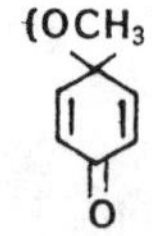 (OCH₃)₂ ... O **30**	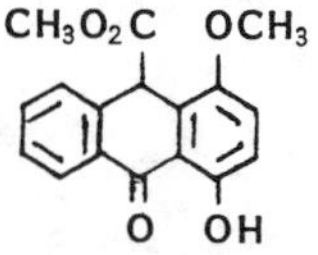 CH₃O₂C OCH₃ ... O OH **35**	60
2	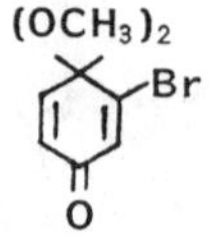 (OCH₃)₂ –Br ... O **31**	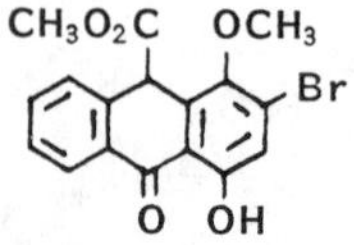 CH₃O₂C OCH₃ –Br ... O OH **36 36**	20
3	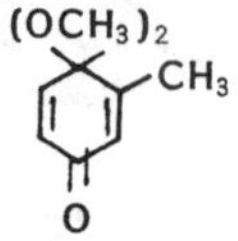 (OCH₃)₂ –CH₃ ... O **32**	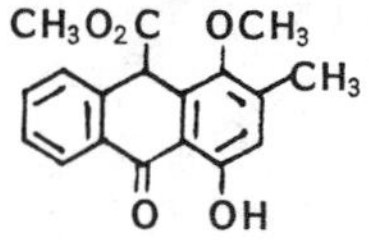 CH₃O₂C OCH₃ –CH₃ ... O OH **37**	40
4	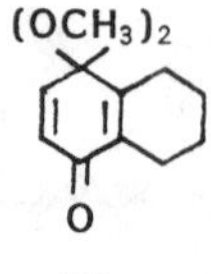 (OCH₃)₂ ... O **33**	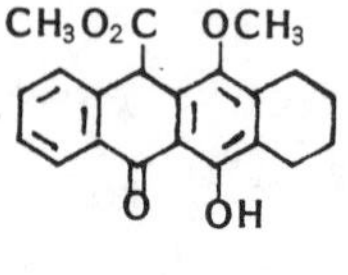 CH₃O₂C OCH₃ ... O OH **38**	60
5	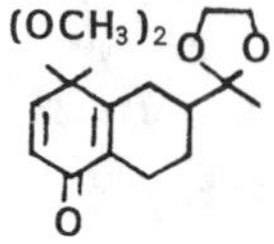 (OCH₃)₂ ... O **34**	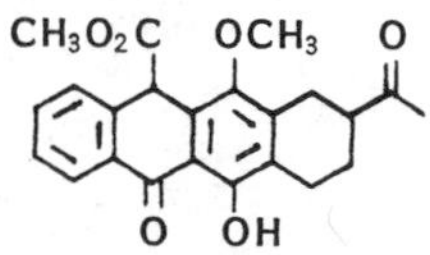 CH₃O₂C OCH₃ O ... O OH **39**	41

^{a}*Yield of recrystallized product, not optimized.*

mild conditions was examined since this readily available compound was judged a convenient model for the desired conversion in the final A-ring-substituted molecule. Unfortunately, attempts at effecting the **38 → 40** conversion under conditions we

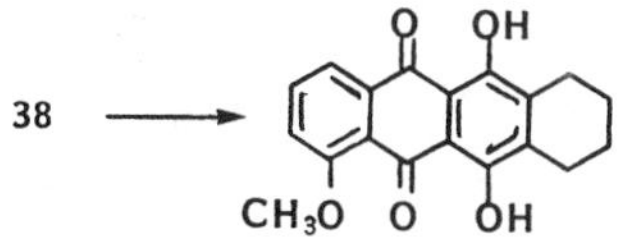

$$38 \longrightarrow$$

O OH

CH$_3$O O OH

40

felt would be compatible with a fully oxygenated A-ring gave little indication that such a conversion would be possible. Thus, we next investigated **27** as our 1,4-dipole equivalent since the required B-ring quinone functionality was formed directly in the annelation reaction.

The annelation chemistry of the Hauser system **27** was examined with the model quinone monoketal **33**. When **27** was reacted sequentially with base and then **33**, the anthraquinone **41** was

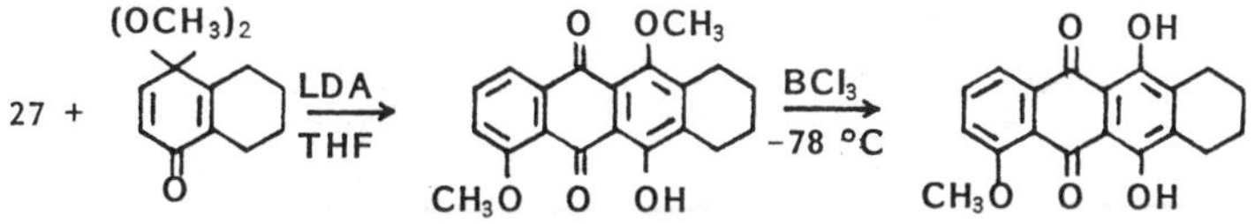

$$27 + \quad \text{(OCH}_3\text{)}_2 \quad \xrightarrow[\text{THF}]{\text{LDA}} \quad \xrightarrow[-78\ ^\circ\text{C}]{\text{BCl}_3}$$

33

O OCH$_3$

CH$_3$O O OH

41

O OH

CH$_3$O O OH

42

isolated in 45% recrystallized yield. Furthermore, boron trichloride was found to specifically hydrolyze the 11-methyl ether to give **42** (90%). Thus, the difficulty attendant with selective demethylation of methyl ethers at C$_6$ and C$_{11}$ in the presence of a C$_4$ methyl ether in a trimethoxylated system is easily overcome in the demethoxy system such as **41** (27,28). Presumably this selective demethylation of **41** arises because initially the boron trichloride reacts with the C$_6$-hydroxyl group, generating **43**. With the C$_5$-keto group complexed, the carbonyl

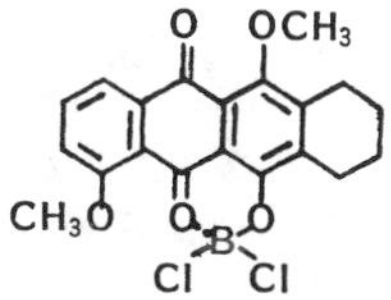

O OCH$_3$

CH$_3$O O O
B
Cl Cl

43

facilitated demethylation of the C_4-methyl ether is inoperative. However, the carbonyl-assisted demethylation of the C_{11}-methoxy ether is still effective, and this leads to the production of **42**. Thus, this sequence affords the daunomycinone tetracyclic system with the oxygen functionality of the B-, C-, and D-rings properly substituted. There remains now the synthesis of the required AB-ring system for daunomycinone itself.

Synthesis of the AB-Ring System

A key aspect in the successful implementation of the annelation chemistry to a regiospecific synthesis of the rhodomycinone aglycons was an efficient route to a quinone monoketal such as **45**. We had extensively studied the regiochemistry of

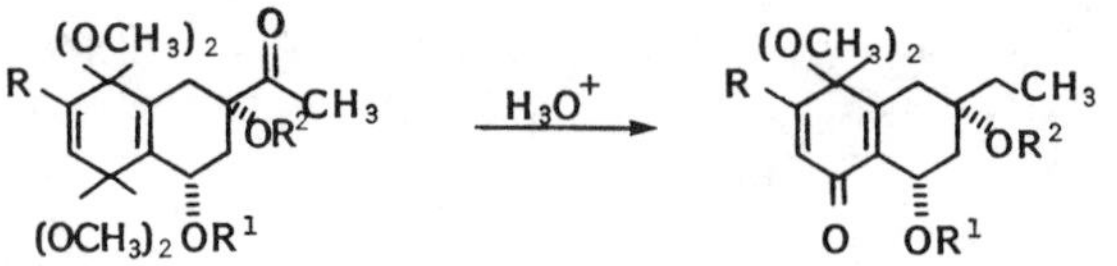

44a, R = Br
 b, R = H

45

bisketal hydrolysis and knew that a bromo substituent such as in **44a** would specifically yield **45a** (20a). Thus, some appropriate species akin to **44a** would be available from the chemistry described earlier (Scheme VI), and **45a** could presumably be reduced to **45b**. This approach was not only esthetically displeasing but entailed three extra synthetic operations to prepare the brominated bicyclic system relative to the hydrogen compound and some reduction procedure for the **44a** → **45b** conversion. In our earlier studies on benzoquinone bisketal hydrolysis, a high regioselectivity of hydrolysis was noted for a number of substituents (Table 3). Somewhat surprisingly at the time, a system having an allylic methoxy group, 46f,

TABLE 3. *Regioselectivity of Monohydrolysis of Selected Benzoquinone Bisketals*

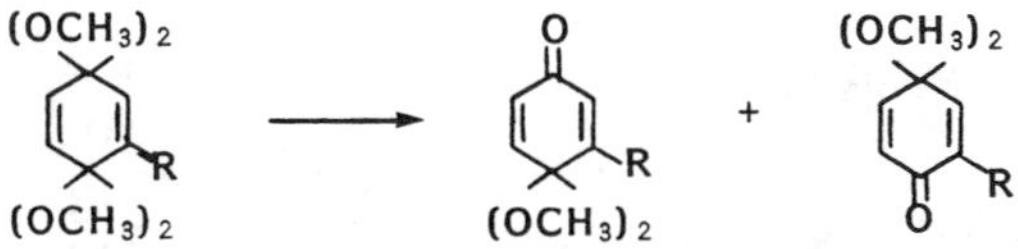

	46		47		48
a, R = Br			95	:	5
b, R = CH$_3$			85	:	5
c, R = OCH$_3$			>98	:	<2
d, R = SCH$_3$			>95	:	<5
e, R = NHCCH$_3$ (O)			>95	:	<15
f, R = CH(CH$_3$)OCH$_3$			73	:	27

showed less selectivity than similarly substituted molecules. While the difference was not overwhelming, it was reasoned that in a system in which the methoxy orientation relative to the ketal linkage was fixed and in which the positions adjacent to the bisketal carbon were substituted, the oxygen might exert a synthetically useful directive effect on the bisketal hydrolysis.

The importance of the neighboring methoxy group on the regiochemistry of bisketal hydrolysis was readily assessed by

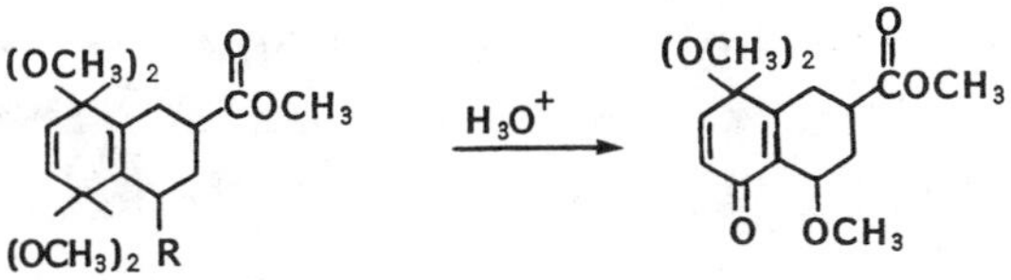

49a, R = H
  b, R = OCH$_3$

50

examining the model systems **49a** and **49b**. Whereas **49a** afforded a ca. 1:1 mixture of regioisomers as determined by 200 MHz-^{1}H-NMR spectroscopy, **49b** gave a single monoketal eventually assigned as **50** in 90% yield. Similarly, anodic oxidation of **51** followed by monohydrolysis afforded **52** in good yield.

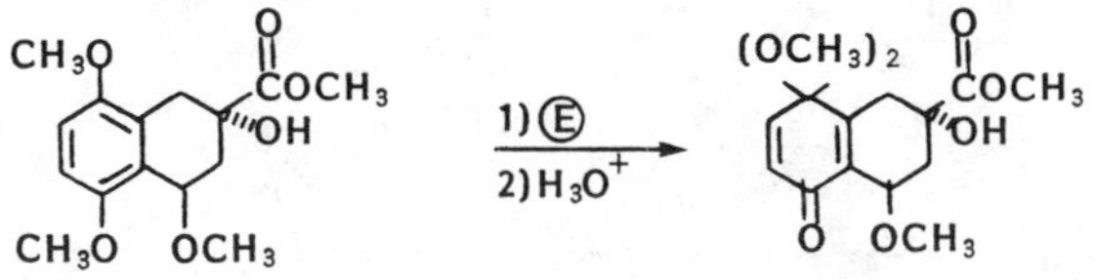

51   52 (78%)

There remained one additional question concerning the utility of this annelation reaction in the synthesis of fully functionalized rhodomycinones: the compatibility of the C_7- and C_9-oxygen functions with the reaction conditions. The availability of **50** and **52** allowed this point to be readily examined. While

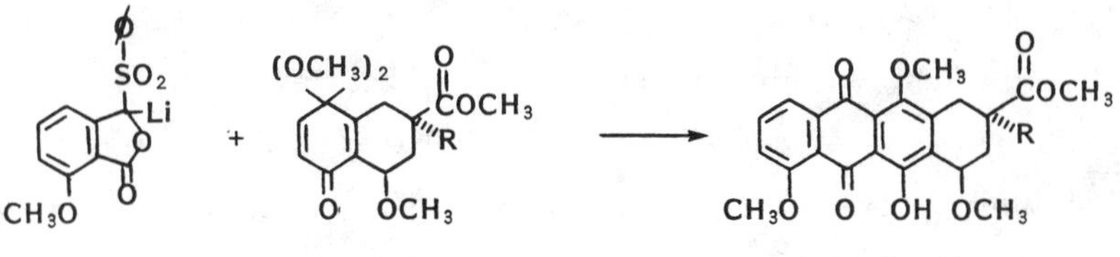

53   50, R = H   55a, R = H
                52, R = OH   b, R = OH
                54, R = OSi(CH$_3$)$_2$

50 underwent clean reaction with the Hauser anion affording **55a**, demonstrating the C_7-methoxy group was compatible with the sequence, **52** gave poor yields of tetracyclic product. However, use of the trimethylsilyl ether **54** led to clean cyclization to **55b**. Thus, the final synthetic target was an A-ring with the C_7- and C_9-hydroxyl groups blocked and the C_{12}-carbonyl group protected (unpublished observations indicated an unprotected carbonyl group gave lower yields in the electrochemical step).

The ketone 56 available via a route analogous to that shown in Scheme VI was the logical starting material for preparing the required protected system (29). A number of combinations of groups were explored to protect both the C_9-hydroxyl and C_{13}-carbonyl group without success. Even the mild ketalization conditions developed for the brominated system 8 gave low yields when applied to 56. Since little success had been observed in blocking both the hydroxyl and carbonyl group of 56, the idea of blocking the hydroxyl group with a bulky group was explored. The premise here was that a suitably large group on the C_9-oxygen would protect the adjacent carbonyl linkage during the electrolysis step. The reaction sequence 56 → 58 proceeded in excellent yield; thus, 58 was available for the annelation step.

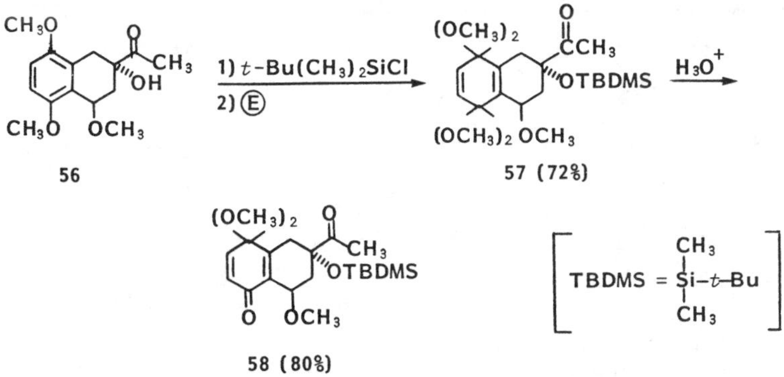

Daunomycinone

The coupling chemistry of 58 and 27 produced 59b in 50% recrystallized yield (29). While the majority of our annelation studies with the Hauser anions were performed in tetrahydrofuran with lithium diisopropylamide as base, improved yields

$$27 + 58 \xrightarrow[\text{2)BCl}_3]{\text{1)CH}_3\text{SOCH}_2\text{Li}}$$

59a, R = CH$_3$
b, R = H

were noted in some systems when the reaction was conducted in dimethyl sulfoxide/tetrahydrofuran (homogeneous conditions) using dimsyl anion as the base. In this manner reaction of **27** with **58** followed by demethylation gave **59b** in 48% recrystallized yield. Treatment of **58b** with trifluoroacetic acid affords a good yield of a mixture of daunomycinone and epi-daunomycinone.

This chemistry serves as an excellent regiospecific route to rhodomycinone aglycons and analogues which are highly functionalized in the A-ring. An especially attractive feature of the synthesis, relative to the daunomycinone/adriamycinone system, is the facile regiospecific demethylation of the C_{11}-methoxyl group without the complications usually associated with demethylations when C_6 and C_{11} both bear methoxyl groups. Furthermore, deoxygenation of these annelation products at C_6 would afford an entry into 6-deoxyrhodomycinone and citromycinone aglycons. Finally, the availability of a wide range of quinone monoketals together with the known 1,4-dipole equivalents presents a versatile and general entry into anthraquinone-type ring systems.

A STEREOSPECIFIC ROUTE TO THE FULLY FUNCTIONALIZED AB-RING SYSTEM

For most of our studies, we have employed an AB-ring system (e.g., **15, 56**) wherein the oxygen functions at C_7 and C_9 have the trans relationship. This requires that at a later stage in the synthesis, the C_7-C_9 oxygen linkages be changed from trans to cis. This can be done by epimerization of the C_7-oxygen function as mentioned earlier. However, the separation of (±) 4-deme-thoxydaunomycinone from its epi-isomer is tedious, and in our experience the analogous separation of (±) daunomycinone from its epi-isomer is even more difficult. Thus, we have been interested in a stereospecific route to the fully functionalized AB-ring system.

This route began with the ketoacid **60** which was transformed to **61** in 85% yield without purification of the intermediate keto-ester. Again, the most troublesome step in the sequence is

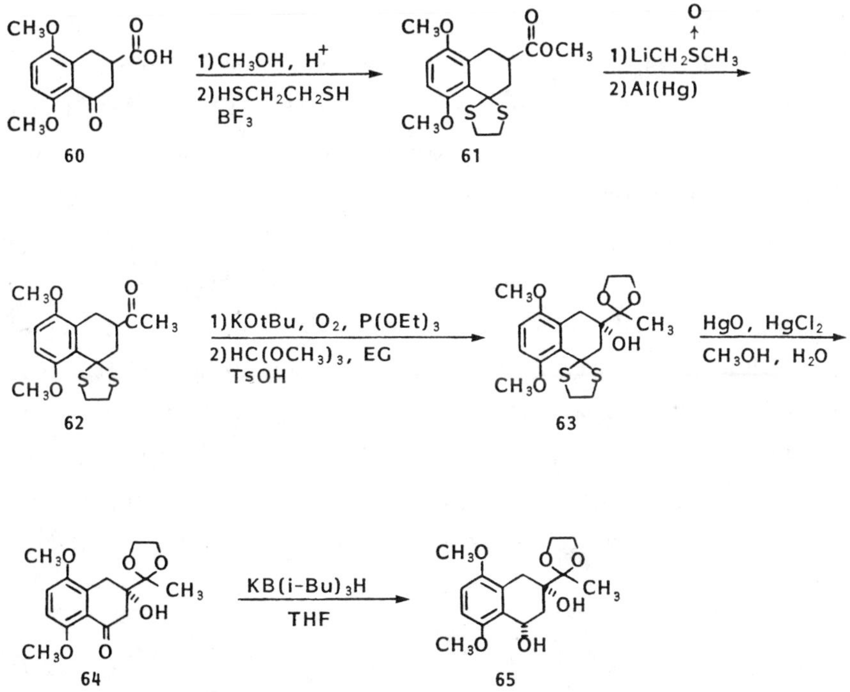

introduction of the oxygen at what eventually will be C_9 of the anthracyclinone. Reaction of the enolate of **61** with $MoO_5 \cdot Py \cdot HMPA$, as employed in the **13 → 14** conversion, gave a complex mixture of products. Perhaps this was due to competing oxidation of the sulfurs in the thioketal with the ester enolate oxygenation.

Introduction of oxygen into the ester **61** having been unsuccessful under our previously utilized conditions, the ester **61** was converted into the ketone **62** (> 80%). Oxidation of **62** under standard conditions afforded the hydroxy ketone in 50% yield after chromatography. Ketalization of this hydroxyketone to afford **63** (93%) was best accomplished at 45 °C under conditions previously used for ketalization of **15**. The stage was now set for deblocking of the thioketal and reduction of the resulting ketone.

The hydrolysis of **63** proceeded smoothly to give **64** which could be isolated as a white crystalline solid. We had expected **64** to be quite susceptible to β-elimination of the hydroxyl group with subsequent aromatization to afford the naphthalene nucleus. However, **64** was quite stable in neutral media and could even be sublimed largely unchanged at 140 °C (bath)/10^{-4} mm. Now there remained the stereospecific reduction of **64** to the cis-diol **65**. While sodium borohydride reduction of **64** gave two alcohols as ascertained by TLC analysis, reduction with K-selectride gave one major product which was isolated pure by recrystallization. Our assignment of the cis stereochemistry to the product must be considered tentative. However, the high-field region of the 300 MHz NMR spectrum of **65** is nearly identical with that of 4-demethoxydaunomycinone and appreciably different than that of the epi-isomer. Studies to optimize reaction conditions for the preparation of **65** and to obtain **65** of proper absolute configuration are in progress.

SUMMARY

The two approaches studied here involve mild annelation conditions for joining a CD-ring segment and an AB-ring segment to form the tetracyclic-ring system of the anthracyclinone. A prime virtue of this type of approach is that all functionality is present when the tetracyclic-ring system is formed. It is our experience that the bromination/solvolysis procedure for introduction of benzylic oxygen functions in the A-ring of anthracyclinones works poorly with (±) daunomycinone.[3] In the 6-deoxyrhodomycinone series, we have never been able to isolate C_7-hydroxyl products from the bromination/ solvolysis sequence (30). Only with the 11-deoxyrhodomycinone systems have good yields been reported for this method of benzylic oxygen introduction (31-33). Thus, in these former two

Scheme X. Generalizations Regarding Success of Bromination/Solvolysis Route for Introduction of C_7-Hydroxyl

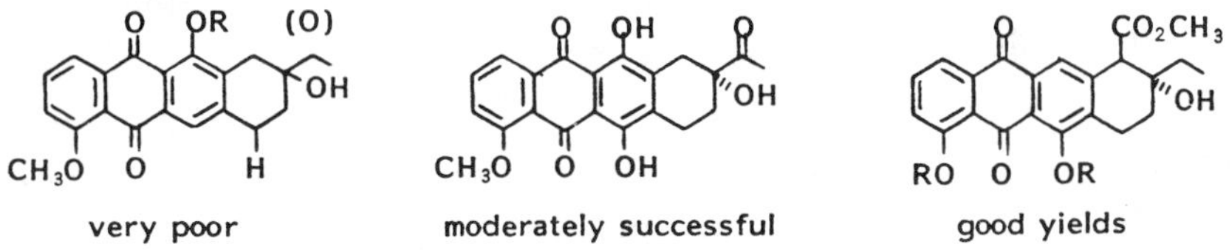

very poor   moderately successful   good yields

systems either a better procedure for functionalization at C_7 of the tetracyclic-ring system is required or else the C_7 oxygen must be present when the tetracyclic-ring system is formed.

There remains one major problem to be solved before the chemistry described herein will lead to a truly convenient synthesis of rhodomycinone aglycons. As noted earlier, separation of isomers at C_7 when the anthracyclinone system is equilibrated with trifluoroacetic acid is time consuming and sometimes difficult if performed on a reasonable scale (> 1-g. amounts). Furthermore, the aglycon / glycon coupling requires an optically active aglycon unless an adequate separation method can be devised for the diastereomers formed in this reaction. Thus,

[3]*Apparently in 4-demethoxydaunomycinone, the bromination/ solvolysis sequence can be utilized more effectively (4a).*

the synthesis of an optically active AB-ring segment functionalized so that the protecting groups on the C_7- and C_9-hydroxyl
functions can be cleaved without disturbing the cis C_7,C_9 stereochemistry is required. Studies reported in the previous section
indicate substantial progress toward solving this last problem.

ACKNOWLEDGMENTS

The author gratefully acknowledges his coworkers who not
only performed the majority of the experimental work but in
several instances made major contributions to the direction of
the work.

REFERENCES

1. Sartorelli, A. C., ed. "Cancer Chemotherapy" American
   Chemical Society Symposium Series No. 30, American Chem-
   ical Society, Washington, D. C. (1976).   Arcamone, F.
   "Topics in Antibiotic Chemistry" (P. G. Sammes, ed.),
   Vol. 2. Chapter 3, Halsted Press, New York (1978).
   Arcamone, F. "Anticancer Agents Based on Natural Product
   Models" (J. M. Cassady, J. D. Douros, eds.), Chapter 1,
   Academic Press, New York (1980).
2. Marsh, J. P.; Iwamoto, R. H.; Goodman, L. *Chem. Commun.*,
   589-590 (1968). Penco, S. *Chem. Ind. (London) 50*, 908
   (1968). Acton, E. M.; Fujiwara, A. N.; Henry, D. W. *J.
   Med. Chem. 17*, 659-660 (1974).
3. For a comprehensive listing of work in this area, see:
   Kelly, T. R.; Vaya, J.; Ananthasubramanian, L. *J. Am.
   Chem. Soc. 102*, 5983-5984 (1980).
4. (a) Wong, C. M.; Schwenk, R.; Popien, D.; Ho, T. L.
   Can. J. Chem. 51, 466-467 (1973).   (b) Arcamone, F.;

Bernardi, L.; Patelli, B.; DiMarco, A. German Offen
2 601 785 (1976). (c) Kende, A. S.; Tsay, Y.-G.; Mills,
J. E. *J. Am. Chem. Soc.* *98*, 1967-1969 (1976). (d) Smith,
T. H.; Fujiwara, A. N.; Henry, D. W.; Lee, W. W. *ibid.*
1969-1971. (e) Smith, T. H.; Fujiwara, A. N.; Lee, W. W.;
Wu, H. Y.; Henry, D. W. *J. Org. Chem.* *42*, 3653-3660 (1977).
(f) Kende, A. S.; Mills, J. E.; Tsay, Y.-G. U. S. Patents
4 021 457 (1977) and 4 070 382 (1978).

5. Brockmann, H.; Niemeyer, J. *Chem. Ber.* *100*, 3578-3587
   (1967).

6. (a) Krohn, K.; Tolkiehn, K. *Tetrahedron Lett.* 4023-4026
   (1978); *Idem Chem. Ber.* *112*, 3453-3471 (1979). (b) Garland,
   R.B.; Palmer, J. R.; Schulz, J. A.; Sollman, P. B.; Pappo,
   R. *Tetrahedron Lett.* 3669-3672 (1978).

7. Jackson, D. K.; Narasimhan, L.; Swenton, J. S. *J. Am.
   Chem. Soc.* *101*, 3989-3990 (1979).

8. ^{14}C-side-chain-labeled adriamycin has been prepared by
   three groups: Penco, S.; Vacario, G. P.; Angelucci, A.;
   Arcamone, F. *J. Antibiot.* *30*, *773-775 (1977).* Vishniwajjala,
   B. R.; Kataoka, T,; Kazer, F. D.; Witiak, D. T.; Malspeis,
   L. *J. Labelled Compd, Radiopharm.* *14*, 77-82 (1978). Chen,
   C. P.; Tan Tong, M.; Fujiwara, A. N.; Henry, D. W.;
   Leaffer, M. A.; Lee, W. W.; Smith, T. H. *Ibid.* *14*, 111-
   117 (1978).

9. (a) Raynolds, P. W.; Manning, M. J.; Swenton, J. S.
   Tetrahedron Lett. 2383-2386 (1977). (b) Swenton, J. S.;
   Raynolds, P. W. *J. Am. Chem. Soc.* *100*, 6188-6195 (1978).

10. (a) Cava, M. P.; Muth, K. *J. Am. Chem. Soc.* *82*, 652-656
    (1960). (b) Cava, M. P.; Napier, D. R.; Pohl, R. J. *Ibid.*
    85, 2076-2080 (1963). (c) Cava, M. P.; Stein, R. P. *J. Org.
    Chem.* *31*, 1866-1869 (1966). (d) Stansfield, F.; Amupitan,
    J. O. *J. Chem. Soc., Perkin Trans.* *1*, 1949-1951 (1974).

11. For examples of t-butyllithium acting as a stronger kinetic base towards bromine than a carboxylic acid proton, see Stein, C. A.; Morton, T. H. *Tetrahedron Lett.*, 4933-4936 (1973). Boatman, R. J.; Whitlock, B. J.; Whitlock, H. W. *J. Am. Chem. Soc. 99*, 4822-4824 (1977).

12. Henton, D. R.; McCreery, R. L.; Swenton, J. S. *J. Org. Chem. 45*, 370-378 (1980), and references cited therein.

13. (a) Cava, M. P.; Napier, D. R. *J. Am. Chem. Soc. 79*, 3606 (1957). (b) Brown, R. F. C.; Solly, R. K. *Aust. J. Chem. 19*, 1045-1057 (1966). (c) Forster, D. L.; Gilchrist, T. L.; Rees, C. W.; Stanton, E. *J. Chem. Soc., Chem. Commun.*, 695-696 (1971). (d) McOmie, J. F. W.; Perry, D. H. *Ibid.* 248-249 (1973).

14. The reduction of cyclic ketones by metal-hydride-reducing agents suggests that polar substituents on the ring tend to produce a higher proportion of cis alcohols (15). However, the temperature dependence of the stereochemistry of the reactin does not appear to have been noted.

15. (a) House, H. O. "Modern Synthetic Reactions," pp. 60-61. W. A. Benjamin, Inc., Menlo Park, CA (1972). (b) Katsui, N.; Matsunaga, A.; Imaizumi, K.; Masamune, T. *Tetrahedron Lett.* 83-86 (1971). *Idem Bull. Chem. Soc. Jpn. 45*, 2871-2877 (1972). (c) Violland, R.; Violland-Duperret, N.; Pachero, H.; Ghazarian, M. *Bull. Soc. Chim Fr.* 307-311 (1971).

16. Chenard, B. L.; Slapak, C.; Anderson, D. K.; Swenton, J. S. *J. Chem. Soc., Chem. Commun.* 179-180 (1981).

17. The use of silver tetrafluoroborate to effect Kornblum oxidation on bromides is known: Lemal, D. M.; Fry, A. J. *J. Org. Chem. 29*, 1673-1676 (1964).

18. Kim, K. S.; Vanotti, E.; Suarato, A.; Johnson, F. *J. Am. Chem. Soc. 101*, 2483-2484 (1979), and references cited therein.

19. The lower yields in this system may result from the *trans*-diaxial relationship of the C_7-hydroxyl group and a C_6-hydrogen facilitating elimination as a side reaction.

20. (a) Henton, D. R.; Anderson, D. K.; Manning, M. J.; Swenton, J. S. *J. Org. Chem. 45*, 3422-3433 (1980), and references cited therein. (b) Dolson, M. G.; Swenton, J. S. *Ibid. 46*, 177-178 (1981).

21. Eisenmuth, W.; Renfroe, H. B.; Schmid, H. *Helv. Chim. Acta 48*, 375 (1965).

22. (a) Hauser, F. M.; Rhee, R. P. *J. Am. Chem. Soc. 99*, 4533-4534 (1979); *ibid. 101*, 1628-1629 (1979). (b) Russell, R. S.; Warrener, R. N. *J. Chem. Soc., Chem. Commun.*, 108-110 (1981).

23. Broom, N. J. P.; Sammes, P. G. *J. Chem. Soc., Chem. Commun.*, 162-163 (1978).

24. Kraus, G. A.; Sugimoti, H. *Tetrahedron Lett.* 2263-2266 (1978).

25. Parker, K. A.; Kang, S. *J. Org. Chem. 45*, 1218 (1980).

26. Chenard, B. L.; Anderson, D. K.; Swenton, J. S. *J. Chem. Soc., Chem. Commun.* 932-933 (1980).

27. Wong, C. M.; Schwenk, R.; Popein, D.; Ho, T. *Can. J. Chem. 51*, 466-469 (1973).

28. See also Kim, K. S.; Vanotti, E.; Suarato, A.; Johnson, F. *J. Am. Chem. Soc. 101*, 2483-2484 (1979).

29. Dolson, M. G.; Chenard, B. L.; Swenton, J. S. *J. Am. Chem. Soc. 103*, 5263-5264 (1981).

30. Unpublished results of T. Haag.

31. Kimball, S. D.; Walt, D. R.; Johnson, F. *J. Am. Chem. Soc. 103*, 1560-1561 (1981); Confalone, P. N.; Pizzolato, G. *Ibid. 103*, 4250-4253; Kende, A. S. *Ibid.*, 4247-4248.

32. For less acceptable brominations, see: Kende, A. S.; Rizzi, J. *Tetrahedron Lett.* 1779-1782 (1981); Kende, A. S.; Boettger, S. D. *J. Org. Chem. 46*, 2799-2800 (1981).

33. For an especially useful route to aklavinone, see: Pearlman, B. A.; McNamara, J. M.; Hasan, I.; Hatakeyama, S.; Sekizaki, H.; Kishi, Y. *J. Am. Chem. Soc.* *103*, 4258-4251 (1981).

GLYCON- AND C-14-MODIFIED,
ANTITUMOR DOXORUBICIN ANALOGS

Derek Horton
Waldemar Priebe

Department of Chemistry
The Ohio State University
Columbus, Ohio

I. INTRODUCTION

The broad goals of our work on modified anthracycline
glycosides have been the chemical synthesis of analogs of the
clinically effective antitumor agents daunorubicin, adriamycin,
and carminomycin. It is well known that neither the glycon
nor the aglycon of these antibiotics is effective on its own
as an antineoplastic agent; indeed the aglycons display
carcinogenic activity. Our program was designed to evaluate
the effect on antitumor activity and toxicity of structural
modifications in the glycon, together with the effect of
introducing different substituents at position 14. The
general methodology involves initial synthesis of stereochemical and substitutional variants of the daunosamine
component, followed by coupling of these sugars to the
corresponding aglycon. For the C-14 substituted analogs, the
methodology has generally involved structural modification at

[1]Supported in part by NIGMS Grant No. 11976.

R′=H ; R^2= Me , daunorubicin

R′=OH; R^2= Me , adriamycin

R′=H ; R^2= H , carminomycin

position 14 after attachment of the sugar component. In
particular, the work set out to provide a factual basis to
substantiate or reject the rather generally held dogma that
an amino group at the 3' position is essential for biological
activity, and that substitution at the 2' position leads to
loss of activity.

The range of structural variants in the glycon portion was
designed to furnish a suitably comprehensive series of
stereochemical and substitutional variants in the daunosamine
moiety and provide anthracycline glycosides synthesized in
sufficient quantity for antitumor evaluation in the NCI P388
mouse screen. These products were expected to allow the
development of structure—activity relationships with respect
to the following daunosamine modifications: replacement of
the terminal methyl group by aminomethyl or hydroxymethyl
groups, stereochemical variation to include the D sugars as
well as the L enantiomers, stereochemical variation at position
3 of the sugar ring, compounds of inverted stereochemistry at
the anomeric center, and also compounds in which the nitrogen
atom at position 3 is replaced by oxygen or sulfur.

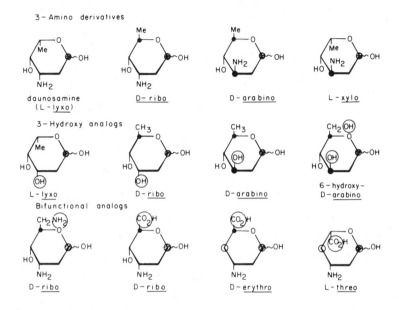

3 - Amino derivatives

daunosamine (L - lyxo)   D - ribo   D - arabino   L - xylo

3 - Hydroxy analogs

L - lyxo   D - ribo   D - arabino   6 - hydroxy - D - arabino

Bifunctional analogs

D - ribo   D - ribo   D - erythro   L - threo

The specific target-sugars proposed as the basis of this
program included particularly the stereovariants of daunosamine epimeric at the 5 position (D-ribo), at the 3 position
(L-xylo), at the 3 and 5 positions (D-arabino), together with
the 3-hydroxy analogs of the natural L-lyxo configuration,
and also the 5-epimer (D-ribo), the 3,5-diepi analog (D-
arabino) and various 6-hydroxy analogs. Further variants
included bifunctional derivatives additionally substituted by
an amino group at C-6, and analogs in which the terminal methyl
group is oxidized to carboxyl, in various stereochemical
series.

II. SYNTHESIS OF THE SUGARS

The structure and stereochemistry of daunosamine itself
was established early in Arcamone's laboratory (1), and its
glycosidic coupling to daunomycinone was demonstrated by Acton
and coworkers (2), who showed that an appropriately protected

glycosyl bromide of daunosamine could be coupled to the
aglycon, and the product deprotected, to reconstruct the
parent antibiotic daunorubicin in a reaction that proceeds
with evident high or complete anomeric specificity to give
the correct α-L linkage. The fact that the aglycon enters
trans to all of the substituents on the sugar ring is probably
an important factor in determining the anomeric specificity
of this reaction, a factor that is not generally so favorable
when sugar derivatives of different stereochemistry are
employed.

Daunosamine has been synthesized by several groups (3),
and a synthesis developed in our laboratory (4) was designed
to provide a high-yielding, practical synthesis of this
otherwise difficultly accessible amino sugar that would at the
same time offer a route, by way of common intermediates, to
give the desired substitutional and stereochemical modifications in high yield. The synthesis sets out from D-mannose
and affords daunosamine in ~40% net yield in few steps, and
without the necessity of chromatographic procedures that would
be an impediment in conducting the preparations on a large
scale.

The methyl α-glycoside of D-mannose was converted into its
2,3:4,6-dibenzylidene acetal, which in reaction with
butyllithium at low temperature gives the 2-deoxy-3-keto
compound indicated through attack at only the dioxolane ring.
The oxime of this ketone undergoes stereoselective reduction,
and N-acetylation of the amino group gives a readily separable
mixture of the non-crystalline, major product having the D-
ribo stereochemistry, separable by filtration from the
crystalline and almost completely insoluble, minor isomer
having the D-arabino stereochemistry. The latter product

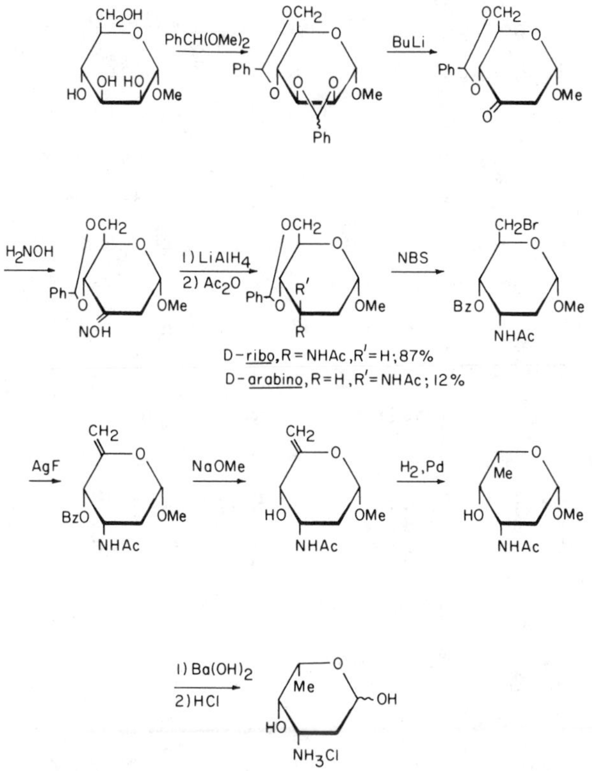

provides the starting point for stereochemical analogs of
daunosamine. Opening of the 4,6-benzylidene acetal ring with
N-bromosuccinimide, by Hanessian's convenient procedure (5),
affords the 6-bromide-4-benzoate, which may be reduced at C-6
to give the protected amino sugar in the D-ribo series, which
constitutes the 5-epimer of daunosamine. Conversion of the 6-
bromide by the action of silver fluoride into the corresponding
5,6-unsaturated derivative, most conveniently through the 4-
debenzoylated product, gives the key intermediate for the D
to L interconversion step. The enol ether undergoes stereospecific reduction by hydrogen in the presence of palladium to

give the N-acetylated methyl glycoside of daunosamine, which
may be readily converted, if desired, into the free amino
sugar.   Physical data for this sugar, and for its 5-epimer
are in excellent accord with the literature (4).

   This general sequence thus leads from the methyl glycoside
of D-mannose, with few isolated steps, to 3-amino-2,3,6-
trideoxy-L-lyxo-hexose (daunosamine). The general synthesis
also provides access to several stereovariants of this sugar,
including the D-ribo compound already mentioned and, in
principle, also the D-arabino and L-xylo products (6).
Furthermore, analogs having additional functionality may be
obtained from the 6-bromide intermediate, as illustrated in
the transformations leading to the 3,6-diamino sugar having
the D-ribo stereochemistry (7), and the corresponding 6-

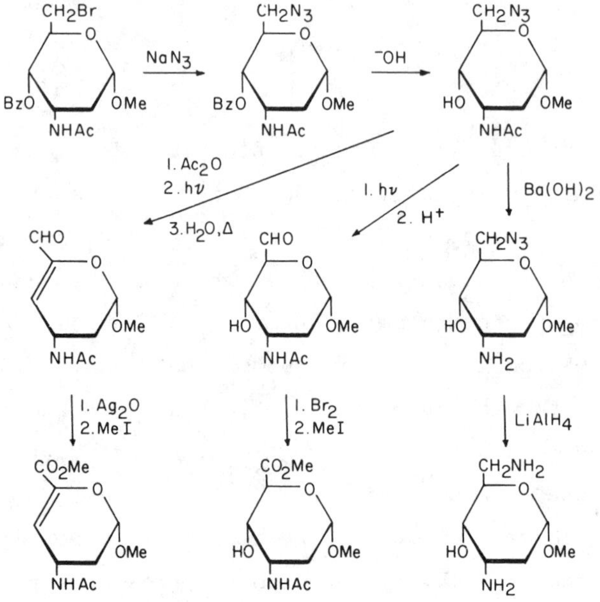

aldehyde obtained photochemically from the azide (8). This
aldehyde may be readily converted into the corresponding
carboxylic acid derivative to provide an amino sugar analog
that is simultaneously an amino acid. Generation of the
carboxyl functionality at C-6 may also be conducted in such a
way as to remove the substituent at C-4 and provide a 4,5-
unsaturated amino sugar uronic acid (8).

For access to the $\underline{L}$-$\underline{xylo}$ amino sugar, the silver fluoride-
mediated elimination from the bromide precursor was not found
satisfactory because of the intervention of an epimine that is
formed readily when the 3-substituent is on the same side of
the ring as the departing bromide group (6). However, a
suitable alternative synthesis of 3-amino-2,3,6-trideoxy-$\underline{L}$-
$\underline{xylo}$-hexose may be accomplished by way of the 3-ketone produced
in the second step of the daunosamine synthesis. Reduction of

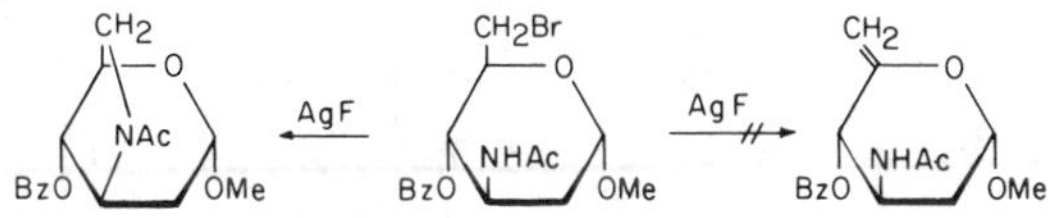

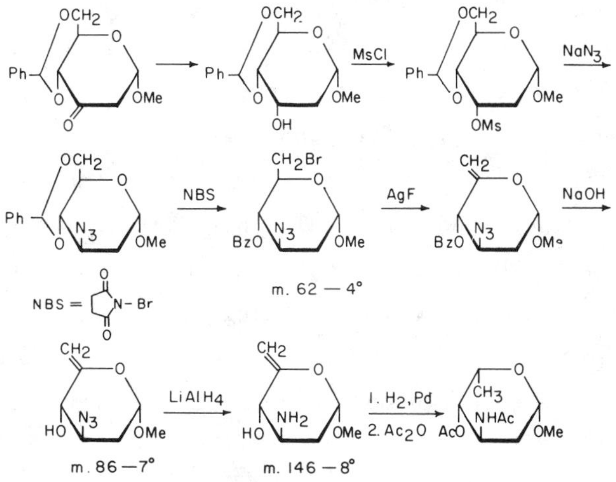

this ketone gives almost exclusively the alcohol having the
D-ribo stereochemistry, whose methanesulfonate undergoes
displacement by azide in high yield to give a product that may
then be carried through the sequence of reactions involving
deoxygenation at C-6 with inversion at C-5 to give the desired
L-xylo amino sugar in good net yield (6).

The same starting alcohol as used in the preceding
sequence also conveniently provided two of the sugar analogs
that are hydroxylated rather than aminated at C-3. These
products are the known deoxy sugars digitoxose and 2,6-dideoxy-
L-lyxo-hexose (which might be termed, albeit incorrectly,
2-deoxy-L-fucose) (9).

III. COUPLING OF THE MODIFIED SUGARS TO ANTHRACYCLINONES

The procedure for coupling the sugar analogs to daunomycinone and other anthracyclinones involved initial preparation of a suitably protected and glycosidically activated
derivative of the sugar. These coupling precursors are
typically N-trifluoroacetylated, and protected at the hydroxyl
groups by such substituents as acetate, trifluoroacetate, or p-
nitrobenzoate, and the anomeric position is activated for
coupling either by way of the glycosyl halide or as the glycal.
The outcome of such glycosidation reactions parallels general
experience in carbohydrate chemistry in that the reaction
course is variable and frequently unpredictable; specific
conditions and protecting groups need to be worked out with
each sugar. No standardized coupling procedure is uniformly
effective when the stereochemistry and substitution mode of
the sugar is varied. In most instances, however, the coupling
method used involved one of the modifications of the
standardized Koenigs—Knorr reaction, or the glycal procedure,

or coupling of the halide mediated by silver trifluoromethane-
sulfonate. In most instances, the reactions afforded not a
single anomer but an anomeric mixture of glycosides linked
through position 7 of the aglycon. Separation of these
glycosides proved frequently tedious, and sometimes impossible,
by available methodology. Recourse had frequently to be made
to repetition of the reaction with different protecting groups
to alter the anomeric ratio or permit a better separation of
the anomers. The final step of deprotection of the sugar
could usually be accomplished uneventfully, but, in a
significant number of instances, difficulties were encountered
in removing all of the protecting groups without simultaneously
causing cleavage of the sugar from the aglycon.

A. Coupling of Amino Sugar Analogs to Daunomycinone

The 3',5' diepimer of daunorubicin was prepared by
coupling a 3-amino-2,3,6-trideoxy-$\underline{D}$-arabino-hexose derivative
to daunomycinone (7). The glycosyl chloride, trifluoro-
acetylated at N-3 and O-4, underwent coupling with
daunomycinone to give an anomeric mixture favoring the α-$\underline{D}$
product; separation of the anomers was difficult. In an
alternative synthesis employing the corresponding glycosyl
halide protected at O-4 by $\underline{p}$-nitrobenzoyl, the α anomer
(NSC 299554) again preponderated, but separation was more
readily achieved, permitting the isolation of both anomers of
this daunorubicin analog; removal of the protecting group from
the sugar was accomplished without difficulty. The favored
formation of the α anomer is explicable on the basis that the
incoming group enters from the side of the ring opposite the
substituents at positions 3 and 5.

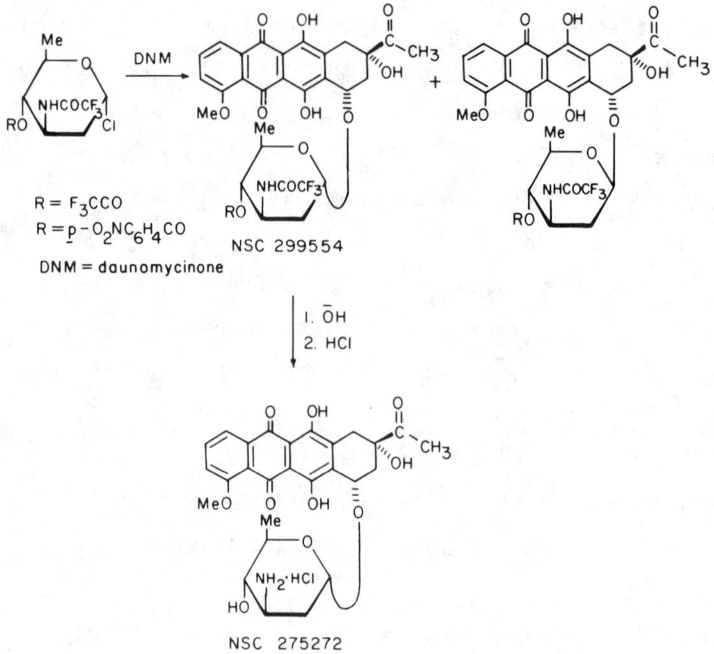

Me

O

DNM

RO   NHCOCF₃   Cl

R = F₃CCO
R = p-O₂NC₆H₄CO
DNM = daunomycinone

MeO

NHCOCF₃

RO

NSC 299554

+

MeO

NHCOCF₃

RO

1. ŌH
2. HCl

MeO

Me

O

NH₂·HCl

HO

NSC 275272

Attempted use of similar strategy for production of the 5'-
epimer of daunorubicin from the D-ribo amino sugar was not
successful as the glycosyl halide proved to be very labile.
The N-trifluoroacetylated, 4-0-p-nitrobenzoylated amino sugar,
as its 1-acetate, decomposed on attempts to convert it into
the corresponding halide, but the elements of acetic acid were
eliminated by heating this compound in the presence of silica
gel to furnish the corresponding glycal. This enol ether
readily underwent coupling to daunomycinone in benzene
solution, in the presence of a trace of p-toluenesulfonic
acid (10). Subsequent deprotection proceded uneventfully,
but the reaction gives stereospecifically the α anomer (NSC
309694) in which the incoming group is situated trans to the
C-5 substituent. The α anomer in the D series has the
opposite relative geometry from that in the parent antibiotics,
and this product was considered less desirable as a model
analog than the corresponding β anomer. However, a successful

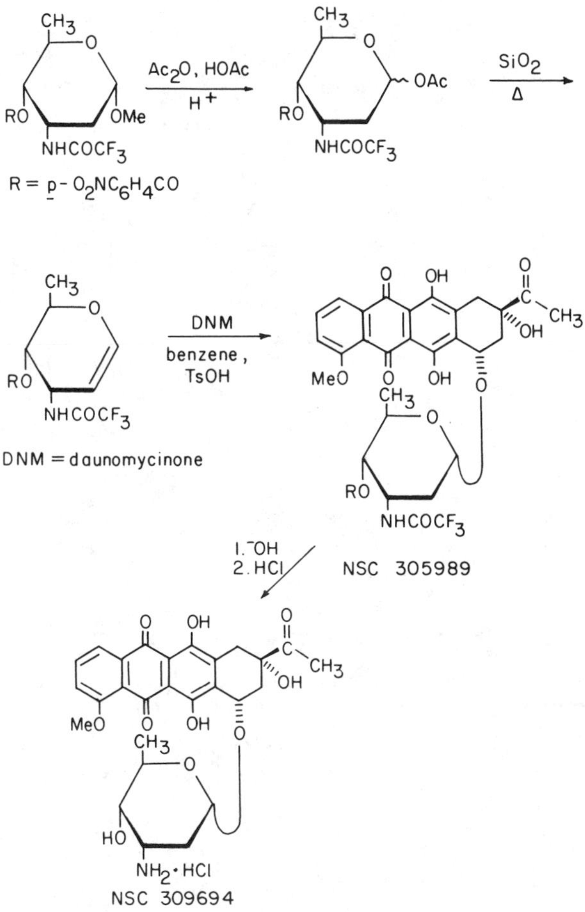

route affording the latter in good yield was not accomplished.

Similar control of anomeric specificity was encountered in attempts to couple 3,6-diamino-2,3,6-trideoxy-$\underline{D}$-$\underline{ribo}$-hexose to daunomycinone (7). The amino sugar, protected at nitrogen by trifluoroacetyl and at oxygen by acetate, did not give a stable glycosyl halide but did afford the corresponding glycal. Coupling of the latter to daunomycinone, followed by depro- tection, gave the 6-amino-5-epi analog of daunorubicin (NSC 302048), but of the α-$\underline{D}$ configuration. Changing the 4

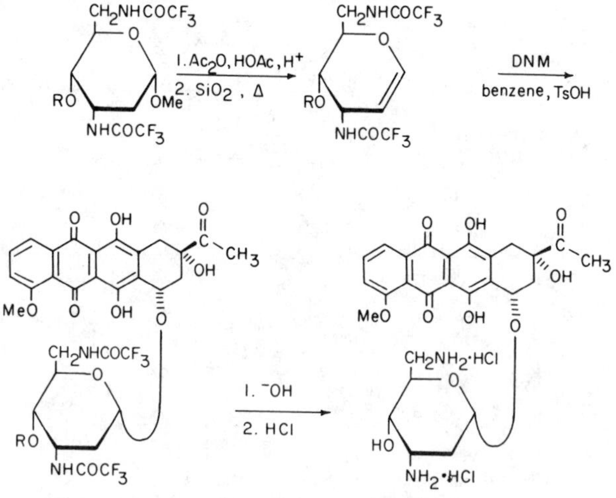

R = Ac ; NSC 293851
R = p - O₂NC₆H₄ ; NSC 302049
DNM = daunomycinone

NSC 302048

substituent to $\underline{O}$-(p-nitrobenzoyl) also led to the same net
result, and the coupling reaction again gave the α-$\underline{D}$ product
(NSC 302049).

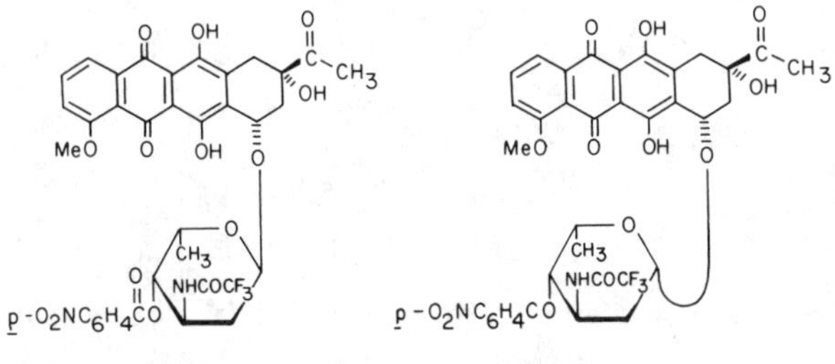

NSC 305992   NSC 305993

In the case of 3-amino-2,3,6-trideoxy-$\underline{L}$-xylo-hexose (11),
the appropriately protected glycal of the sugar reacted with
the aglycon stereoselectively rather than stereospecifically,
and led to the α-$\underline{L}$ anomer (NSC 305992) as the major product,
but the β-$\underline{L}$ anomer (NSC 305993) was also formed in lower

yield (12). The directing effect of the methyl group in promoting attachment of the aglycon to the opposite side of the ring is again evident, but in this instance the glycal route favored formation of the more desirable anomer, having identical stereochemistry to the parent daunorubicin except for epimerization at C-3.

B. Synthesis of 3-Oxy Analogs of Daunorubicin

The readily available deoxy sugar, 2-deoxy-$\underline{\underline{D}}$-$\underline{arabino}$-hexose, was coupled to daunomycinone by way of the $\underline{p}$-nitrobenzoylated glycosyl chloride and the Koenigs—Knorr

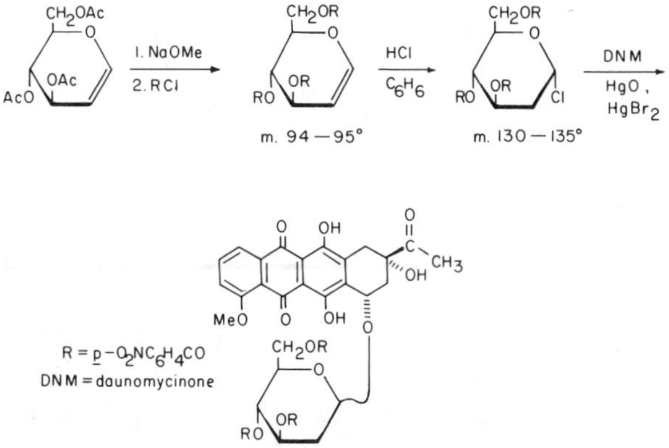

m. 94—95°   m. 130—135°

R = $\underline{p}$-O$_2$NC$_6$H$_4$CO
DNM = daunomycinone

α; NSC 305990 ; 27% , m. 240—244°
β; NSC 305991 ; 51% , m. 188 — 190°

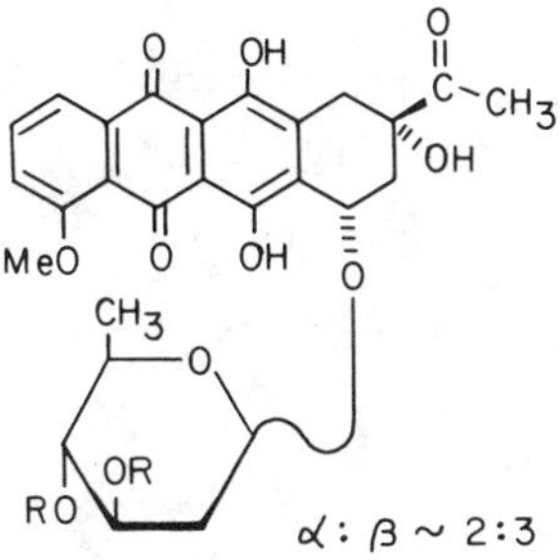

α : β ~ 2:3

R=H ; NSC 299555
R=Ac; NSC 333862

procedure to give a mixture of anomers in which the β-$\underline{\underline{D}}$ anomer (NSC 305991) preponderated (13). Repetition of this procedure with the corresponding 6-deoxy sugar of the same configuration likewise gave a mixture of anomers (NSC 299555; NSC 333862), in this instance, in approximately equal

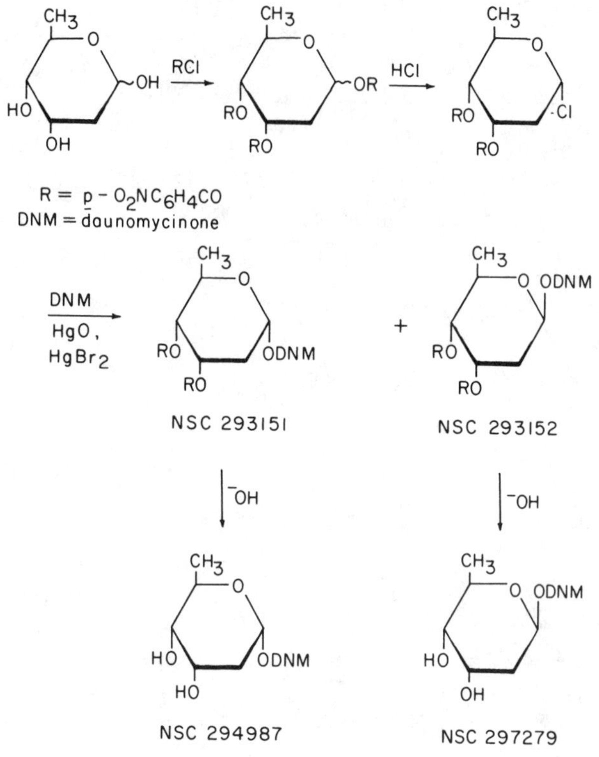

CH_3 $\xrightarrow{RCl}$ CH_3 $\xrightarrow{HCl}$ CH_3

HO ... OH → RO ... OR → RO ... Cl

R = $\underline{p}$ - $O_2NC_6H_4CO$
DNM = daunomycinone

$\xrightarrow[HgBr_2]{\substack{DNM \\ HgO,}}$

CH_3 RO ... ODNM   + CH_3 O ODNM   RO

NSC 293151   NSC 293152

$\downarrow$ $^-$OH $\downarrow$ $^-$OH

CH_3 HO ... ODNM HO CH_3 O ODNM HO OH

NSC 294987   NSC 297279

proportion. The starting point for the $\underline{\underline{D}}$-$\underline{ribo}$ 3-oxygenated analog was the deoxy sugar digitoxose previously mentioned, and it was coupled by way of its $\underline{p}$-nitrobenzoylated glycosyl chloride, again to give a 5:3 mixture of anomers (NSC 293151 and NSC 293152) of the coupled product; these were not readily resolved by chromatography (14).

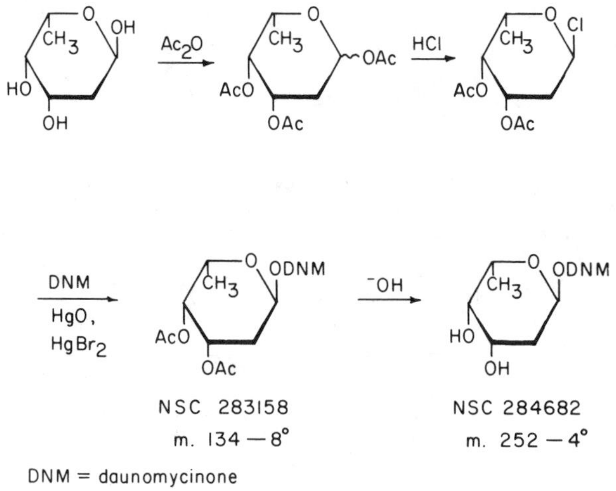

NSC 283158
m. 134 — 8°

NSC 284682
m. 252 — 4°

DNM = daunomycinone

Systematic mention of biological activity of these
compounds has not been made thus far, as data for practically
all of the glycon-modified analogs from this program are
discussed in detail elsewhere in this volume (15); specific
mention is made here when compounds displayed notably high
activity in the in vivo P-388 mouse assay. The next compound
to be described is, in fact, such an example; it is the 3'-
hydroxy analog of daunorubicin, which may also be termed
deaminodaunorubicin (14). The starting point for this
synthesis was 2,6-dideoxy-L-lyxo-hexose ("2-deoxy-L-fucose").
The triacetate of this compound is readily converted into the
corresponding glycosyl chloride, which may be coupled in high
yield and with complete stereospecificity to give a compound
(NSC 284682) identical with daunorubicin in all respects
except for the replacement of the amino group by hydroxyl. As
the rationale for the biological activity of daunorubicin has
frequently invoked a key role for the amino group, this
compound might be expected to have little activity. However,

in comparative tests with daunorubicin and adriamycin, the
3-hydroxyl analog, and also its 3',4'-diacetate (NSC 283158),
displayed very good activity in the P-388 assay, albeit at
dose levels considerably higher than those used with the
parent drugs. As these compounds are tolerated by the animals
at much higher dose-levels than the parent drugs, they have
much lower acute toxicity. The fact that the diacetate (NSC
283158) shows activity comparable to that of the free hydroxy
compound (NSC 284682) suggests that the diacetate may simply
act as a pro-drug for the deacetylated derivative, undergoing
hydrolysis of the acetate groups by nonspecific esterases in
the animal tissues. Indeed, such esters may be more effective
than the deprotected compounds. However, as the comparative
table of activities of these various daunorubicin analogs
indicates, no activity was observed in any of the products in
which such large acyl groups as p-nitrobenzoyl are present.

The α-D-arabino analog of daunorubicin (1,3,5-triepi-
daunorubicin, NSC 275272) displays marginal activity, but the
6-amino-5-epi analog is essentially inactive, as are the D
compounds in general, except for the D-arabino analogs (7).
It should be noted that the β-D-ribo analog might adopt a
conformation favorable for mimicking the parent structure.
Until this compound has been tested, it would be unwise to
make a firm conclusion that the D sugar analogs are invariably
inactive. However, general conclusions at this stage indicate
that stereochemical change at C-1' or at C-3' leads to
decrease of activity. Stereochemical inversion at position 4'
leads in many instances, as has been shown by the work from Dr.
Arcamone laboratory (16), to analogs having activity comparable
to the parent compound and displaying lower toxicity. It
appears that additional functional groups at C-6 may be undesirable, as illustrated by the 6-hydroxy and the 6-amino

Biological Activity of Daunomycinone Glycosides on P388 Lymphocytic Leukemia in Mice (intraperitoneal injections at day 5, 9, and 13) (R = daunomycinone)

NSC. No.	Structure	Dose Level	T/C (%)	NSC. No.	Structure	Dose Level	T/C (%)
275272	Me, NH₂, HO, OR, x HCl	12.5 100.5	123 125	283158	Me, OR, AcO, AcO	50.0 200.0 100.0	125 186 155
299554	Me, O, COCF₃, NH, R'O, OR, R' = COC₆H₄NO₂	25.0	104	284682	Me, OR, HO, HO	50.0 200.0 50.0 50.0*	150 192 183 146
						*B-16 Melanocarcinoma	
302648	Me, O OR, NH₂, HO, x HCl	50.0	110	293151	Me, O, R'O, OR, R'O, R' = COC₆H₄NO₂	12.5	110
293851	H₂CNHCOCF₃, O, AcO, OR, NHCOCF₃	12.5	108	293152	Me, OR, R'O, R'O, R' = COC₆H₄NO₂	25.0	106
302049	H₂CNHCOCF₃, O, R'O, OR, NHCOCF₃, R' = COC₆H₄NO₂	50.0	100	294987	Me, O, HO, OR, HO	25.0	101
302048	H₂CNH₂, O, R'O, OR, NH₂ x 2HCl	50.0 12.5 6.25	103 103 103	297279	Me, O OR, HO, HO	50	102
				299555	Me, O, OH, OR, HO	50.0 31.3	100 100

analogs, which have low activity, but replacement of the 3-amino group by an oxygenated substituent, either hydroxyl or acetoxyl, leads to compounds which retain high activity, when administered at larger dose-levels.

IV. ANALOGS MODIFIED AT THE 14 POSITION

The well-documented higher activity of adriamycin in
comparison with daunorubicin prompted synthesis of the analog
of adriamycin in which the 3'-amino group is replaced by an
oxy substituent, displayed here as the 3',4'-diacetate (17).
Following the rationale of the transformation of daunorubicin
by way of its 14-bromide into adriamycin, it was considered
that a similar sequence might be used with the corresponding
3'-oxy analog of daunorubicin. However, all attempts to
brominate this compound at C-14 invariably resulted in loss
of the glycon, and it appears that the amino group in the
parent natural antibiotic must play an important role in
permitting this reaction to take place without loss of the
sugar. An alternative approach considered utilized a
protected derivative of adriamycinone bearing a methoxytrityl

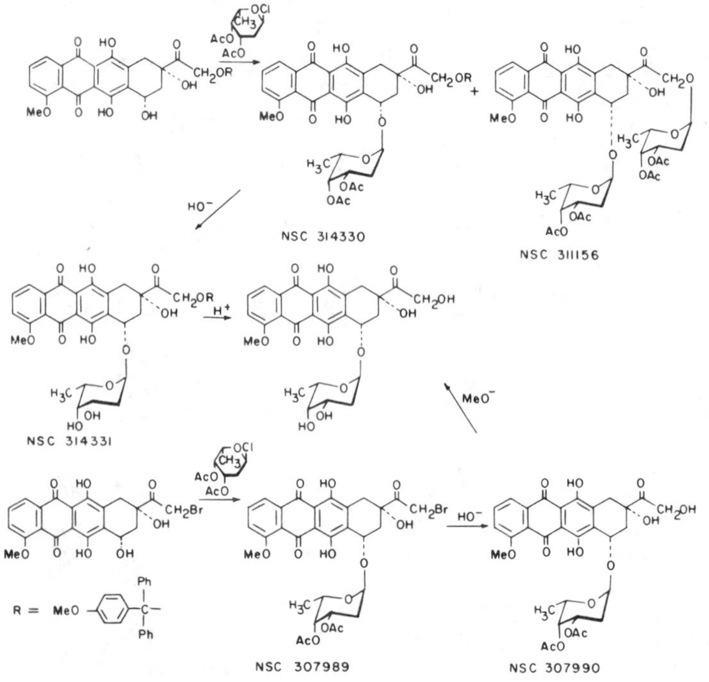

group at 0-14. This compound underwent condensation with the acylated glycosyl chloride obtained from 2,6-dideoxy-$\underline{L}$-$\underline{lyxo}$-hexose to give the desired coupled product (NSC 314330), together with a small proportion of a bis(glycosylated) product (NSC 311156) evidently resulting from loss of the protecting group and subsequent glycosylation at 0-14. The 3',14-bis(glycosylated) derivative was not active. The protecting groups could be removed from the monoglycosylated product to give the desired 3'-hydroxy adriamycin analog, but the overall yields were extremely poor as much difficulty was encountered in the deprotection step. The protected compound is much more labile toward loss of the glycon than any of the other compounds encountered in this study.

An excellent, high-yielding synthesis of the desired product, as its 3',4'-diacetate (NSC 307990), was, however, accomplished by initial bromination of daunomycinone, obtained from daunorubicin by hydrolysis, followed by the glycosylation step to give the corresponding coupled 14-bromide (NSC 307989), which may be converted readily, through replacement of the bromine atom by hydroxyl, into the 3',4'-diacetate of 3'-hydroxyadriamycin (NSC 307990). This compound shows excellent activity throughout most of the series of detailed in vivo tests (17) conducted by the National Cancer Institute, as illustrated in the table. In the P-388 screen, a T/C index of 269 was exhibited at a dose level of 50 mg/kg and corresponding high activity was observed in the other tests. In comparison with the corresponding daunorubicin analog, the adriamycin analog was clearly superior throughout all of the tests (17). This compound is one of the most promising agents resulting from the study reported here.

ANTITUMOR EVALUATIONS^a, IN MICE, OF 7-O-(3,4-Di-0-acetyl-2,6-dideoxy-α-$\underline{L}$-lyxo-hexopyranosyl)adriamycinone (NSC 307 990)

Tumor	T/C (%)	Dose (mg/kg)	Mouse strain	Route^b	Schedule^c	Parameter^d
P388 lymphocytic leukemia	269	50.00	CD_2F_1	I.p.	5,9,13	M.s.t.
L-1210 lymphoid leukemia	203	12.50	CD_2F_1	I.p.	1-9	M.s.t.
B-16 melano-carcinoma	195	25.00	$B_6C_3F_1$	I.p.	1	M.s.t.
Colon 26	150	300.00	CD_2F_1	I.p.	1,8(so)	M.s.t.
LX-1 lung xenograft	53	25.00	Nu/Nu-BALB/C (nude mouse)	I.r.i.	1-10	Delta
$CD8F_1$ mammary tumor	6	12.50	$CD8F_1$	S.c.	1,8,15, 22,29	M.t.w.
CX-1 colon xenograft	35	25.00	Nu/Nu Swiss (nude mouse)	I.r.i	1-10	Delta
Colon 38	124	250.00	$B_6D_6F_1$	S.c.	1,8,15	M.t.w.
Lewis lung carcinoma	338	12.00	$B_6D_2F_1$	I.v.	1-9	M.s.t.
MX-1 breast xenograft	82	6.25	Nu/Nu Swiss (nude mouse)	I.r.i.	1-10	Delta

^{a}*Data obtained under the auspices of the National Cancer Institute, Division of Cancer Treatment, Drug Research and Development Branch.* ^{b}*I.p., intraperitoneal; i.r.i., intrarenal inoculation or subrenal capsule; s.c. subcutaneous; i.v. intravenous.* ^{c}*P, q, r.: injections on day p, q, and r; 1-n: injections on each day of days 1-n; 1:1 injection; 1,8(so): injections on days 1 and 8 (solution);* ^{d}*M.s.t., median survival time; Delta, change in average tumor diameter between day 0 and day of final evaluation; M.t.w., median tumor weight estimated from tumor diameter.*

The availability of 14-bromodaunomycinone having the 2,6-dideoxy-$\underline{L}$-$\underline{lyxo}$-hexopyranosyl substituent attached at position 7 (NSC 307989) provided an attractive starting point for synthesis of a range of different 3'-oxyadriamycin analogs produced by appropriate nucleophilic replacement of the bromine atom at C-14. These compounds included the 14-azido, the 14-thiocyanato, and the 14-acetylthio compound in one comparative series (18). Reaction with various carboxylate salts likewise afforded the corresponding acetate, propanoate, and a series of higher fatty acyl-substituted homologs at the 14-position (19). The third tabulation shows the biological test-data for the different 14-substituents in the series hydrogen, bromide, azide, thiocyanate, thioacetate, hydroxyl,

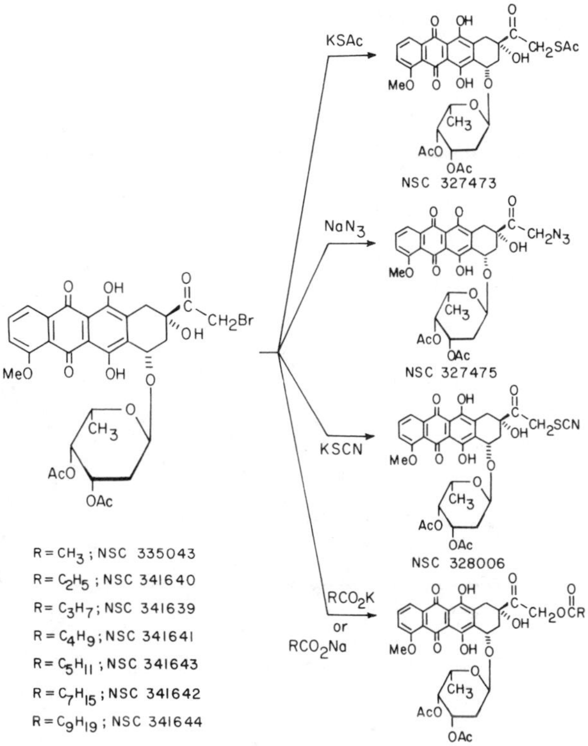

R = CH$_3$; NSC 335043
R = C$_2$H$_5$; NSC 341640
R = C$_3$H$_7$; NSC 341639
R = C$_4$H$_9$; NSC 341641
R = C$_5$H$_{11}$; NSC 341643
R = C$_7$H$_{15}$; NSC 341642
R = C$_9$H$_{19}$; NSC 341644

KSAc → NSC 327473

NaN$_3$ → NSC 327475

KSCN → NSC 328006

RCO$_2$K or RCO$_2$Na

IN VIVO ANTITUMOR ACTIVITIES
(Mouse P-388) of GLYCON AND
C-14 MODIFIED ADRIAMYCIN ANALOGS

R	NSC No.	T/C^a	$Dose^b$
H [c]	284682	192	200
Br	307989	109	50
N_3	327475	124	125
SCN	328006	123	200
SAc	327473	100	125
OH	307990	269	50
OAc	335043	261	50
OCOEt	341640	160	50
OCOPr	341639	221	50
OCOBu	341641	198	50
$OCOC_5H_{11}$	341643	183	50
$OCOC_7H_{15}$	341642	202	100
$OCOC_9H_{19}$	341644	174	100
Adriamycin	123127	174	16

[a] *Ratio of median survival time expressed as percent of untreated controls.*

[b] *CDF_1 mice were injected i.p. with 10^6 P-388 lymphocytic leukemia cells on day 0 and treated i.p. on day 5, 9, and 13 with the drug dose specified. Toxic deaths were not observed in any of the tests.*

[c] *3',4'-0-deacetylated analog.*

and 14-esters. The data show a high T/C index for the
daunorubicin analog at a dose level of 200 mg/kg, but clearly
superior behavior, with a T/C index of 269 at the lower dose
level of 50 mg/kg for the corresponding 14-hydroxyl
(adriamycin, NSC 307990) analog. It is remarkable that the 14-
bromide appears to be completely inactive, and the azide and
thiocyanate show only marginal activity, as does the
thioacetate. In contrast, the 14-acetate shows excellent
activity (18), comparable to that of the corresponding 14-
hydroxyl compound, and this compound may, in fact, serve as a
pro-drug for the fully deacetylated compound acting in vivo.
The other 14-(fatty acyl) derivatives also all show activity,
although a slight decreasing trend appears evident as chain
length increases.

The use of an allylic rearrangement reaction with glycals
as described by Priebe and Zamojski (20) provided convenient
access to daunorubicin analogs having alkylthio-group
replacement at the 3'-position. Thus, starting from di-0-
acetyl-D-fucal, there was obtained the 3'-(methylthio)-3'-epi
analog of daunorubicin (21,22) and a similar sequence from di-
0-acetyl-L-rhamnal afforded the 3'-(methylthio)-4'-epi analog
of daunorubicin (21,22). As already noted (15), these two
compounds do show activity, in particular the latter product,
but not to a level as high as that displayed by the 3'-hydroxy
or 3'-acetoxy analogs. It will be of interest to determine
whether a free thiol group at the 3' position would lead to a
compound of high activity.

The last major area of interest concerns compounds in
which a substituent is introduced at C-2 of the glycon (19,22).
Following the rationale already established up to this point,
the alkoxyiodination reaction of Thiem (23), applied to the
acetylated glycals of L-fucose and L-rhamnose, appeared

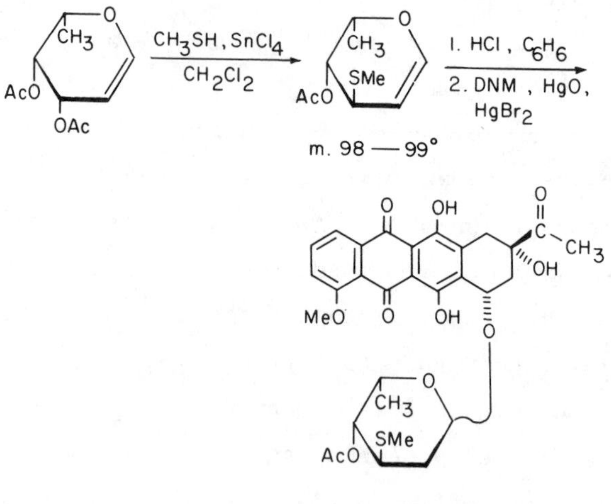

m. 98 — 99°

NSC 314333

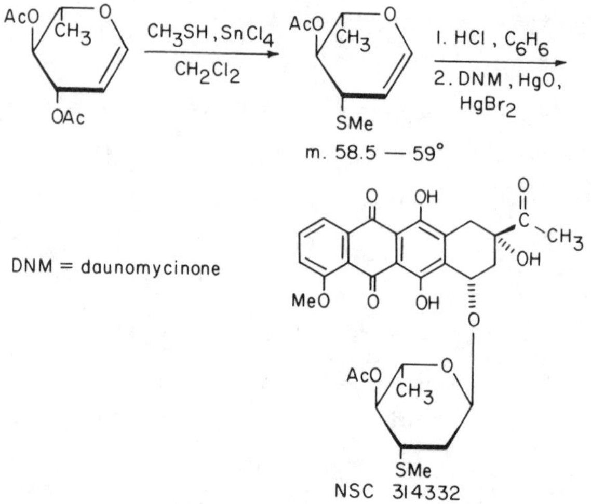

DNM = daunomycinone

m. 58.5 — 59°

NSC 314332

attractive. Indeed, application of this reaction with daunomycinone afforded in good yield the indicated 2'-iodo derivatives (NSC 327472 and NSC 331962) (19) that are structurally identical with the diacetates of 3'-hydroxy daunorubicin and its 4'-epimer, respectively, except for the introduction of an iodine atom in the illustrated stereochemical configuration at C-2'. As already noted

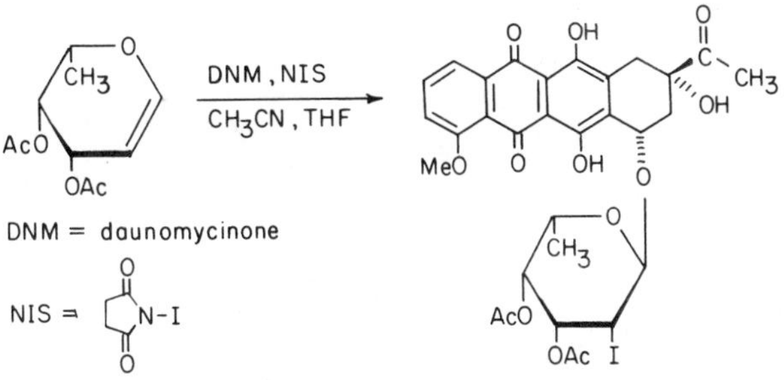

DNM = daunomycinone

NIS =

NSC 327472
m. 131°

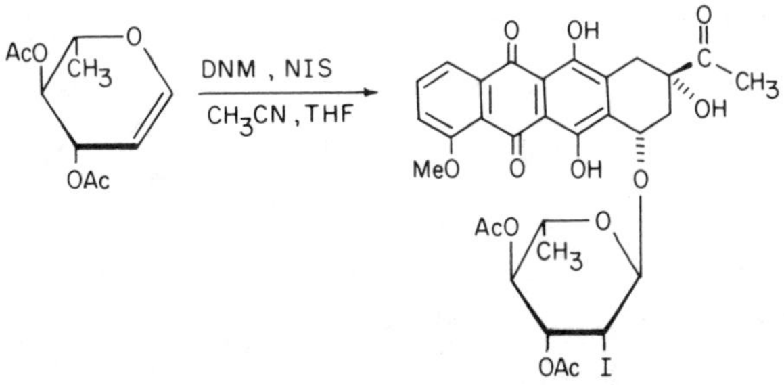

NSC 331962
m. 142 −144°

elsewhere (15), the former compound (NSC 327472) shows good
activity, with a T/C index of 172 at 12.5 mg/kg, and the
compound derived from L-rhamnal (NSC 331962) shows still
higher activity, with T/C 247 at a similar dose-level. This
result is impressive, and also unexpected in the light of
prior assumptions that would suggest that substitution at
C-2' should lead to inactivation. These compounds, especially
NSC 331962, are of considerable interest as potential
antineoplastic agents. It is well known that 2-haloglycosides
are hydrolyzed much more slowly than the 2-deoxy analogs, and
this stabilization may be therapeutically advantageous,
minimizing metabolic inactivation and possibly permitting oral

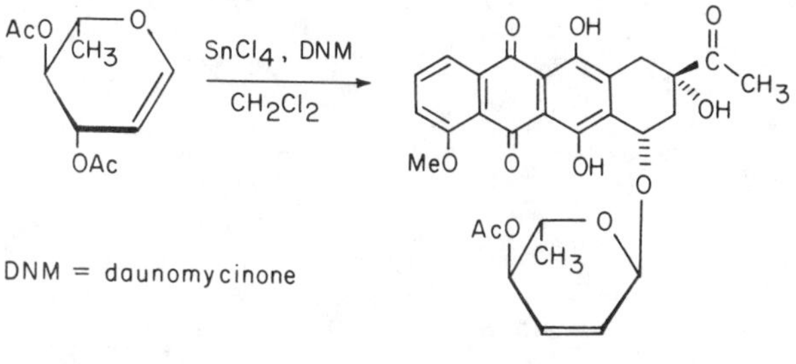

NSC 335645
m. 142 — 4°

DNM = daunomycinone

use. Furthermore, reduction of the iodo derivatives with incorporation of deuterium or tritium offers a potential route to isotopically labeled analogs for metabolic studies.

A final compound in this series that may be mentioned is the unsaturated analog (NSC 335645), prepared by way of an allylic displacement-reaction (24), followed by coupling to daunomycinone (19); its detailed testing is still in progress.

V. SUMMARY CONCLUSIONS

This study set out to evaluate the effect on antitumor activity of structural modifications in daunorubicin and adriamycin analogs modified in the glycon and at C-14. In particular, the work challenged existing hypotheses that the presence of 3'-amino group and the absence of substituents at the 2'-position are essential for activity. The project has provided a versatile synthetic route to substitutional and stereochemical modifications of daunosamine, and has explored coupling methodology and the question of anomer distribution and separation as a function of stereochemical and substitutional variation in the sugar. Of the analogs synthesized, approximately 50 have been evaluated in vivo in the murine P-388 screen. In general, high activity was observed in compounds having the α-<u>L</u>-<u>lyxo</u> or the α-<u>L</u>-<u>xylo</u> stereochemistry in the glycon. The hypothesis that the 3'-amino group is essential is found untenable, as the 3'-hydroxy and 3'-acetoxy analogs of daunorubicin and adriamycin show good activity. Furthermore, examples incorporating an axial 2'-iodo group also show high activity, indicating that an unsubstituted 2'-position is not essential for activity. The activity of the 3'-oxy daunorubicin analogs is increased by introduction of a hydroxyl group at C-14 to generate the corresponding adriamycin analogs. Acylation at this position does not lead to inactivation, but most other substituents introduced at this position lead to diminution or total loss of activity.

REFERENCES

1. Arcamone, F., Cassinelli, G., Orezzi, P., Franceschi, G., and Mondelli, R., J. Am. Chem. Soc. 86, 5335 (1964).

2. Acton, E. M., Fujiwara, A. N., and Henry, D. W., J. Med. Chem. 17, 659 (1974).

3. Wovkulich, P. M., Uskoković, M. R., J. Am. Chem. Soc. 103, 3956 (1981), and references cited therein.

4. Horton, D., and Weckerle, W., Carbohydr. Res. 44, 227 (1975); U. S. Pat. 4,024,333, May 17, 1977.

5. Hanessian, S., Carbohydr. Res. 2, 86 (1966).

6. Cheung, T. M., Horton, D., Sorenson, R. J., and Weckerle, W., Carbohydr. Res. 63, 77 (1978).

7. Fuchs, E. F., Horton, D., Weckerle, W., and Winter, B., J. Antibiot. 32, 223 (1979).

8. Horton, D., Weckerle, W., and Winter, B., Carbohydr. Res. 70, 59 (1979).

9. Cheung, T. M., Horton, D., and Weckerle, *Carbohydr. Res.*, *58*, 139 (1977); *Methods Carbohydr. Chem.* *8*, 195, 201 (1980).

10. Horton, D., Nickol, R. G., Weckerle, W., and Winter-Mihaly, E., *Carbohydr. Res. 76*, 269 (1979).

11. Cheung, T. M., Horton, D., and Weckerle, W., *Carbohydr. Res. 74*, 93 (1979).

12. Cheung, T. M., Horton, D., and Turner, W. R., *unpublished results*.

13. Horton, D., Priebe, W., and Turner, W. R., *unpublished results*.

14. Fuchs, E. F., Horton, D., Weckerle, W., and Winter-Mihaly, E., *J. Med. Chem. 22*, 406 (1979); Horton, D., Weckerle, W., Fuchs, E. F., Cheung, T. M., Winter, B., and Sorenson, R. J., *U. S. Pat. 4,201,773*, May 6, 1980.

15. Naff, M. B., Chapter 1, in "Anthracycline Antibiotics", *ACS Symp. Series*.

16. Arcamone, F., Penco, S., Vigevani, A., Redaelli, S., Franchi, G., Di Marco, A., Cassazza, A. M., Dasdia, T., Formelli, F., Necco, A., and Soranzo, C., *J. Med. Chem. 18*, 703 (1975).

17. Horton, D., Priebe, W., and Turner, W. R., *Carbohydr. Res. 94*, 11 (1981).

18. Horton, D., Priebe, W., *J. Antibiot. 34*, 1019 (1981).

19. Horton, D., and Priebe, W., *Abstr. Pap. Am. Chem. Soc. Meet.* 182, CARB-11 (1981).

20. Priebe, W., and Zamojski, A., *Tetrahedron 36*, 287 (1980).

21. Horton, D., *Jpn. J. Antibiot. 32 Suppl.* S 145 (1979).

22. Horton, D., and Priebe, W., *Abstr. Pap. Sec. Chem. Congr. North American Continent* CARB-22 (1980).

23. Thiem, J., Karl, H., and Schwentner, J., *Synthesis 9*, 696 (1978).

24. Grynkiewicz, G., Priebe, W., and Zamojski, A., *Carbohydr. Res. 68*, 33, (1979).

SYNTHESIS OF SUGAR MODIFIED DAUNORUBICIN ANALOGS ; APPROACHES TO ACLACINOMYCIN ANALOGS

C. Monneret, J. Boivin, A. Martin and M. Païs

Institut de Chimie des Substances Naturelles,
91190 Gif-sur-Yvette, France

The amino sugar moiety of daunorubicin (1,2), adriamycin (3) and carminomycin (4), namely daunosamine (3-amino-2,3,6-trideoxy-L-lyxo-hexose) and its D-enantiomer have been the subject of numerous syntheses, either by transformation of abundant and natural sugars (5-11), or by means of total synthesis (12-19).

On the other hand, in order to obtain structure-activity relationships or to decrease the toxicity of natural compounds, different other sugars of very similar structure were also synthesized in view of linking to the aglycon.

The results which were obtained in our laboratory during the past five years when we began to be interested in the synthesis of daunorubicin analogs by modification of the sugar moiety can be subdivided in three parts :

- A first part with classical syntheses of 3-amino-2,3,6-trideoxy-L or D-hexopyranoses which have been subjected to coupling to daunomycinone under a new method available for 2,6-dideoxy-hexoses.

- A second part in which glycals will be presented as useful intermediates to yield, following a convenient and short route, some analogs of daunorubicin such as 4'-epi or 3',4'-diepi-daunorubicin.

ANTHRACYCLINE ANTIBIOTICS

225

1 DAUNOSAMINE *L lyxo* 2 ACOSAMINE *L Arabino* 3 RISTOSAMINE *L Ribo* 4 3-EPI-DAUNO *L Xylo*

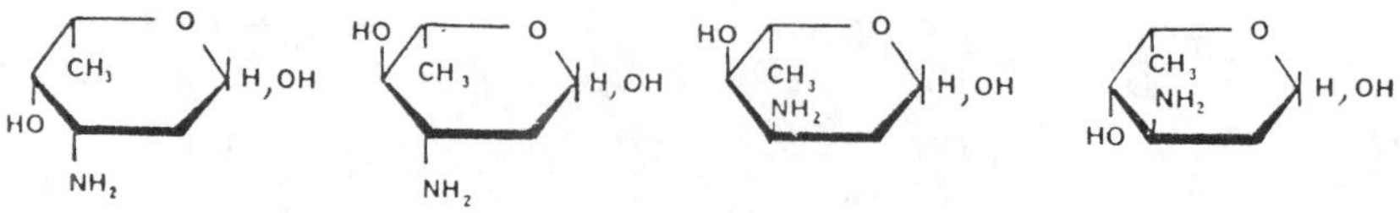

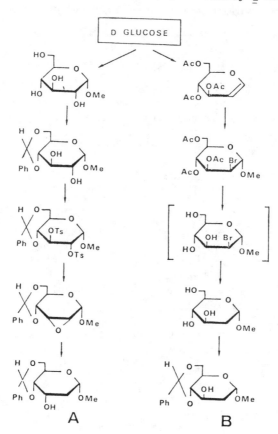

Figure 1 3-amino-2,3,6-trideoxy-*L*-hexoses

Figure 2 Synthesis of the Synthons A and B

- At last, in a third part will be discussed
the synthesis of disaccharides naturally occurring
in anthracycline antibiotics and their glycosidation
with daunomycinone.

Thus at first the aim of this work was to synthesize isomeric analogs of daunosamine. Among the
three isomers of daunosamine 1 of L-configuration
(Figure 1) two of them were already known, acosamine
(20), 2, a component of actinoidin antibiotic, and
ristosamine (21) 3, a component of the ristomycin A
antibiotic. For its part, the amino-sugar of L-xylo
configuration (3-epi-daunosamine), 4, was unknown in
nature and had not yet been synthesized in either
enantiomeric form.

We decided to start a general program aimed at
the synthesis of this sugar as well as the synthesis
of the corresponding D-enantiomers of daunosamine,
acosamine and ristosamine.

To this end, two useful intermediates were
prepared from the very inexpansive D-glucose, the
methyl 4,6-O-benzylidene-2-deoxy-α-D-ribo-hexopyra-
noside A and its 3-epimer of D-arabino-configuration,
B (figure 2).

The synthon A was obtained from methyl α-D-
glucopyranoside in four steps following a classical
sequence of reactions (22,23) benzylidenation, di-
tosylation, epoxidation and then reduction with lithium aluminium hydride (24) with an overall yield
of 40-45 % from methyl α-D-glucopyranoside.

For its part the synthon B was prepared via
the synthesis of per-O-acetyl-D-glucal and functiona-
lisation of the double bond with methanol in presence of N-bromosuccinimide (25). Hydrogenolysis of the
crude product in presence of sodium methanolate
afforded in a one-pot reaction, without isolation of
the bromo derivative, the methyl glycoside of 2-deo-
xy-D-glucose which was then treated with α,α-dime-
thoxytoluene in presence of p-toluenesulfonic acid
according to the procedure of Evans (26). Thus the
intermediate B was easily prepared with 60 % overall
yield from per-O-acetyl-D-glucal in three steps
without any chromatography since pure α anomer was
separated in the final step by crystallization (27).

Using the same sequence of reactions and starting from A or B we have been able to easily synthesize different diastereoisomers of L- and D-daunosamine.

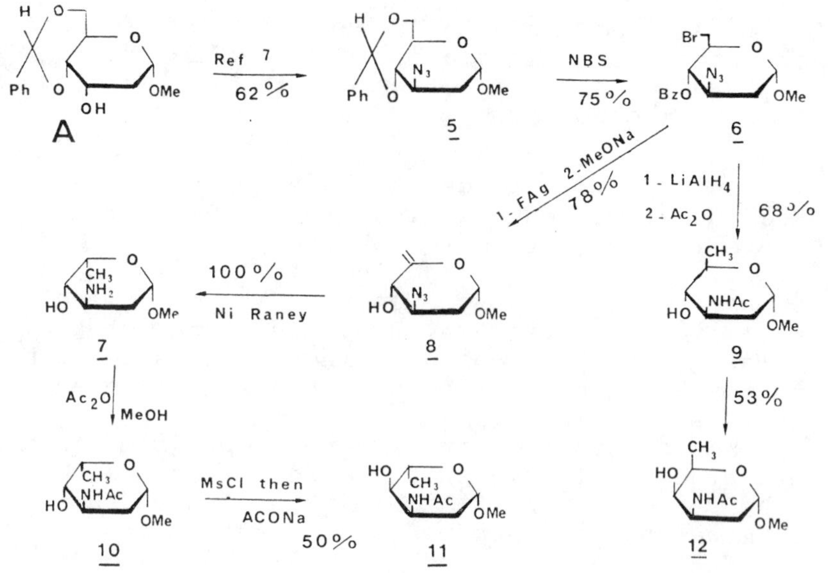

Figure 3   *Synthesis of methyl 3-amino-2,3,6-trideoxy-L-xylo,*
           L-ribo and D-arabino, D-lyxo-hexopyranosides, 7,11,9,12

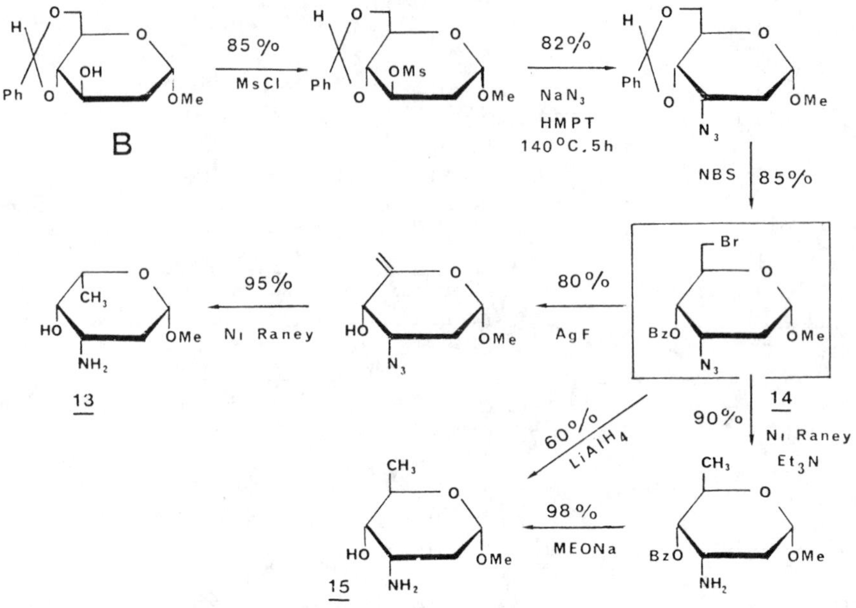

Figure 4   *Synthesis of methyl 3-amino 2,3,6-trideoxy-L-lyxo and*
           D-ribo-hexopyranosides, 13 and 16

At first the Synthon A was transformed into 5 (figure 3) according to Richardson (7). After ring opening of the benzylidene acetal with N-bromo-succinimide (NBS) (28), reduction of the product 6, with lithium aluminium hydride followed by N-acety-lation afforded the methyl glycoside of the N-acetyl 4-epi-D daunosamine (D-acosamine) 9. Inversion of configuration at C-4 according to Richardson (7) led to the D-daunosamine derivative, 12. Access to the L-series was achieved via the well known, now, eli-mination-inversion sequence at C-5 (6,29). After several unsuccessful attempts to reduce the enose 8, we found that a good result was obtained with Raney nickel in ethanol. This afforded stereospecifically (98 %) the methyl glycoside of 3-epi-L-daunosamine, our first target, 7. After N-acetylation, and inver-sion of configuration at C-4, the N-acetyl deriva-tive of methyl L-ristosaminide 11 was isolated (overall yield 50 %).

The same kinds of reactions applied to the synthon B provided the 3-amino sugar of D-ribo configuration (D-ristosamine), 15 (figure 4) and then, after inversion of configuration at C-5, the methyl glycoside of L-daunosamine, 13 (30). Azido sugar 14 was also used as intermediate in the syn-thesis of a disaccharide (vide infra).

In order to also synthesize (31) the corres-ponding deamino 2,6-dideoxy-hexoses, the synthon A was acetylated and treated with N-bromosuccinimide. Direct reduction of the 6-bromo compound with LiAlH$_4$

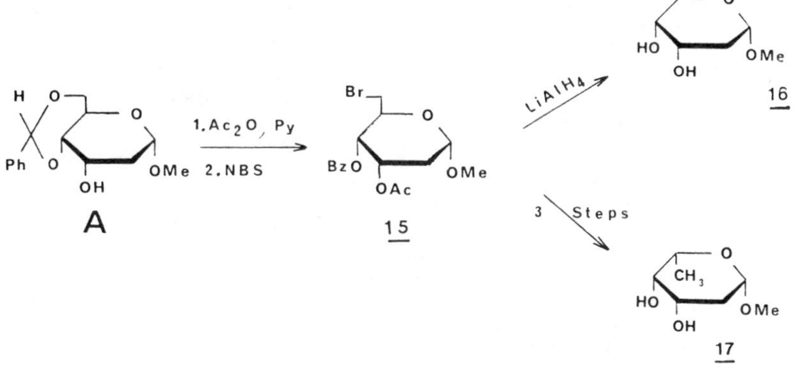

Figure 5   Synthesis of methyl D-digitoxoside and 2-deoxy-L-fucoside, 16 and 17

gave the methyl glycoside of digitoxose, 16 (figure 5) while removal of bromine followed by catalytic hydrogenation afforded stereospecifically the methyl glycoside of 2-deoxy-L-fucose, 17, a sugar present as a natural component in many oligosaccharide - containing anthracyclines. Very closely related syntheses of 16 and 17 were simultaneously reported by Horton's group (32).

   The problem at this stage of our work was to realize the glycosidation of the amino sugars of L-xylo, 7, D-arabino, 9 and D-lyxo 12, configurations, since, to our knowledge, such anthracycline anti-biotics had not yet been prepared. We first lent our attention to the glycosidation of the 3-amino sugar of L-xylo configuration, 7.

   After protection of the amino group as a tri-fluoroacetamide and of the hydroxyl group as a p-nitrobenzoate, the glycosidic bond was hydrolysed and, in order to use the Koenigs-Knorr conditions, different attempts were made to prepare the halogeno sugar derivative from 18 (figure 6) via the 1-O-p-nitrobenzoyl or trifluoroacetyl or acetyl hexose. The two former derivatives could not been isolated, their great reactivity leading to decomposition products while the latter, the 1-O-acetyl hexose 19 could be characterized but invariably led to the reducing sugar 18 when treated with anhydrous hydrogen chloride in dry dichloromethane or ether.

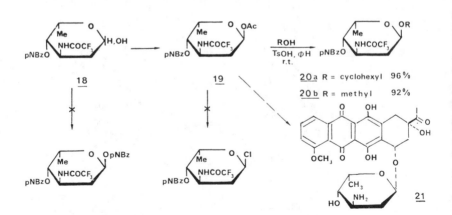

Figure 6   Glycosidations of 1-O-acetyl-2,3,6-trideoxy-L-xylo-hexopyranose

Following these observations we found that the acetyl was a suitable leaving group in the case of 2,6-dideoxy hexoses and preparation of the corresponding glycosides in the presence of one mole of alcohol and of a protic acid whose conjugate base was not too nucleophilic, was investigated (33).

Thus the 1-O-acetyl derivative of the aminosugar of L-xylo configuration, 19, reacted in benzene with cyclohexanol or methanol and p-toluenesulfonic acid as catalyst, at room temperature to give the corresponding glycosides, 20a or 20b in high yield. Furthermore the α L-anomers were stereospecifically formed. Coupling 19 with daunomycinone led also stereospecifically to an α-anomer, 21 after deprotection (∿ 50 % yield) (Figure 6).

That this method can also been used for the glycosidation of deamino 2,6-dideoxy-sugars is demonstrated by the glycosidations of digitoxose, 22, 2-deoxy-L-fucose, 23 and 2-deoxy-L-rhamnose 24 with methanol and cyclohexanol (Figure 7). Isolation of mixtures of α and β anomers was not surprising since in other experiments we have shown that the reaction proceeds via an enoxonium ion (30).

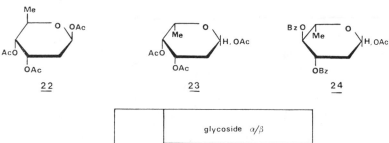

sugar	glycoside α/β	
	cyclohexanol	methanol
22	30/70	45/55
23	80/20	40/60
24	40/60	40/60

yields 60-80%

Figure 7   Glycosidations of 1-O-acetyl digitoxose, 2-deoxy-L-fucose and 2-deoxy-L-rhamnose

However, better yields were obtained in glycosidation of suitably protected (N-trifluoroacetamido
and O-p-nitrobenzoyl) D-daunosamine, 25,D-acosamine,
26 and D-ristosamine, 27, derivatives,with alcohols
of low molecular weight. Higher stereoselectivity
toward the formation of α anomer was also observed
(Figure 8).

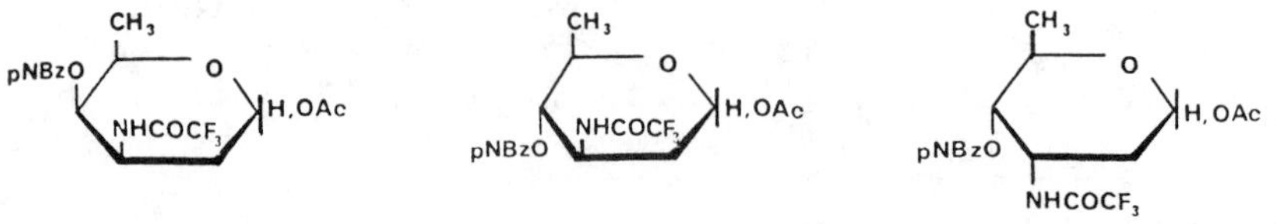

D Daunosamine   D Acosamine   D Ristosamine

25   26   27

	sugar	glycoside α/β	
		cyclohexanol	methanol
yields 80-95%	25	70/30	60/40
	26	70/30	52/48
	27	90/10	66/33

*Figure 8   Glycosidations of 1-O-acetyl derivatives of D-daunosa-
mine, D-acosamine and D-ristosamine*

Finally, after successful glycosidation of the
amino sugar of L-xylo configuration, 19 with daunomycinone, the method was extended to L-daunosamine
and also, as already published (34), to D-acosamine
and D-daunosamine, respectively 26 and 25.
These 1-O-acetyl-hexoses were reacted with
daunomycinone in the presence of p-toluenesulfonic
acid as catalyst and afforded the glycosides 28, 29
and 30 in 50 to 83 % yield (Figure 9). As expected,
both α and β anomers were formed in all cases but
comparison of the ratio of these anomers between L
and D daunosamine 28 and 30 shows a substantial difference. This suggests an important asymmetric induc-
tion exerted by the bulky aglycon.
Before leaving this chapter we would like to
report some of the results we have obtained in the
synthesis of 4-amino-2,4,6-trideoxy-hexoses and

their glycosidation with daunomycinone.

28

α/β = 90/10

29

α/β = 58/42

30

α/β = 55/45

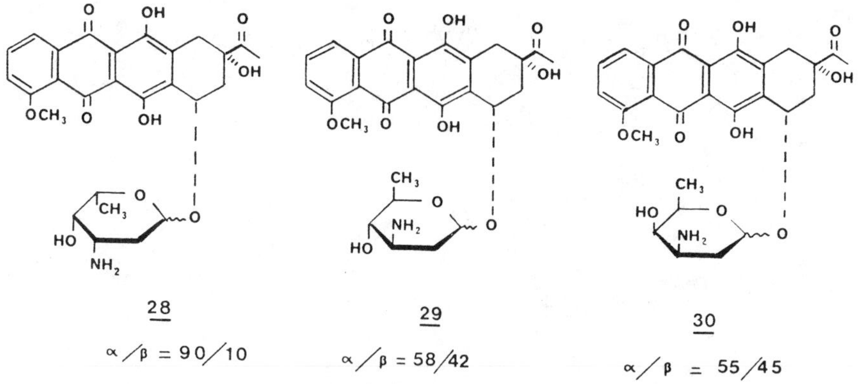

Figure 9 *Synthesis of daunorubicine 28, 4'-epi-D-daunorubicine*
29 and D-daunorubicine 30

The isomeric compound of L-lyxo and L-xylo
configuration 33 and 34 have been prepared from
methyl 2-deoxy-rhamnoside 31a, the former according
to a route recently reported in the literature (35)
with regiocific benzoylation of the starting material, giving the intermediate 31c, the latter via
the methyl 3,4-anhydro-2,6-dideoxy-α-L-ribo-hexopy-
ranoside 32. The same anhydrosugar 32 has been previously used in our laboratory in order to prepare
the 4-epi-holantosamine 35 (29). These three amino-
sugars were suitably protected and transformed into
1-O-acetyl-hexoses as represented in figure 10. Glycosidation with daunomycinone in presence of p-toluenesulfonic acid led to new anthracycline glycosides. The biological activity of these new compounds
is now under investigation.

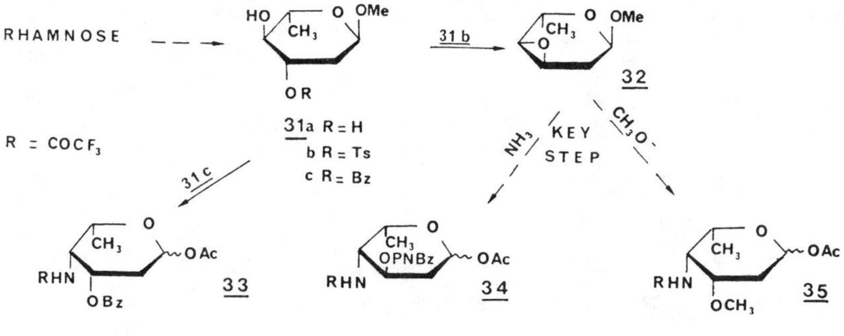

Figure 10 *Synthesis of 4-amino-2,4,6-trideoxy-hexopyranoses*

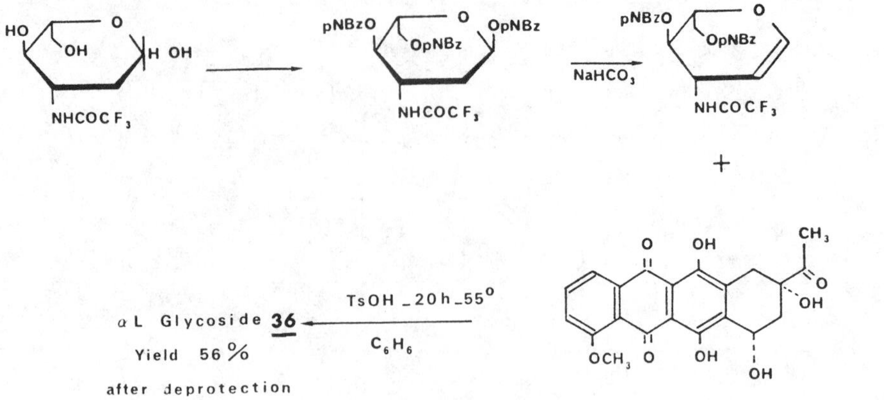

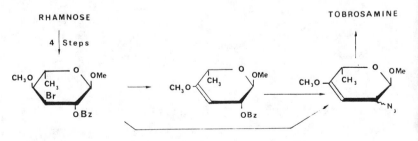

Figure 11 Stereocontrolled synthesis of 4'-epi-6'-hydroxy-dau-norubicine

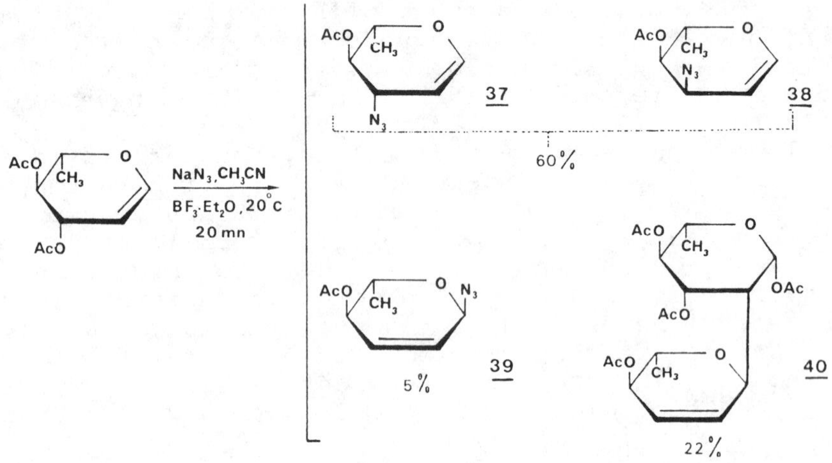

Figure 12 Azidolysis of di-O-acetyl-L-rhamnal

Figure 13 Key step of synthesis of tobrosamine

In the second part of this talk will be discussed the results we have obtained in the synthesis
of anthracycline analogs by transformation of glycals into 3-amino-3-deoxy-glycals and after suitable
protection by their glycosidation with daunomycinone.
This approach was based on two principal observations :

- First of all, among the different syntheses
previously that were reported in the literature concerning the glycosidation of sugars with daunomycinone, one of them retained our attention. This was
the stereocontrolled synthesis of 4'-epi-6'-hydroxy-
daunorubicine, 36 reported by Arcamone and co-workers (36) who used a suitably protected 3-amino-3-
deoxy-glycal as starting material for the sugar
moiety. This led,in a stereospecific way, to the α
anomer with a rather good yield (Figure 11). Although
this route seemed particularly interesting, it was,
in the field of anthracycline antibiotics, the only
example of such a glycosidation, and moreover synthesis of the glycal itself required a particular
sequence of reactions.

However if 3-amino-3-deoxy glycals could be
readily prepared from available D-glucal or L-rhamnal for example, such a route would become more general. For this purpose, the allylic alcohol group
present at C-3 of the glycal would have to be replaced with an azide function and the latter reduced
into amino group. This route seemed reasonable since
Heyn's group (37,38) had already obtained by reacting sodium azide and di-O-acetyl-L-rhamnal under
boron trifluoride catalysis, compounds 37 and 38
with simultaneous formation of small amounts of
pseudorhamnal 39 and of the dimeric compound 40
(Figure 12).
We also had succeeded (39) in a synthesis of
tobrosamine, in replacing a benzoate ester derivative of an allylic alcohol with sodium azide in HMPT
solution at high temperature (140°) (Figure 13).
Thus the general synthetic strategy as represented in figure 14 includes three principal steps :

1. Introduction of an azido group at C-3.
2. Reduction of the azido group into amino
function and protection of the two groups at C-3 and
C-4.
3. Coupling of the suitably protected 3-amino-
3-deoxy glycal with daunomycinone.

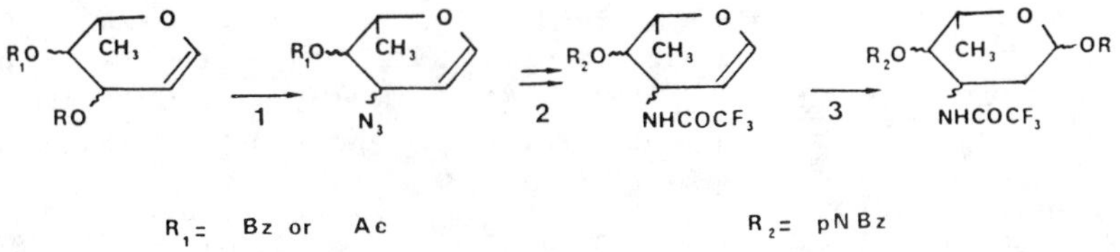

R₁ = Bz or Ac   R₂ = pNBz

Figure 14   General synthetic scheme for the synthesis of suitably
protected 3-amino 3-deoxy glycals and their glycosi-
dation

Following this scheme (40), the dibenzoate derivative of L-rhamnal was treated under NaN₃-DMF
conditions or NaN₃-BF₃ etherate conditions and the
results are shown in figure 15. L-rhamnal reacted to
give a mixture of 4 products well resolved by HPLC
and fully characterized by 240 MHz NMR spectroscopy.

2 azido-glycals 41 and 43 and
2 unsaturated glycosylazides 42 and 44.

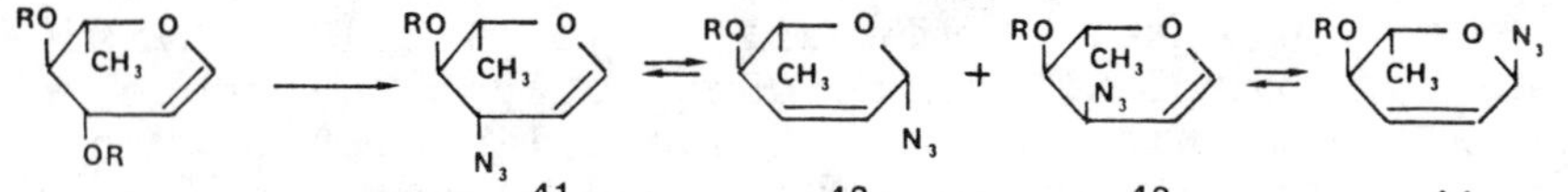

	41	42		43	44
NaN₃ – DMF 140°	38 %	6 %		40 %	16 %
		44 %		56 %	
NaN₃-BF₃ [12 eq] 5mn -0°	25 %	4 %		51 %	20 %
		30 %		70 %	

Figure 15   Azidolysis of di-O-acyl-L-rhamnal derivatives

The azido-glycals 41 and 43 could be separated
by HPLC but they quickly rearranged to give, respectively, a mixture of 41 and 42 and 43 and 44. The
equilibrium was reached within 8 h at 20°C and the
equilibrium value ratios are indicated in figure 15.
Isomerisation of allylic azides have been well studied and are generally believed to proceed via an
intramolecular rearrangement. Thus these equilibria
do not depend upon the presence of sodium azide in
the mixture.

In contrast, transformation of each product into the general mixture required the initial conditions to be present. When such an experiment was carried out in the presence of boron trifluoride, as a degradation of starting material was observed it became hasardous to conclude to a thermodynamic equilibrium.

No traces of dimers as reported by Heyn's group (37) could be detected but as shown by Guthrie and co-workers (41) their competitive formation depends on the reaction conditions - time, temperature, quality and amount of sodium azide and boron trifluoride - .

In any case, in order to synthesize the 3-amino-3-deoxy-glycals, the crude mixtures were reduced with lithium aluminium hydride in ether to give exclusively (figure 16) with 70 % yield, the corresponding 3-amino-3-deoxy-glycals 45 and 46, easily separated by column chromatography. The ratio of 45/46 was exactly the same as the equilibrium ratio of 41 + 42/43 + 44. The α-unsaturated glycosylamines could not be detected but the only reported compound of this type was shown to be very unstable (42).

Finally the amino and hydroxy groups were protected as shown in figure 16 by means of successive treatment with trifluoroacetic anhydride in presence of triethylamine, with methanol and then with p-nitrobenzoyl chloride in pyridine.

In subsequent scaled-up preparations of 47 and 48, the procedure was slightly modified in that isolation of the intermediates 41-44 or 45 and 46 was avoided so that column chromatography was required exclusively in the final step.

The glycals of L-acosamine and L-ristosamine, 47 and 48, were thus obtained in three principal steps in an overall yield of respectively, 17 % and 22 % by the DMF-method, or 13 % and 33 % by the BF₃-etherate method. The total yield of the fully protected 3-amino-3-deoxy-glycals was approximately 40-45 %.

The glycosidation of 47 and 48 with daunomycinone was carried out under conditions closely similar to those previously used for the 1-O-acetyl hexoses, 2 molar-equivalents of sugar, 1 molar-equivalent of daunomycinone and 0.5 molar-equivalent of TsOH in a mixture of benzene-dichloromethane at r.t. for 47 and 50° for 48. This gave 46 % of 49 and 42 % of 50 (figure 16).

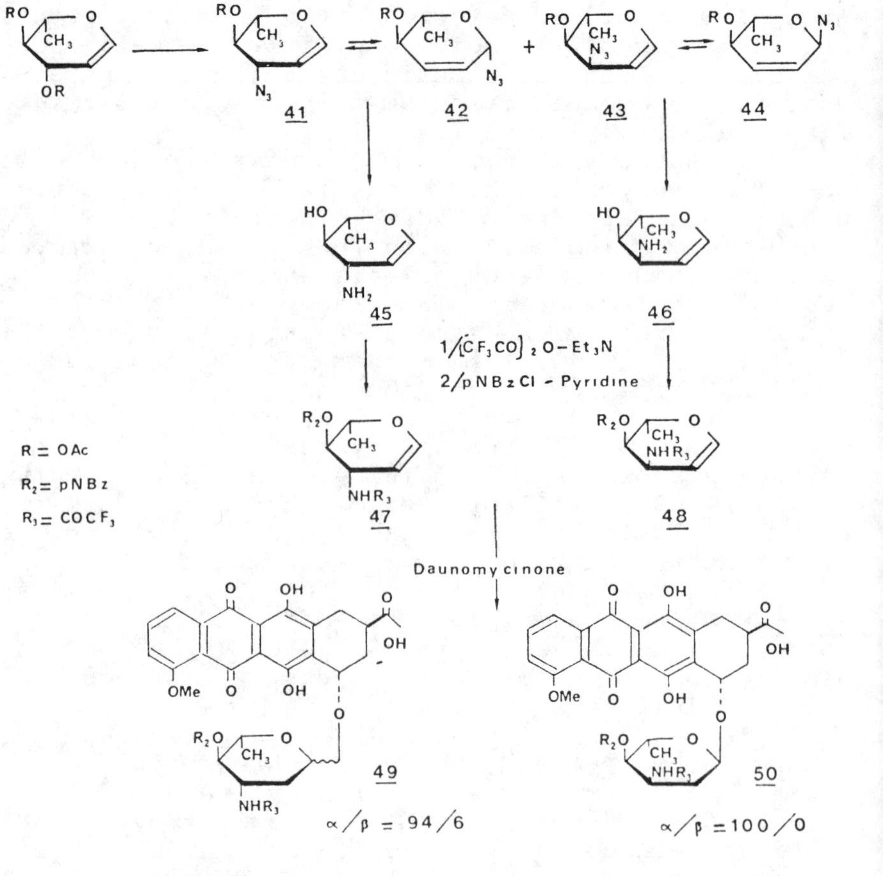

Figure 16   Synthesis of 4'-epi and 3', 4'-epi-daunorubicines 49 and 50

Following the same route as before, the corresponding D-enantiomers were also prepared (34)
(figure 17). As it was found that the 4-O-acetyl-
pseudo rhamnal, 52 gave exactly the same product as
the D-rhamnal derivative 51 under NaN₃-BF₃-etherate
conditions, we epimerized the allylic 4-OH of 52
to access to 53 in order to synthesize the glycals
of suitably protected 3-epi-D-daunosamine 56 and D-
daunosamine, 57. In fact in this latter case, only
one isomeric 3-amino-3-deoxy glycal was found after
azidolysis, reduction and protection. No traces of
the glycal of D-daunosamine, 57 could be detected,
even after several attempts to epimerize.

Stereospecificity (α anomers) was observed
during glycosidation of glycals of D-ristosamine, 54
and of 3-epi-D-daunosamine, 56 with daunomycinone
while a mixture of α and β anomers resulted from the
glycosidation of the glycal of D-acosamine, 55 (figure 17).

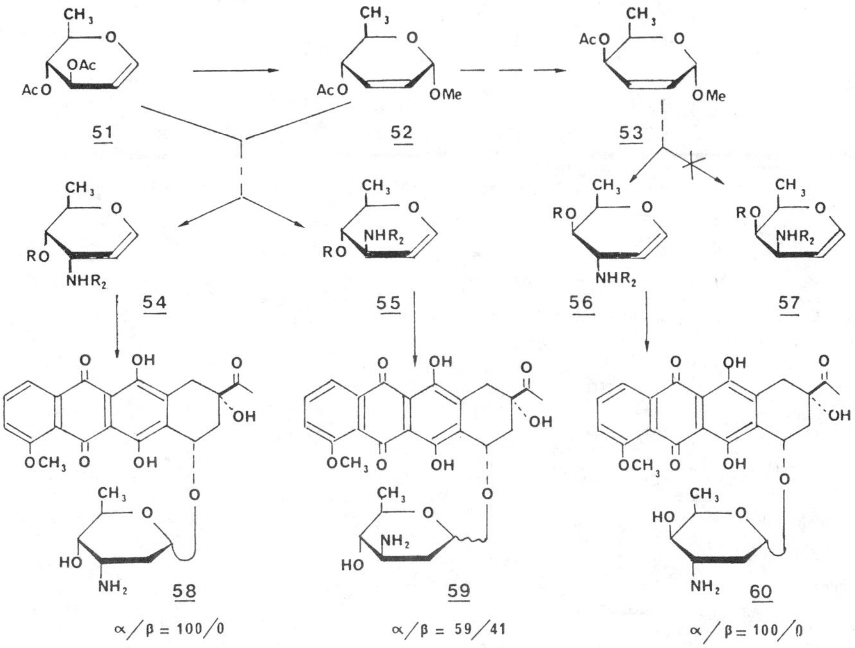

Figure 17   Synthesis of 3',4'-diepi, 4'-epi and 3'-epi-D-
daunorubicines, 58, 59 and 60

During the last decade, several anthracycline antibiotics which exist in the form of oligosaccharide glycosides have been found. Among them, one of the most interesting is undoubtly Aclacynomicine A (43), 61, which has a potent antitumor activity against various experimental tumors and a low cardiac toxicity (figure 18).

Aklavinone was shown to be the aglycon of Aclacinomycin A while the sugar sequence was shown to consist of L-rhodosamine-2-deoxy-L-fucose and L-cinerulose A.

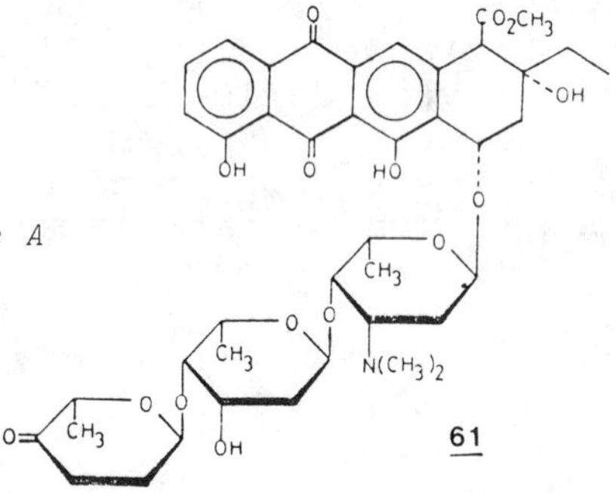

Figure 18   Aclacinomycine A

This trisaccharide has provided challenging problems to organic chemists. Although such a compound was our target, we decided first to investigate the synthesis of a disaccharide-containing anthracyclin such as represented in figure 19 with the anthracycline antibiotic, daunosaminyl-daunorubicine (44), 62 or musettamycine (45), 63 by coupling the disaccharide, 2-deoxy-α-L-fucosyl (1→4) daunosamine with daunomycinone.

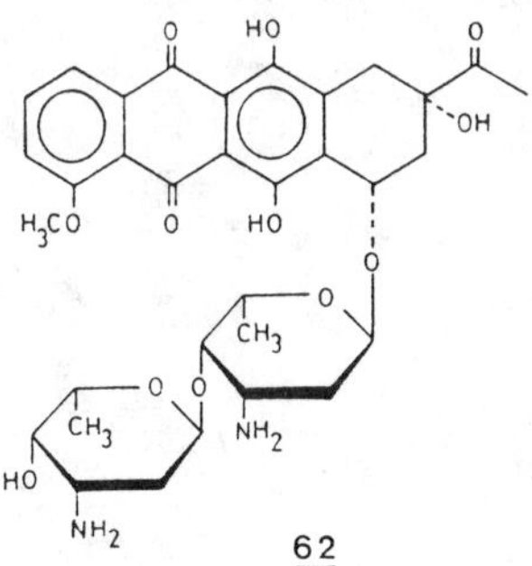

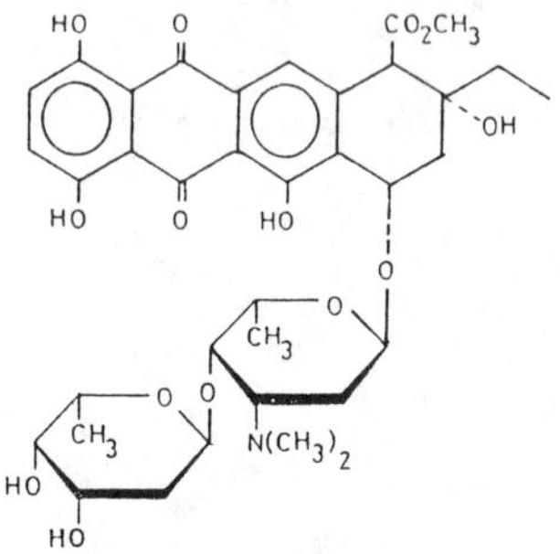

Figure 19   Daunosaminyl-daunorubicine and musettamycine 62 and 63

Two principal approaches can be used for the synthesis of such disaccharide-containing anthracyclines. The first of them would be through the reaction of the 2-deoxy-fucosyl halide with the N-trifluoroacetyl derivative of daunorubicine for example. The other, more general, would be through the synthesis of the disaccharide then through its glycosidation with daunomycinone.

In fact, the first approach invariably results, as reported by El Khadem (46), in transglycosylation or gives as reported by Arcamone's group (47) the desired compound in rather low yield, our attention was turned toward the second approach.

As we have already synthesized the per-O-acetyl-2-deoxy-L-fucose, 64 and the methyl glycosides of L-rhodosamine, 65a, N-trifluoroacetyl daunosamine 65c and of N-acetyl daunosamine, 65b, the easiest route according to this approach would consist in realizing the glycosidation in presence of p-toluenesulfonic acid as catalyst. In fact such attempts (figure 20) failed in that the reactions led to inseparable mixtures of products that were not investigated further. The same observation was made with the corresponding deamino sugar 66.

The lack of success with the above reactions led us to turn to other possible routes for preparing the disaccharide. Since this failure seemed to be due to the L-lyxo configuration of the amino sugar moiety rather than to the amino group at C-3, a 2-deoxy-hexose with the same configuration as daunosamine at C-3 and C-4 but of opposite configuration at C-5 was selected as starting material. As an amino group at C-3 or an azido group must be also already present in this precursor, this was the azido sugar of D-ribo configuration, 14a, intermediate during the synthesis of daunosamine.

The presence of a bromine at C-6 allowed access to the 6-deoxy-L-amino sugar moiety by the classical elimination-inversion sequence at C-5 after glycosylation.

When reacted with per-O-acetyl-2-deoxy-fucose 64, in benzene during 2 h at room temperature in presence of TsOH as catalyst the azido compound 14a gave stereoselectively the disaccharide 67 in 60 % yield. Removal of hydrobromic acid by means of silver fluoride in pyridine afforded the exocyclic unsaturated derivative 68. This enose underwent stereospecific reduction with hydrogen in the presence

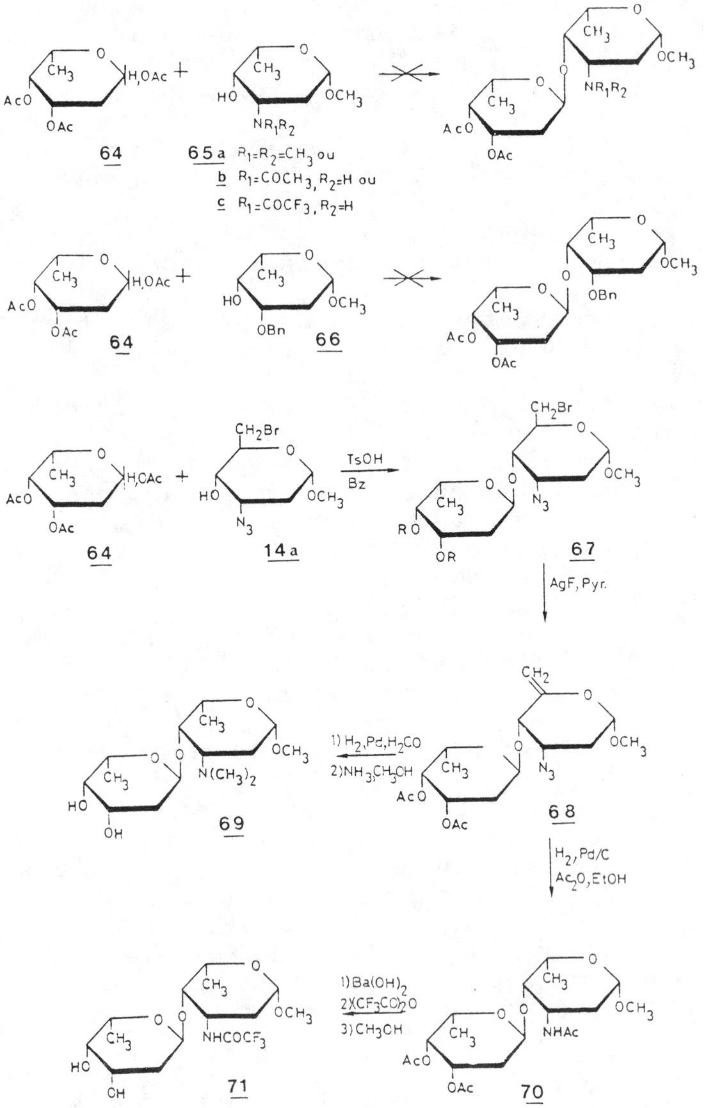

Figure 20   Synthesis of the methyl 2-deoxy-α-L-fucosyl (1-4)-
N-trifluoroacetyl-daunosaminide

of palladium and formaldehyde to give the N,N-dime-
thyl-disaccharide 69, the methyl glycoside of the
disaccharide naturally occurring in antitumor anthracyclin antibiotics. The corresponding N-acetyl
derivative 70 was isolated when hydrogenation was
carried out in presence of acetic acid instead of
formaldehyde. The N-acetyl derivative was also converted into N-trifluoroacetyl derivative 71 as indicated in figure 20.

The synthesis of a disaccharide-containing anthracycline then required a regiospecific hydrolysis
of the glycosidic bond of the amino sugar moiety in
order to prepare a halogeno or an acetyl derivative.
This acidic hydrolysis was incompatible with the
fragility of the glycosidic obnd between the two
sugars and even a mild treatment of 71 with aqueous
acetic acid (1:1) led after 2 days at room temperature, and after acetylation of the crude mixture, to
the starting per-O-acetyl-2-deoxy-fucose 64 and to
the β-methyl glycoside of the fully protected daunosamine, 72 (figure 21).

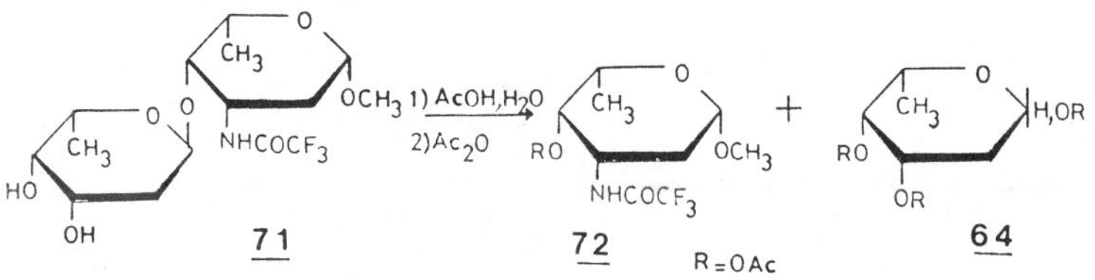

Figure 21   Acidic hydrolysis of 71

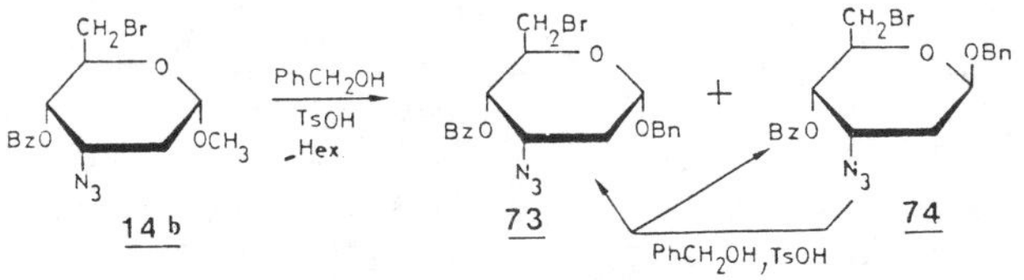

Figure 22   Transglycosidation reaction

For this reason a benzyl glycoside as starting
material should be better than the methyl glycoside
previously used. The fact we had a large amount of
the azido sugar 14b (R=Rz) prompted us to investigate a direct replacement of the methyl group by a

benzyl group. This was achieved by an original transglycosidation reaction (Figure 22). Treatment of a
solution of 14b in hexane with benzylic alcohol and
p-toluenesulfonic acid as catalyst at reflux in a
Dean-Stark apparatus to remove the methanol formed
in the reaction, led after 2 h to a thermodynamic
mixture of the α and β benzyl glycosides, 73 and 74
in a 55/45 ratio. The α D-anomer 73, was isolated as
a pure product by crystallization from dichlorome-
thane-hexane while a further treatment of the mother-
liquors under the same transglycosidation conditions
led to the same thermodynamic mixture. Thus after
three operations, the α D anomer 73 was obtained in
80 % yield as a crystalline compound.

     The disaccharide 76 was then obtained stereo-
specifically in 50 % yield after removal of the benzoyl ester of 73 by transesterification and condensation of 75 with per-O-acetyl-2-deoxy-fucose, 64.
Treatment of 76 with silver fluoride in pyridine
afforded the enose, 77. Hydrogenation was conducted
in two steps in order to avoid the formation of by
products. The azido function was first reduced by
hydrogenation in presence of Raney-nickel for a very
short time (5 to 10 min). Under these particular
conditions the double bond and the O-benzyl ether at
C-1 were not affected. Before completing the hydrogenation the amino function was protected as a tri-
fluoroacetamide to afford 78 (overall yield for the
two steps : 87 %). Then the double bond was hydrogenated and the benzyl group removed in a one-step
procedure by treatment of 78 with hydrogen in the
presence of palladium-on-carbon in ethyl acetate.
This led to the reducing disaccharide 79 and, after
acetylation, to the 1-O-acetyl derivative, 80.

     Then, in view of the afore-mentioned difficul-
ties encountered with the acidic hydrolysis of the
corresponding methyl glycosides, a great problem
remained to be solved. Where would protonation of 80
take place during the glycosidation with daunomycinone in presence of p-toluenesulfonic acid ? Because
of the greater nucleophilic character of the 1-O-
acetyl oxygen compare to that of the oxygen joining
the 2-deoxy-fucosyl and the N-trifluoroacetyl daunosaminyl moieties, we expected that protonation would
take place preferentially at the former position.

     Glycosidation was performed in a mixture of
dichloromethane and benzene under standard conditions and afforded after 30 min a crude mixture

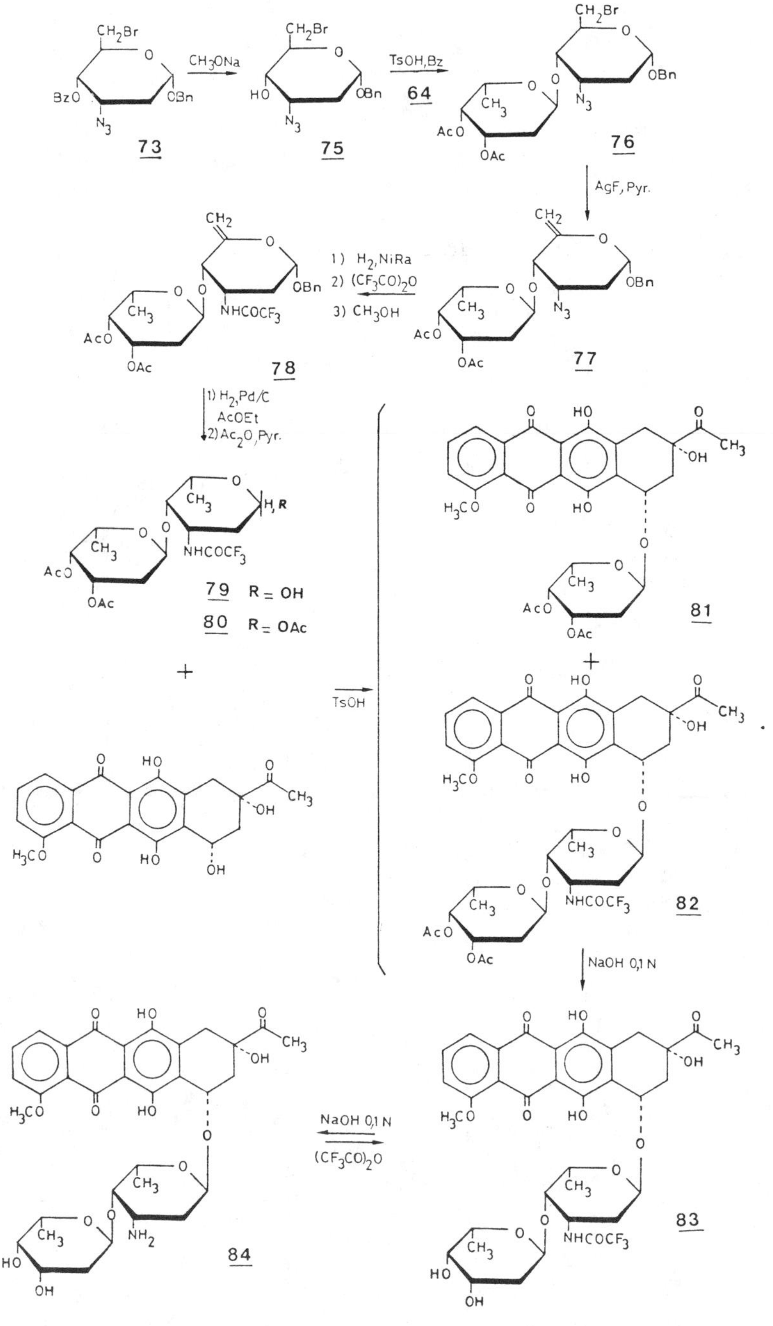

Figure 23   Synthesis of 2-deoxy-fucosyl-daunorubicine

COMPOUNDS	Induction prophage λ	Antitumor activity / Refer.	in vitro tests Cytotoxicity	in vitro tests DNA synth.
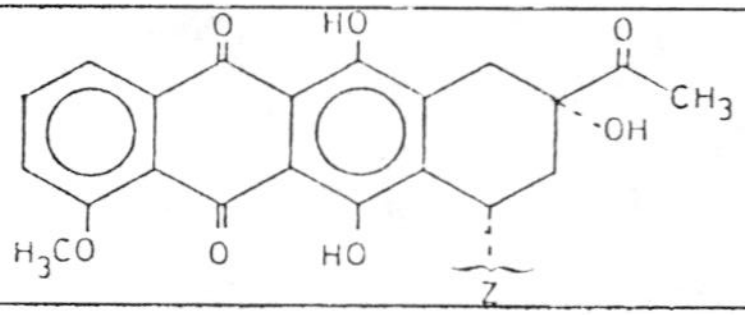				
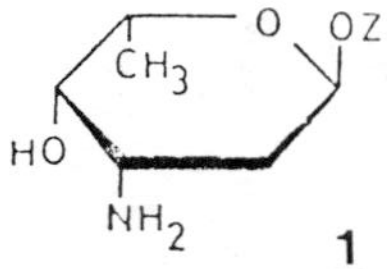 L-daunosamine **1**	+	+	+	0,96-1,75
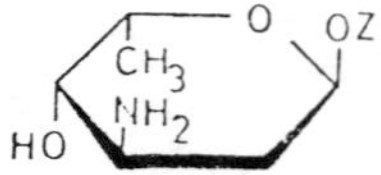 epi-3 L-daunosamine (L"xylo") **28**	−	NT	−	1,8-3,6
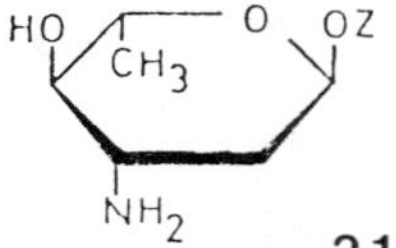 epi-4 L-daunosamine (L-acosamine) **21**	+	+ [51]	NT	NT
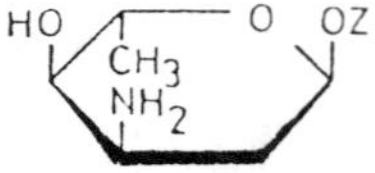 diepi-3,4 L-daunosamine (L-ristosamine) **49**	−	+ [51]	+	NT

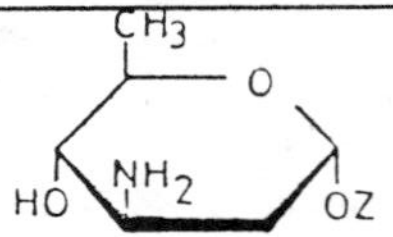

3,6	−	±	−	D-acosamine **29**
NT	NT	± 52	−	D-acosamine **29**
1,13–1,4	+	+ − 53	NT	D-ristosamine **54**
1,13–1,33	−	NT	NT	D-"xylo" **60**
				D-daunosamine **30**

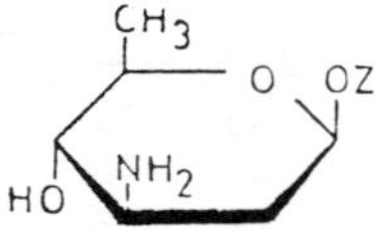

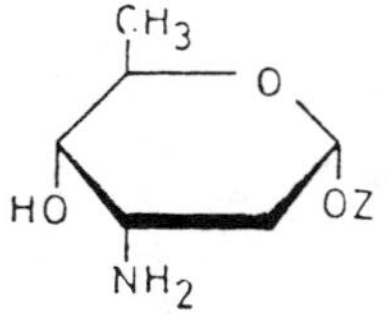

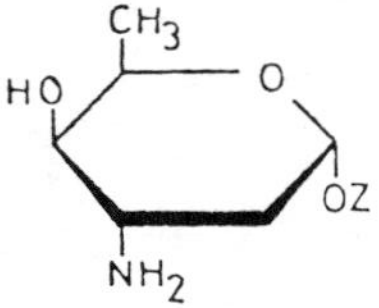

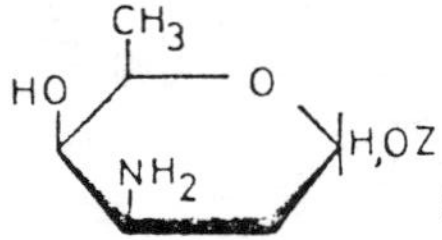

NT = NO TEST

Figure 24   *Biological activity of daunorubicine analogs*

247

which was chromatographied on silica gel. Isolated
successively were 2-deoxy-fucosyl-daunomycinone, 81,
the disaccharide containing anthracycline 82 and unreacted daunomycinone. Monitoring of the reaction by
tlc we showed that 81 and 82 obtained in 7 and 10 %
yield respectively were formed at the same time.
This demonstrates that protonation took place in
part at C-1 with formation of the required glycoside
82 but also, in part between the two sugars affording   82, already synthesized in a different way by
Horton's group (48) (figure 23).
     Alkaline hydrolysis of 82 gave, after 20 min
the N-trifluoroacetyl derivative 83 and after 5 h,
the basic compound 84. The latter must be transformed into its tartrate   or into its N-trifluoroacetyl derivative, 83 since it slowly decomposes.

Biological activity

     Thus by means of classical syntheses or by the
glycal route we have been able to prepare in good
yield the seven diastereoisomers of   daunosamine.
This led after glycosidation to nine daunorubicin
analogs (figure 24).
     Some of these compounds were tested (49) for
their ability to induce prophage λ in *Escherichia
Coli* K12 since preliminary correlation (50) supported the idea that the antineoplastic activity of the
anthracyclines is a consequence of their capacity to
damage DNA.
     The results have shown that for the L-series,
the configuration of the 4' hydroxy group is relatively unimportant for the generation of prophage
inducing lesions in DNA whereas the 3'-amino group
must be trans with respect to the α anomer oxygen in
order for that compound to have a detectable activity.
     With respect to the parent antibiotic, 1, none
of the new derivatives (21, 29, 30, 54, 60) exhibits
a greater or similar activity in "in vitro test"
for cytotoxicity or inhibition of DNA synthesis
except the α glycoside of D-ristosamine 54. In fact
it was previously reported by Horton's group (50)
that this glycoside shows antitumor activity on
P388 comparable to that of daunorubicine but with
higher dose-levels. However as they said in this
publication, more information will be needed in order to assess the pharmacological potential (if any)

of anthracycline glycosides of the $\underline{D}$-series.

Acknowledgments

Financial assistance from the "Centre National de la Recherche Scientifique" and from the "Ligue National contre le Cancer" is gratefully acknowledged. We are also indebted to Rhône-Poulenc laboratories for gifts of daunomycinone.

Literature cited

(1) Grein, A., Spalla, C., DiMarco, A., Canevazzi, G., Giorn.Microbiol. (1963), 11, 109.
(2) Dubost, M., Ganter, P., Maral, R., Ninet, L., Pinnert, S., Preud'homme, J., Werner, G.-H., C.R.Acad.Sci. Paris (1963), 257, 1813.
(3) Arcamone, F., Franceschi, G., Penco, S., Selva, A., Tetrahedron Letters (1969), 1007.
(4) Brazhnikova, M.G., Zbarskii, V.B., Ponomarenko, V.L., Potapova, N.P., J.Antibiotics (1974), 27, 254.
(5) Marsch, J.P., Jr, Mosher, C.W., Acton, E.A., Goodman, L., Chem.Comm. (1967), 973.
(6) Horton, D., Weckerle, W., Carbohydr.Res. (1975) 44, 227.
(7) Richarson, A.C., Ibid. (1967), 4, 422.
(8) Baer, H.H., Capek, K., Cook, M.C., Can.J.Chem. (1969), 47, 89.
(9) Boivin, J., Pais, M., Monneret, C., Carbohydr. Res. (1978), 64, 271.
(10) Yamaguchi, Y., Kojima, M., Ibid. (1977), 59, 343.
(11) Medgyes, G., Kuszmann, J., Ibid. (1981), 92, 225.
(12) Wong, C.M., Ho, T.-L., Niemczura, W.P., Can.J. Chem. (1975), 53, 3144.
(13) Dyong, I., Wiemann, R., Ang.Chem.Int. Ed. Engl. (1978), 17, 682.
(14) Iwataki, I., Nakamura, Y., Takahashi, K., Matsumoto, T., Bull.Chem.Soc. Japan (1979), 52, 273.
(15) Dyong, I., Wiemann, R., Chem.Ber. (1980), 113, 2666.
(16) Fronza, G., Fuganti, C., Grasselli, P., J.C.S., Chem.Comm. (1980), 442.
(17) Hauser, F.M., Rhee, R.P., J.Org.Chem. (1981), 46, 227.

(18) Wovkulich, P.M. , Uskokovic´, M.R. , J.Am.Chem.
     Soc. (1981) <u>103</u>, 3956.
(19) Fuganti, C. , Grasselli, P. , Pedrocchi-Fantoni,
     G. , Tetrahedron Letters (1981), 4017.
(20) Lomakina, N.N. , Spiridonova, I.A. , Yu, I. ,
     Vlasova, T.F. , Khim.Prir.Soedin. (1973), <u>9</u>, 101;
     Chem.Abstr. (1973), <u>78</u>, 148170m.
(21) Bognar, R. , Sztaricskai, F. , Munk, M.E. , Tamas,
     J. , J.Org.Chem. (1974), <u>39</u>, 2971 and references
     cited therein.
(22) Richtmyer, N.K. , Methods Carbohydr.Chem. (1962)
     <u>1</u>, 107 and references cited therein.
(23) Wiggins, L.F. , Ibid. (1963), <u>2</u>, 188.
(24) Rosenthal, A. , Catsoulacos, P., Can.J.Chem.
     (1968), <u>46</u>, 2868.
(25) Tatsuta, K. , Fujimoto, K. , Kinoshita, M. ,
     Umezawa, S. , Carbohydr.Res. (1977), <u>54</u>, 85.
(26) Evans, M.E. , Ibid. (1972), <u>21</u>, 473.
(27) Boivin, J. , These Doctorat d'Etat, Paris-Orsay
     1981.
(28) Hanessian, S. , Carbohydr.Res. (1966), <u>2</u>, 86.
(29) Monneret, C. Conreur, C. , Khuong-Huu, Q. , Ibid.
     (1978), <u>65</u>, 35.
(30) Boivin, J. , Monneret, C. , Pais, M. , Unpublished
     results.
(31) Boivin, J. , Pais, M. , Monneret, C. , C.R.Acad.
     Sci. Paris (1978), <u>286C</u>, 51.
(32) Cheung, T.M. , Horton, D. , Weckerle, W. , Carbo-
     hydr.Res. (1977), <u>58</u>, 139.
(33) Boivin, J. , Monneret, C. , Pais, M. , Tetrahedron
     Letters (1978), 1111.
(34) Boivin, J. , Montagnac, A. , Monneret, C. , Pais,
     M. , Carbohydr.Res. (1980), <u>85</u>, 223.
(35) A.F. Hadfield, Cunningham, L. , Sartorelli, A.C. ,
     Ibid. (1979), <u>72</u>, 93.
(36) Arcamone, F. , Bargiotti, A. , Cassinelli, G. ,
     Redaelli, S. , Hanessian, S. , DiMarco, A. ,
     Casazza, A.M. , Dasdia, T. , Necco, A. , Reggiani,
     P. , Supino, R. , J.Med.Chem. (1976), <u>19</u>, 733.
(37) Heyns, K. , Hohlweg, R. , Chem.Ber. (1978), <u>111</u>,
     1632.
(38) Heyns, K. , Lim, M.-J. , Park, J.I. , Tetrahedron
     Letters (1976), 1477.
(39) Florent, J.C. , Monneret, C. , Khuong-Huu, Q. ,
     Carbohydr.Res. (1977), <u>56</u>, 301.
(40) Boivin, J. , Pais, M. , Monneret, C. , Ibid. (1980)
     <u>79</u>, 193.

(41) Guthrie, R.D. (Gus), Irvine, A.W., Ibid (1980), 82, 207 and 225.
(42) Lemieux, R.U., Bose, R.J., Can.J.Chem. (1966), 44, 1855.
(43) Oki, T., J. Antibiotics (1977), 30, S70.
(44) Arcamone, F., Cassinelli, G., Penco, S., Tognoli, L., Ger.Offen., 1, 923, 885 ; Chem. Abstr. (1970), 72, 131086s.
(45) Bradner, W.T., Misiek, J.Antibiotics (1977), 30, 519 ; Nettleton, D.E., Jr, Bradner, W.T., Bush, J.A., Coon, A.B., Moseley, J.E., Myllymaki, R.W., O'Herron, F.A., Schreiber, R.H., Vulcano, A.L., J.Antibiotics (1977), 30, 525.
(46) El Khadem, H.S., Liav, A., Carbohydr.Res. (1979) 74, 199.
(47) Penco, S., Franchi, G., Arcamone, F., Ger.Offen. 2, 751, 395 ; Chem.Abstr. (1978), 89, 110283q.
(48) Fuchs, E.F., Horton, D., Weckerle, W., Winter-Mihaly, E., J.Med.Chem. (1979), 22, 406.
(49) Anderson, W.A., Boivin, J., Monneret, C., Pais M., Mutation Research (1980), 77, 341.
(50) Anderson, W.A., Moreau, P.L., Devoret, R., Maral, R., Ibid (1980), 77, 197.
(51) Arcamone, F., Llyodia (1977), 40, 45.
(52) Fuchs, E.-F., Horton, D., Weckerle, W., Winter, B., J.Antibiotics (1979), 32, 223.
(53) Horton, D., Nickol, R.G., Weckerle, W., Winter-Mihaly, E., Carbohydr.Res. (1979), 76, 269.

ANTHRACYCLINE ANALOGS MODIFIED IN THE SUGAR MOIETY

H. S. El Khadem, D. Matsuura, D. L. Swartz and R. Cermak

Department of Chemistry and Chemical Engineering
Michigan Technological University
Houghton, Michigan 49931

INTRODUCTION

Anthracyclines constitute a group of antibiotics that comprises several clinically used antineoplastic agents.[1-7] Table I shows the activity of some antineoplastic anthracyclines and their analogs. Anthracyclines are classified into two groups. The first group includes adriamycin (1), daunorubicin (2) and carminomycin (3),[8-22] and the second group comprises more complex molecules such as the cinerubins and the aclacinomycins (4,5), etc.[23-31] These two groups are sometimes designated as class I anthracyclines and class II anthracyclines, respectively.

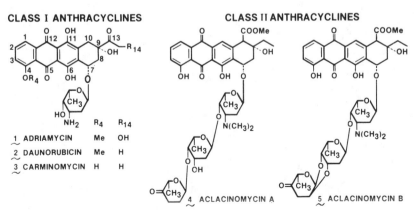

Figure 1. *Examples of class I and class II anthracyclines*

ANTHRACYCLINE ANTIBIOTICS

Table I

ACTIVITY OF ANTINEOPLASTIC ANTHRACYCLINES

ANTHRACYCLINES	(T/C) P388	L1210
DAUNORUBICIN	173	
ADRIAMYCIN	238	
CARMINOMYCIN	177	
11-DEOXY-DAUNORUBICIN	181	
11-DEOXY-ADRIAMYCIN	245	
MARCELLOMYCIN		150
MUSETTAMYCIN		157
RUDOLFOMYCIN		143
PYRROMYCIN		129
ACLACINOMYCIN A	208	213
=N-NHCOPH	276	
=N-NHCOPH-P-CL	209	
=N-NHCOPH-M-NO$_2$	200	
(=N-NHCOCH$_2$-)$_2$	283	
N-TRIFLUOROACETYL-ADRIAMYCIN		533
N-TRIFLUOROACETYL-ADRIAMYCIN-14-VALERATE		545
N-BENZYL-ADRIAMYCIN	185	
N-BENZYL-DAUNORUBICIN	185	
N,N-DIBENZYL-ADRIAMYCIN	175	
N,N-DIBENZYL-DAUNORUBICIN	259	
4'-O-METHYL-DAUNORUBICIN	156	
4'-O-METHYL-ADRIAMYCIN	270	287
4'-EPI-DAUNORUBICIN	200	
3'-4'-EPI-DAUNORUBICIN	251	
4'-DEOXY-DAUNORUBICIN		187
4'-DEOXY-ADRIAMYCIN		177
2'-DEOXY-L-FUCOSE-DAUNORUBICIN	192	
2'-DEOXY-L-FUCOSE-CARMINOMYCIN		186
2'-DEOXY-3',4'-DI-O-ACETYL-L-FUCOSE-ADRIAMYCIN	269	203
2'-DEOXY-3',4'-DI-O-ACETYL-L-FUCOSE-DAUNORUBICIN	186	
2'-DEOXY-3',4'-DI-O-ACETYL-D-RIBOSE-ε-RHODOMYCINONE	125	

Classes I and II anthracyclines differ not only in the structure of their aromatic moieties, but also in the number of sugar units attached to the anthracyclinone. Class I anthracyclines have no substitutient in position 10 of the aromatic moiety, but instead have a carbonyl group in position 13, whereas class II anthracyclines possess a methoxy carbonyl group in position 10 and no carbonyl in position 13. As for the sugar moiety, class I anthracyclines are found naturally linked to a monosaccharide, usually daunosamine, whereas class II anthracyclines possess an oligosaccharide chain, usually a trisaccharide, composed of rhodosamine, the N,N-dimethyl derivative of daunosamine, 2-deoxy-L-fucose and a third saccharide which varies from one antibiotic to the other. The oligosaccharide moiety renders the binding of class I anthracyclines to DNA much less firm than the binding of anthracyclines of class I. This is why class II anthracyclines inhibit less DNA than do class I anthracyclines.[5] It is possible, through chemical modification, to start with a class I anthracycline, attach a group such as an N,N-dibenzyl group to its amino sugar, which weakens the complexation with DNA to obtain an anthracycline which behaves more like a class II anthracycline.[32] The same can be achieved by replacing the amino group of daunosamine by a hydroxyl group. Thus, the 2-deoxy-L-fucosyl carminomycinone (6) prepared by us[33] and the 2-deoxy-L-fucosyl daunomycinone[34] (7) and adriamycinone[35] (8) prepared by Horton exhibit more the properties of class II anthracyclines than those of class I. The structures of compounds 6, 7 and 8 are depicted below in Figure 2.

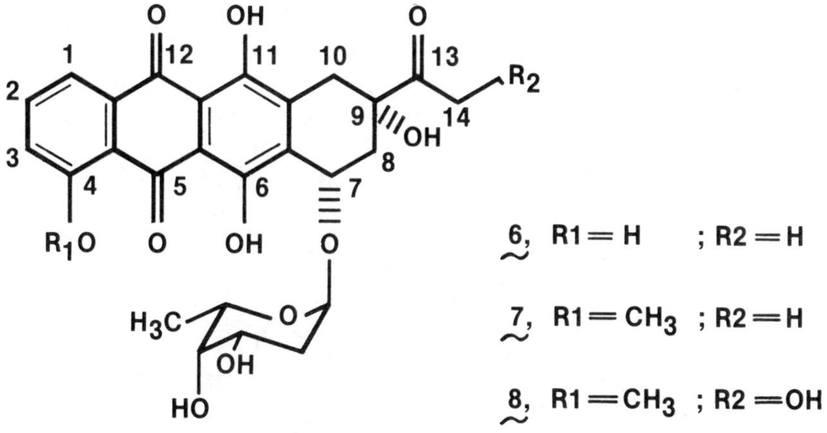

6, R1 = H   ; R2 = H

7, R1 = CH$_3$; R2 = H

8, R1 = CH$_3$; R2 = OH

Figure 2.   *Some active 2-deoxy-L-fucosyl anthracyclinones*

During the past five years we have worked extensively in
the area of anthracyclines and converted several class I anthracyclines into class II anthracyclines. This is because
we believe that the cardiotoxicity of class I anthracyclines
may be decreased by weakening their complexation with DNA.
Although a direct correlation has not been demonstrated between complexation with DNA and cardiotoxicity, one is struck
by the fact that anthracyclines belonging to class II
are usually less cardiotoxic than anthracyclines of
the class I type. Thus, for example, aclacinomycin A is much
less toxic than adriamycin.[6]

Our synthetic work on class II anthracyclines concentrated on two areas: (a) synthesis of monosaccharide derivatives of anthracyclinones that will not bind firmly to DNA,
(b) synthesis of oligosaccharide derivatives of anthracyclinones.

(a) Synthesis of Monosaccharide Derivatives

Early in our work we showed that the methyl group attached
to position 5 of the pyranosyl ring could be substituted with
a hydrogen atom without great change in the activity. This
was demonstrated by comparing the activity of 2-deoxy-L-
fucosyl-ε-rhodomycinone (14) and 2-deoxy-D-ribopyranosyl-ε-
rhodomycinone (15).[36] The latter and its acetate (13) were
more active than the former on P388 lymphatic leukemia in CDF
mice. Thus 2-deoxy-di-O-acetyl-D-ribopyranosyl-ε-rhodo-
mycinone (13) had a T/C of 125 at a dose of 64 mg/kg/day and
110 at a dose of 128 and 32 mg/kg/day. The unblocked glyco-
side(15) had a T/C of 115 at a dose of 13 mg/kg/day, whereas
2-Deoxy-L-fucopyranosyl-ε-rhodomycinone (14) had a T/C of 109
at a dose of 18 mg/kg/day. See figure 3 for a synthetic
scheme of some ε-rhodomycinone glycosides.

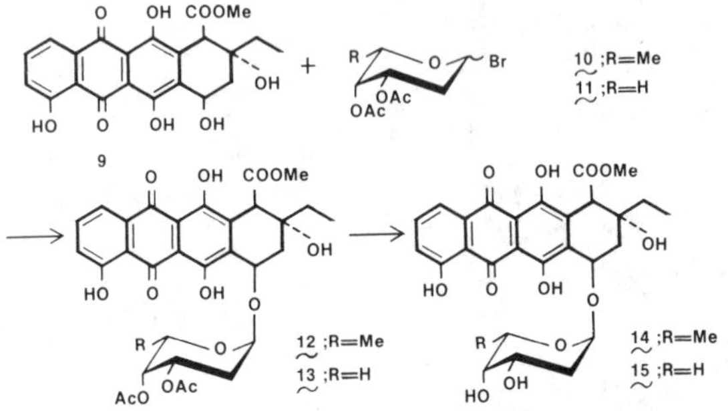

Figure 3. *Synthesis Scheme for ε-rhodomycinone glycosides*

This led us to prepare more 2-deoxy-L-fucopyranosyl and 2-deoxy-D-ribopyranosyl anthracyclinones. These included 2-deoxy-L-fucopyranosyl carminomycinone (6), 2-deoxy-D-ribopyranosyl carminomycinone (24), 2-deoxy-D-ribopyranosyl daunomycinone (25), 2-deoxy-L-fucopyranosyl-ε-pyrromycinone (26) and 2-deoxy-D-ribopyranosyl-ε-pyrromycinone (27). For a synthetic scheme, see Figure 4.

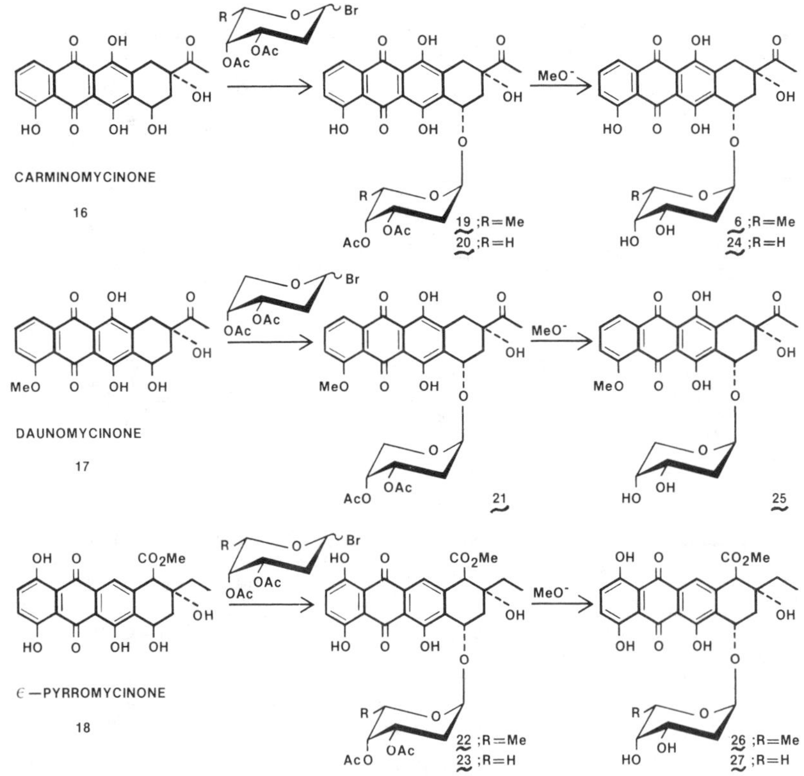

Figure 4. *Synthesis of some 2-deoxy-L-fucopyranosyl and D-ribopyranosyl anthracyclinones*

Screening results of 2-deoxy-L-fucopyranosyl-carminomycinone (6), have shown that this compound possesses a better therapeutic index than the parent carminomycin, but like the analogous 2-deoxy-fucopyranosyl-daunomycinone (7) and adriamycinone (8), its potency was lower than the natural anti-biotic.[33] This was attributed to the fact that these compounds complex more loosely with DNA than the natural aminated anthracycline analogs. Table 2 shows antitumor activity of compound 6 and some of its analogs and table 3 the anti-bacterial activity of these and other compounds.

Table II. Antitumor Screening Results[a]

no.	treatment	tumor	dose, mg/kg	MST, days (% T/C)	av wt. change	survivors, day 5
6	once, day 1 (expt 1)	L1210	12.8	186	−0.4	6/6
			6.4	136	−1.1	6/6
			3.2	114	−0.9	6/6
			1.6	107	−0.8	6/6
			0.8	114	+1.2	6/6
			0.4	107	−0.8	6/6
6	once, day 1 (expt 2)	L1210	51.2	171	−1.9	5/6
			25.6	164	−1.2	6/6
			12.8	136	+0.3	6/6
			6.4	157	+0.7	6/6
			3.2	114	+0.2	6/6
			1.6	129	−0.6	6/6
6	QD 1-9	L1210	12.8	114	−1.6	5/6
			6.4	171	−1.7	6/6
			3.2	157	−0.3	5/6
			1.6	121	+0.6	6/6
			0.8	114	+2.3	6/6
			0.4	114	+0.6	6/6
25	once, day 1	L1210	12.8	107	+2.3	6/6
			6.4	93	+2.4	6/6
			3.2	100	+0.2	6/6
			1.6	86	+2.6	6/6
			0.8	100	+1.8	6/6
			0.4	100	+1.5	6/6
25	every 4th day	P388	50	110	+0.2	6/6
			25	110	−0.5	6/6
			12.5	112	−1.3	6/6
			6.25	100	−1.2	6/6
			3.13	100	−2.0	6/6

[a] Tests done on L1210 were carried out at Bristol Laboratories according to the procedure of R. I. Geran, N. N. Greenberg, M. M. McDonald, A. M. Schumacher, and B. J. Abbott, Cancer Chemotherapy Report, part III, p. 9, 1972. Tests on P388 were carried out in the NCI according to the protocol described in Instruction 14, Screening Data Summary Interpretation and Outline of Current Screen, Drug Evaluation Branch, Drug Research and Development Program Division of Cancer Treatment, National Cancer Institute, Bethesda, Md. Tumor inoculum: 10^6 ascites cells implanted ip into BDF$_1$ female mice. Evaluation: MST = median survival time in days; % T/C = MST treated/MST control × 100. Criteria: % T/C = 125 considered significant antitumor effect.

258

TABLE III. Antibacterial Screening[a]

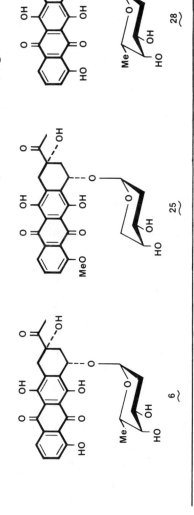

		dose, μg/mL:		inhibition zone, mm				
no.	test organism	50	25	12.5	6.25	3.1	1.6	0.8
6	BS-8[b]	21.5	21.5	21.3	19.5	17.2		
6	ILB[c]	2.3	1.3	1.2	1.1	0.8	0.7	0.8
25	BS-8[b]	18.8	15.8	12.5	10			
25	ILB[c]			0.1	3.3	3.3		
28	BS-8[b]	15	13.8	12.8	10.3			
28	ILB[c]	0.4	1.1	1.1	0.9	0.8		0.8

[a] Compounds 1-5, 7, 9, and 10 showed no reaction in the above tests at 50 μg/mL. [b] When tested for antibiotic activity against B. subtilis ATCC 6633 via a plate assay, carminomycin gave an inhibition zone of 20.2 mm at 12.5 μg/mL. [c] See K. E. Price, R. E. Buck, and J. Lein, Appl. Microbiol., 12, 428 (1964). In this test, carminomycin gave an inhibition zone of 3.5 mm at 6.3 μg/mL.

259

To explore if a completely unsubstituted pyranosyl ring
could impart antitumor activity to an anthracyclinone, we
proceeded to prepare 2-tetrahydropyranyl derivatives of
anthracyclinones. These were prepared from a common starting
material, 2,3-dihydro-4*H*-pyran (29), which was treated with
HCl, and the resulting 2-chlorotetrahydropyran (30) allowed
to react with the chosen anthracyclinones by the usual
Koenigs-Knorr method. The glycosides (31,32) were then
separated from the unreacted sugars by chromatography on
silica gel (see Figure 5). The glycosides shown in Figure 5
proved inactive.[37]

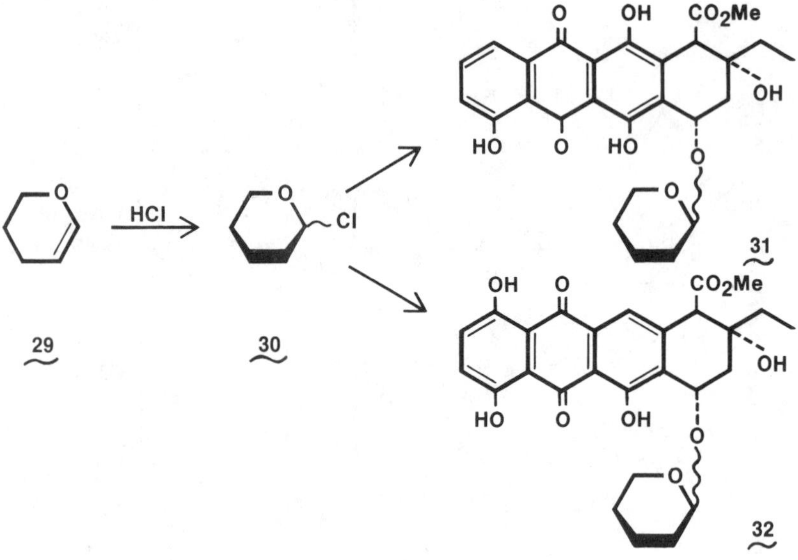

Figure 5. *Synthesis of two tetrahydropyranyl
anthracyclinones*

Since it was found by others that the R and S configuration in position 4 of the pyranose ring did not affect antitumor activity,[38] we also studied the 4-epimers of the monosaccharides linked to anthracyclinones.[36] Accordingly, we
proceeded to synthesize rhodinose, which is 2,3,6-trideoxy-
L-*threo*-hexopyranose and its 4-epimer amicetose, 2,3,6-
trideoxy-L-*erythro*-hexopyranose,[39] which are components of
class II anthracyclines. 3,4-Di-*O*-acetyl-L-rhamnal (33) was
treated with benzyl alcohol in the presence of BF$_3$ etherate;
this caused migration of the double bond affording benzyl
4-*O*-acetyl-2,3,6-trideoxy-L-*erythro*-hex-2-enopyranoside (34),
which was saponified to give benzyl 2,3,6-trideoxy-L-*erythro*-
hex-2-enopyranoside (35), then tosylated and the 4-ester

(36) treated with acetate to afford a 2,3-unsaturated compound (37). The latter was then catalytically hydrogenated
to give the desired benzyl 4-O-acetyl-2,3,6-trideoxy-L-
threo-hexopyranoside (38).

To prepare amicetose, benzyl 4-O-acetyl-2,3,6-trideoxy-
L-erythro-hex-2-enopyranoside (34) was hydrogenated to give
benzyl 4-O-acetyl-2,3,6-trideoxy-L-erythro-hexopyranoside
(40). For a synthesis scheme for rhodinose and amicetose,
see Figure 6.

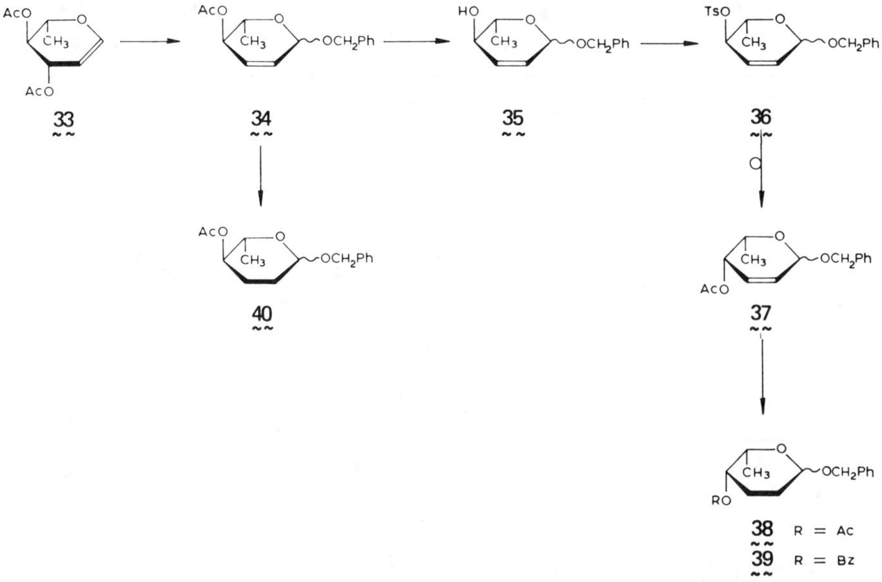

Figure 6. *Scheme for the synthesis of rhodinose and
amicetose benzyl glycosides*

To prepare anthracyclinone glycosides, the benzyl
glycosides 41 and 45 were either refluxed with acetic acid
to give the acetates (42,46) or hydrogenated and then
p-nitrobenzoylated. The esters were then treated with
anhydrous HCl in dichloromethane and the halides coupled with
the anthracyclinone in the usual manner to afford glycosides
43 and 44 from acetate 42 and 47 and 48 from acetate 46.
For a synthetic scheme, see Figure 7.

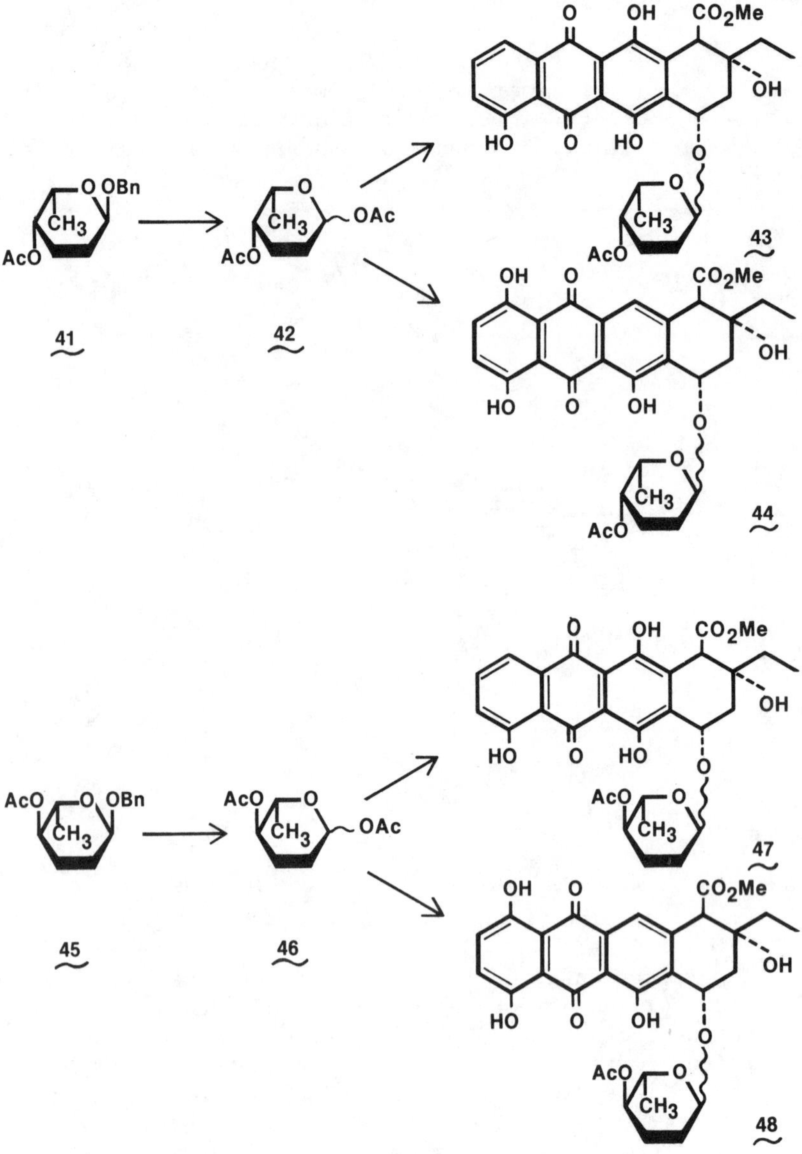

Figure 7. *Synthesis of rhodinose and amicetose anthracyclinone glycosides*

Other monosaccharides prepared were 2,3-dideoxy-D-
glycero-pentopyranose,[40] the demethyl derivative of rhodinose,
as well as 2,4-dideoxy-pentopyranose.[41] The synthesis of the
former started with di-*O*-acetyl-D-xylal (49), which was
treated with benzyl alcohol in the presence of BF$_3$ etherate
to give a mixture of the anomeric benzyl 4-*O*-acetyl-2,3-
dideoxy-α,β-D-*glycero*-pent-2-eno-pyranosides (50,51), which
were separated by chromatography on silica gel. The beta
anomer was then catalytically hydrogenated to benzyl 4-*O*-
acetyl-2,3-dideoxy-D-*glycero*-pentopyranoside (52) and subjected to acetylosis and coupling with the anthracyclinones
to give glycoside 54. For a synthetic scheme, see
Figure 8.

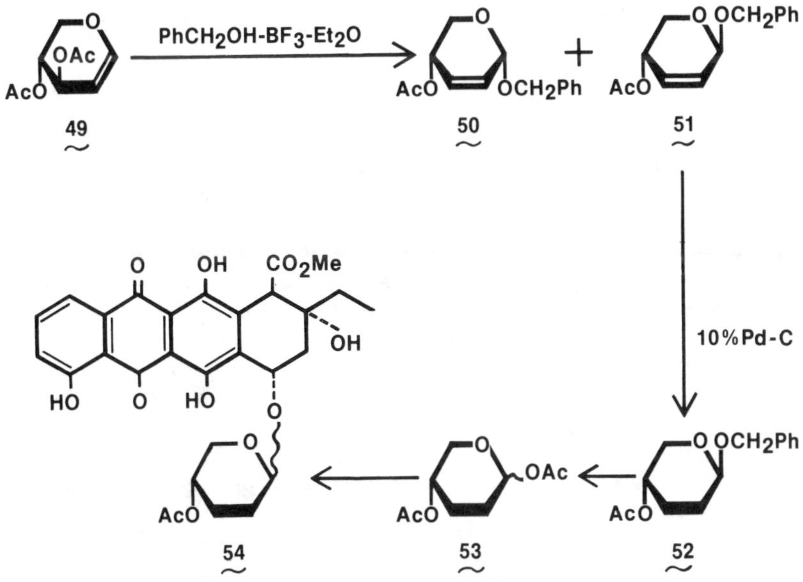

Figure 8. *Synthesis of anthracyclinone glycosides of
2,3-dideoxy-D-*glycero-*pentopyranose*

Compound 57 was obtained by treating 2,3-dihydro-4*H*-
pyran (29) with lead tetracetate, affording the 3-hydroxy
derivatives that include compound 55. This was treated with
HCl without separation affording a mixture containing

4-acetoxy-2-chlorotetrahydropyran (56), which was reacted
with ε-rhodimycinone to afford the desired 4-acetoxy-
tetrahydropyran-2-yl-ε-rhodimycinone (57), after separation
on column chromatography. For a synthetic scheme, see
Figure 9.

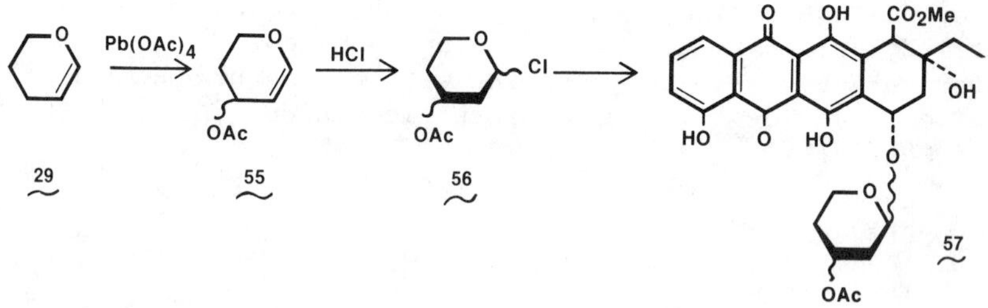

Figure 9. *Synthesis of 4-acetoxy-tetrahydropyran-2-yl-ε
rhodimycinone*

When the previous saccharides were converted to the
anthracyclinone glycosides and screened, it was found that
they all showed no or very little activity. This suggested
that a certain number of polar groups were needed in the
saccharide moiety before antitumor activity could be developed. These polar groups are probably needed to induce
some sort of loose complexation with DNA. It seems that a
sugar having one amino group and one hydroxyl group as, for
example, daunosamine, when linked to an anthracyclinone,
induces strong complexation with DNA and affords a class I
anthracycline, whereas a sugar with two hydroxyl groups as,
for example, 2-deoxy-L-fucose or 2-deoxy-D-ribose complexes
loosely with DNA and results in a class II anthracycline. On
the other hand, one hydroxyl group is not enough for complexation and the resulting glycoside is devoid of activity.
It should be noted that introducing more hydroxyl groups in
position 2 and 6 of the monosaccharide molecules has also a
detrimental effect on antineoplastic activity.[42]

All the naturally occurring mono- and oligosaccharide
anthracycline types have their carbohydrate moieties in the
pyranose form. Very little work was done on anthracycline
analogs having furanose amino sugars, probably due to the
early notion that a stable complexation with DNA is essential
for these antibiotics to exhibit their antitumor activities.[43]
Since the structure and stereochemistry of daunosamine would
be altered drastically in a furanose form, the latter would

not retain the geometrical requirements for a stable
drug-DNA complex. The result could, however, be an anthracycline analog having class II characteristics. It was,
accordingly, decided to prepare anthracyclines with amino
sugar moieties in the furanose form. Two furanosyl amino
sugars, namely 3-amino-2,3,6-trideoxy-L-$lyxo$- and D-$ribo$-
hexofuranose (daunosamine and 4-epidaunosamine) were synthesized and coupled with daunomycinone,[44] as follows:

Starting with the known N-trifluoroacetyl derivative of daunosamine (58), 2,3,6-trideoxy-3-(trifluoroacetamido)-L-$lyxo$-hexose, and treating it with ethanethiol,
afforded the diethyl dithioacetal (59), which was cyclized
with mercuric oxide in methanol to give a mixture of the
α-furanoside (60, 37%), the β-furanoside (61, 29%), the
α,β-pyranosides (7%), and 2,3,6-trideoxy-3-(trifluoroacetamido)-L-$lyxo$-hexose dimethyl acetal (5%), which was
separated by column chromatography. The α- and β-furanosides
(60 and 61) were treated with p-nitrobenzoyl chloride, to
afford the α and β anomers of the 5-p-nitrobenzoates
(62 and 63) in crystalline form. Acetolysis of these
afforded the desired 1-O-acetyl-2,3,6-trideoxy-5-O-(p-nitro-
benzoyl)-3-(trifluoroacetamido)-L-$lyxo$-hexofuranose (64).
The overall yield of compound 64 from N-(trifluoroacetyl)
daunosamine (58) was 42%. Coupling acetate 64 with
daunomycinone in the presence of $SnCl_4$ or p-toluene sulfonic
acid afforded 5-O-p-nitrobenzoyl-2,3,6-trideoxy-3-trifluoro-
acetamido-α-L-$lyxo$-hexofuranosyl daunomycinone (65). The
latter was deblocked in the usual manner to afford the
desired furanose analog of daunorubicin (66). For the
synthetic scheme of the furanose analog of daunorubicin,
see Figure 10.

Reaction of N-acetylepidaunosamine (3-acetamido-2,3,6-
trideoxy-D-$ribo$-hexopyranose) (67) with ethanethiol in concentrated hydrochloric acid afforded the acyclic dithioacetal
68 in 80% yield. Compound 68 could either be used directly
for the next step, or purified by conversion into the
crystalline acetate (69), and this deacetylated with sodium
methoxide, to give pure 68. Cyclization of compound 68 with
mercuric chloride and mercuric oxide in methanol afforded a
mixture of the methyl 3-acetamido-2,3,6-trideoxy-α- and -β-
D-$ribo$-hexofuranosides (70 and 71) in 17 and 35% yield,
respectively, as well as the methyl α- and β-pyranosides in
10% yield, and 3-acetamido-2,3,6-trideoxy-D-$ribo$-hexose
dimethyl acetal in 17% yield, separated in a column of silica
gel eluted with chloroform-methanol. The furanose derivatives (70 and 71) were readily distinguished from the

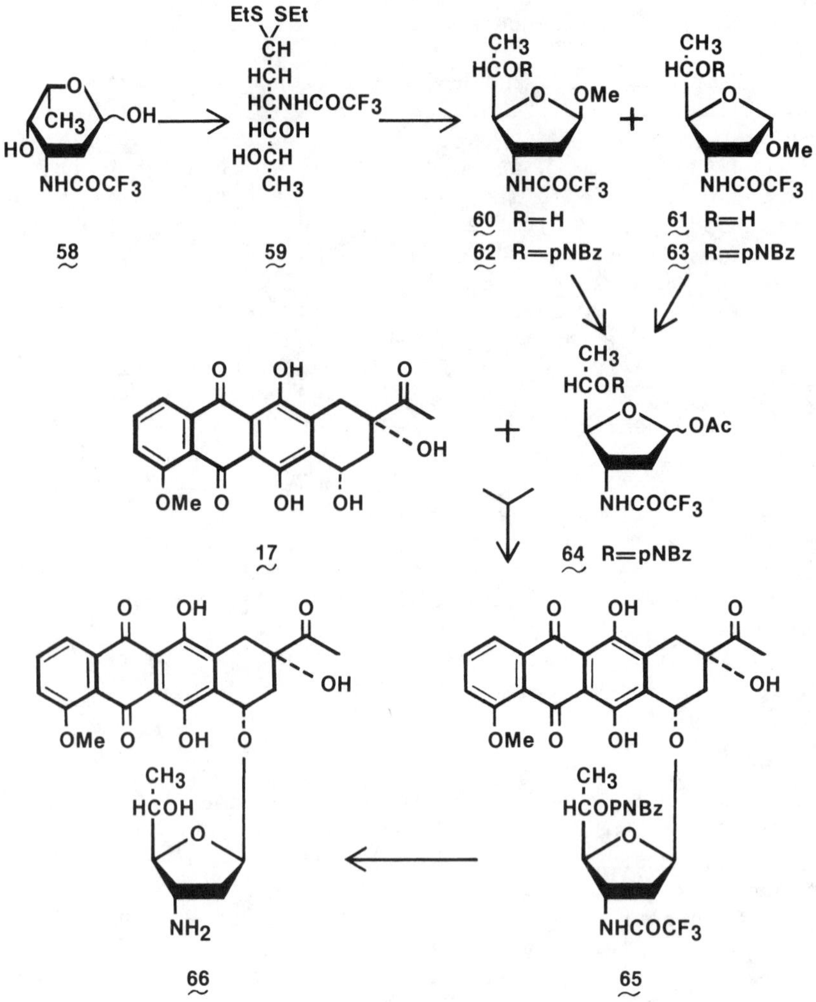

Figure 10. *Synthetic scheme for the furanose analog of daunorubicin*

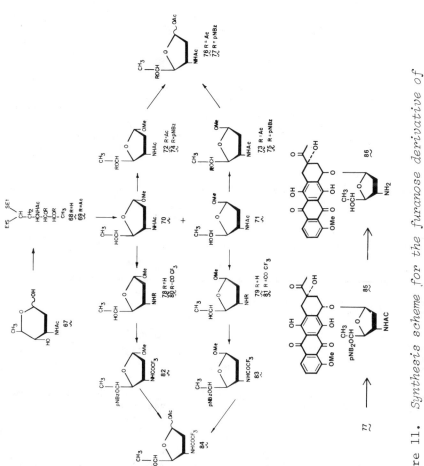

Figure 11. *Synthesis scheme for the furanose derivative of 5'-epidaunosamine*

pyranose derivatives by their n.m.r. spectra, which showed
the anomeric protons of the furanose derivatives at lower
field (δ5) than those of the corresponding pyranose derivative (δ4.6). The anomeric configuration of compound 70 and
71 was established by comparison of their optical rotations,
using Hudson's Rule. After protecting 0-5 with an acetyl
group, to give compounds 72 and 73, or a *p*-nitrobenzoyl
group, to give compounds 74 and 75, the protected methyl
α- and β-furanosides were subjected to acetolysis, to give
3-acetamido-1,5-di-*O*-acetyl-2,3,6-trideoxy-D-*ribo*-hexo-
furanose (76) from compounds 72 and 73, and 3-acetamido-1-*O*-
acetyl-2,3,6-trideoxy-5-*O*-(*p*-nitrobenzoyl)-D-*ribo*-hexo-
furanose (77) from compounds 74 and 75. The acetolysis of
compounds 72 and 73 proceeded in low yield, and was accompanied by considerable degradation. As this could effect the
integrity of the furanose ring, we have recommended the use
of compound 77 for glycoside formation, which may be performed either directly, or after conversion into the halide.

As it is easier to remove a trifluoroacetyl group than
an acetyl group, it was decided also to prepare *N*-trifluoro-
acetyl epidaunosamine furanosides. For this purpose, compounds 70 and 71 were deacetylated by treatment with barium
hydroxide, to afford the methyl α- and β-methyl glycosides
78 and 79. These reacted with trifluoroacetic anhydride to
give first di-trifluoroacetylated compounds, which were
treated with anhydrous methanol to afford the desired methyl
2,3,6-trideoxy-3-(trifluoroacetamido)-α- and -β-D-*ribo*-hexo-
furanosides (80 and 81). Treatment with *p*-nitrobenzoyl
chloride gave the anomeric 5-*p*-nitrobenzoates (82 and 83),
which were subjected to acetolysis to give 1-*O*-acetyl-2,3,6-
trideoxy-5-*O*-(*p*-nitrobenzoyl)-3-(trifluoroacetamido)-D-*ribo*-
hexofuranose (84). For a synthetic scheme, see Figure 11.

In the above synthesis, it was found that small amounts
of the pyranose sugar, as well as the dimethyl acetal of
epidaunosamine were always formed. A synthesis was,
therefore, developed which eliminates completely the formation of both of these byproducts. Treating *N*-acetyl-4-*O*-
benzoyl-epidaunosamine (86) in the pyranose form with ethyl-
mercaptan afforded the acyclic dithioacetal (87). This was
successively treated with dihydropyran to block the five
position, and with sodium methoxide to remove the benzoyl
group. The resulting molecule (89) was now left with only
0-4 deblocked, so that upon cyclization only the furanose
ring could be formed. To prevent formation of the dimethyl
acetal, which was the second byproduct in previous syntheses,
the cyclization was carried out in water instead of methanol,

to afford furanose the sugar, N-acetyl-5-O-tetrahydropyranyl-epidaunosamine (90). This was acetylated to give 3-N-acetyl-1-O-acetyl-5-O-tetrahydropyranyl epidaunosamine (91), which can readily be made to react with an anthracyclinone in BF_3 or $SnCl_4$.

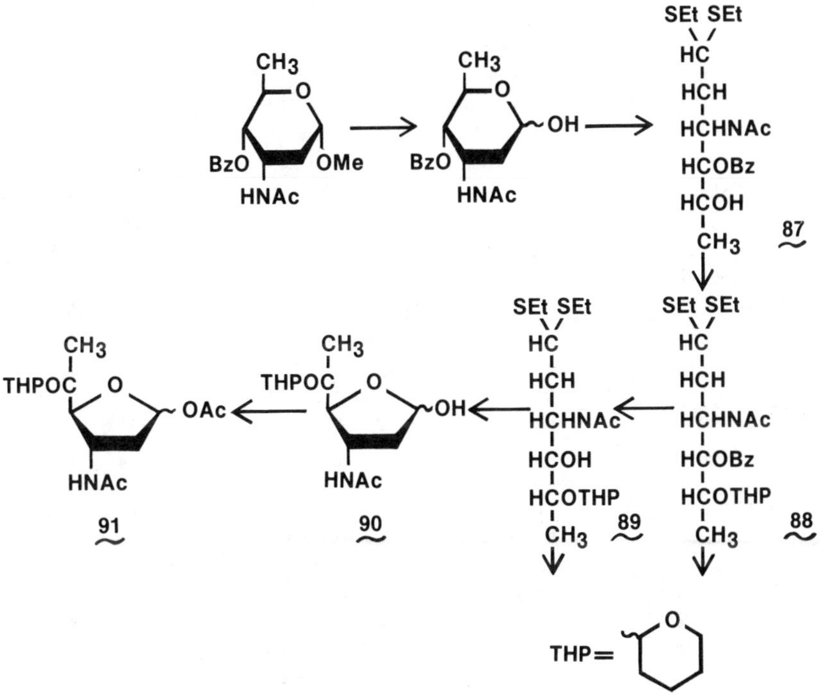

Figure 12. *Synthetic scheme for the furanose derivative of epidaunosamine*

(b) Synthesis of Disaccharide Derivatives

The remarkable improvement in activity which accompanies an increase in the number of carbohydrate units in the side chains of class II anthracyclines,[5] such as aclacinomycins,[6] prompted us to synthesize oligosaccharide glycosides of daunorubicin to impart to it the characteristic biological activities inherent to class II anthracyclines, such as increased potency, selective inhibition of nuclear RNA synthesis, and reduced cardiotoxicities.[6]

Attempts to increase the length of carbohydrate side
chains of daunorubicin and adriamycin are not unprecedented.
Although carminomycins are known to exist as oligosaccharide
glycosides (carminomycin II and III),[20] which are biologically
active, the oligosaccharide glycosides of the clinically
important daunorubicin and adriamycin are not found
naturally. In search for new anthracyclines with higher
therapeutic indeces, Oki and coworkers attempts to convert
various biologically inactive anthracyclinones, including
daunomycinone and adriamycinone into active glycosides by
adding them to a culture of an aclacinomycin negative mutant
KE303, which did not produce aklavinone.[46] Both daunomycinone
and adriamycinone were not glycosidated. It seemed that the
presence of both of the methoxyl group at C-4 and a carbonyl
group at the C-13 positions blocked the glycosidation of these
anthracyclinones. However, from Streptomyces coeruleorubidus
ME130-A4, Oki isolated daunomycin analogs with extended
carbohydrate side chains at C-4.[31,47] For example,
baumycin A has a pseudo-saccharide linked to the daunosamine
moiety and shows a 10 fold increase in potency. Umezawa and
coworkers synthesized 4'-O-tetrahydropyranyl adriamycin.[48]
The compound is less potent, but much less cardiotoxic than
either aclacinomycin A, N-trifluoroacetyl adriamycin
14-valerate (AD-32).[49]

A preparation of daunosaminyl daunomycin was described
in the literature, but it was obtained in very low yields.[50]
In our laboratory attempts to prepare the oligosaccharide
glycosides of anthracyclinones by reacting the natural
anthracyclines with glycosyl halides invariably resulted in
transglycosidation and formation of a new monosaccharide
glycosides of the anthracyclinone. Therefore, it was
decided to prepare first the oligosaccharides and then
combine these with the desired anthracyclinones. Several
disaccharides containing the sugars daunosamine,[51] 2-deoxy-L-
fucose and L-rhodinose[39] were synthesized. The first group
had the sugars in the unnatural sequence, i.e. 2-deoxy-L-
fucose or daunosamine were linked to rhodinose or 2-deoxy-D-
ribose (and not the reverse, which is the natural sequence).
In principle, the synthesis of such a disaccharide would
involve the reaction of a daunosamine derivative possessing
a good leaving-group on C-1 with a deoxy sugar having only one
free hydroxyl group. Since the resulting disaccharide is
needed for glycosylation, the protecting group attached to
C-1 of the disaccharide must be of such a nature that it can
be removed without effecting the glycosidic bond linking the
two monosaccharides.

In our laboratory, we have prepared benzyl-2,3-dideoxy-
D-*glycero*-pentopyranoside, an excellent candidate for the
aforementioned disaccharide synthesis; it has one free
hydroxyl group, and possesses on O-1 a benzyl group that,
after formation of the disaccharide, can be removed by
hydrogenolysis without affecting the glycosidic bond. As
regards the choice of the needed daunosamine derivative
possessing a good leaving-group on C-1, we avoided the use of
halides, because these compounds are not crystalline, are
relatively unstable, and cannot be prepared in high yields.

The ester 92 readily underwent nucleophilic substitution
when treated with benzyl 2,3-dideoxy-D-*glycero*-hexopyranoside
(93) in the presence of *p*-toluenesulfonic acid as the
catalyst. It should be noted that, although compound 93 has
only one free hydroxyl group available for linkage with the
daunosamine moiety, two reaction-products were obtained. The
major one was identified as the previously prepared benzyl
2,3,6-trideoxy-4-O-(*p*-nitrobenzoyl)-3-(trifluoroacetamido)-
L-*lyxo*-hexopyranoside (94), evidently formed by transglycosylation. Careful chromatography of the reaction products
yielded, in addition, a small proportion of the desired
disaccharide (96). For a synthetic scheme, see Figure 13.

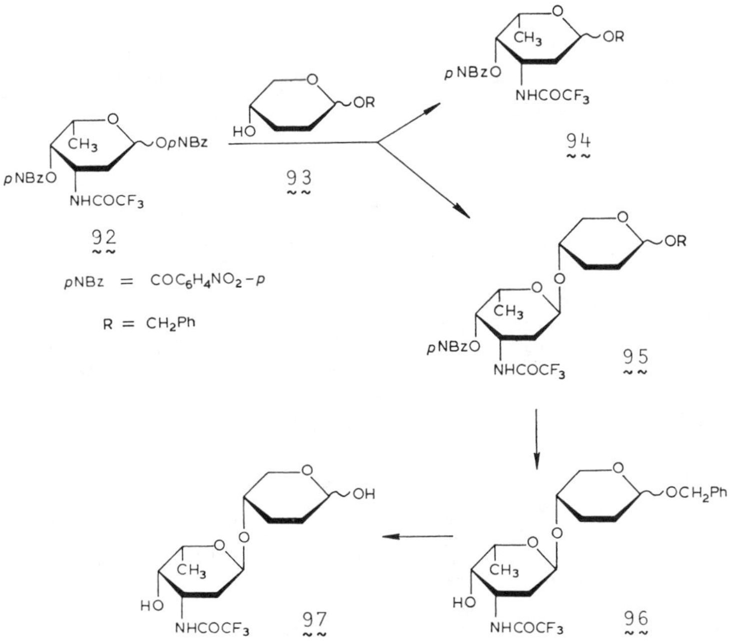

Figure 13. *Synthetic scheme for the synthesis of a*
daunosamine containing disaccharide

Other disaccharides prepared were the benzyl glycosides
of 2-deoxyfucosyl rhodinose (101) and amicetose (104), as
well as those of 4-amicitosyl amicetose (105), tetrahydropyranyl amicetose (106). The first two disaccharides,
namely benzyl 4-*O*-(3,4-di-*O*-acetyl-2-deoxy-α-L-rhodinose (101)
and amicetose (104), were obtained by reacting 3,4-*O*-di-*O*-
acetyl-L-fucal (98) with benzyl rhodinoside (99) and benzyl
amicetoside (102), respectively, using *p*-toluene sulfonic
acid as a catalyst. The yield in both reactions could be
improved by carrying out the reaction with NIS to afford the
2'-iodo disaccharides 100 and 103, which were then hydrogenated to give the desired benzyl glycosides (101 and 104).
For a synthetic scheme, see Figure 14.

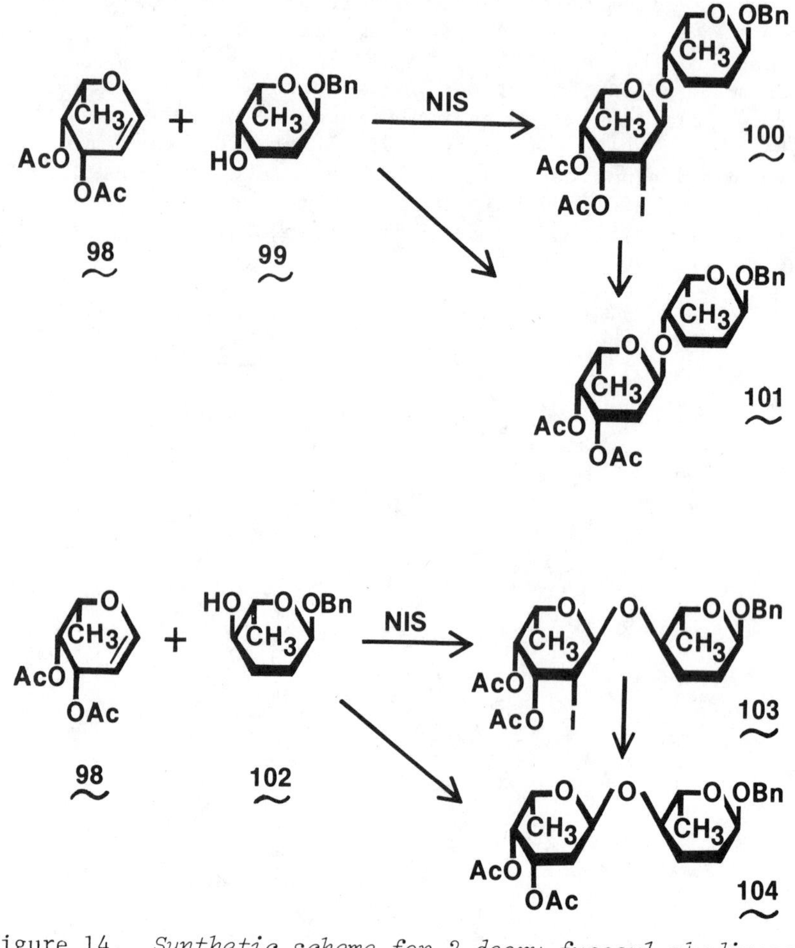

Figure 14. *Synthetic scheme for 2-deoxy-fucosyl rhodinose
            and amicetose*

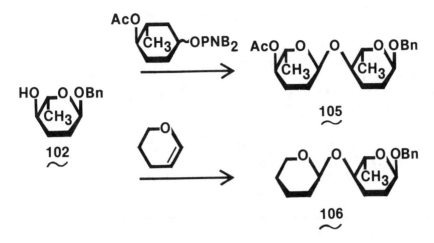

Figure 15. *Synthetic scheme for tetrahydropyranyl*

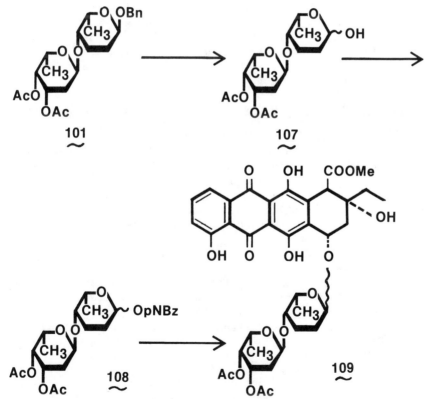

Figure 16. *Synthetic scheme for 2-deoxy-fucopyranosyl rhodinosyl ε-rhodomycinone*

The last two disaccharides, namely benzyl 4-*O*-(4-*O*-acetyl-L-aceamicetosyl)-L-amicetose (105), and 4-*O*-tetrahydro-pyranyl amicetose (106), were prepared in 35% yield by react-ing benzyl α-amicetoside (102) with *p*-nitrobenzoyl-4-*O*-acetyl-L-amicetose or dihydropyran using *p*-toluene sulfonic acid or the pyridinium salt of *p*-toluene sulfonic acid as a catalyst. For a synthetic scheme, see Figure 15.

To prepare the disaccharide glycosides of the anthra-cyclinone, the benzyl glycosides of the disaccharides were hydrogenated to give the reducing disaccharide. The latter were the *p*-nitrobenzoylated and reacted with the anthra-cyclinones in the presence of *p*-toluene sulfonic acid. The reaction is exemplified by the preparation of the disaccharide glycoside of ε-rhodimycinone (109). For a synthetic scheme, see Figure 16.

Later an attempt was made to synthesize disaccharides having daunosamine and 2-deoxy-L-fucose in the sequence found naturally in class II anthracyclines. The first target disaccharide selected was methyl 4-*O*-(3',4ᴸ-di-*O*-acetyl-2',6ᴸ-dideoxy-α-L-*lyxo*-hexopyranosyl)-2,3,6-trideoxy-3-trifluoro-acetamido-β-L-*lyxo*-hexopyranoside (112).[52] The starting material for the synthesis was 2-deoxy-L-fucopyranosyl chloride (10), which was treated with methyl β-L-daunosa-minide *N*-trifluoroacetate (110) (a sugar that has only one unprotected position through which it can be linked, namely *O*-4) in the presence of mercuric bromide and yellow mercuric oxide,[53] to afford the desired disaccharide (112) in 35% yield. This compound was accompanied by some di-*O*-acetyl-L-fucal, formed by elimination of H-2 from the L-fucopyranosyl chloride. In addition, a disaccharide, di-*O*-acetyl-2-deoxy-α-L-α-fucopyranosyl-di-*O*-acetyl-2-deoxy-α-L-fucopyranoside, was isolated in small yield. The structure ot disaccharide (112) was confirmed by n.m.r. spectroscopy and mass spectrometry.

Attempts to convert the disaccharide methyl glycoside (112) prepared into a glycosyl halide either directly or via an acetolysis resulted in degradation and formation of mono-saccharide derivatives. It was, therefore, decided to repeat the synthesis using a benzyl protecting group on the dauno-samine moiety.[44] The resulting benzyl glycoside of the disaccharide prepared could later be hydrogenated without fear for the integrity of the interglycosidic bond. The free disaccharide could then be readily converted to an acetyl derivative capable of coupling with anthracyclinones.

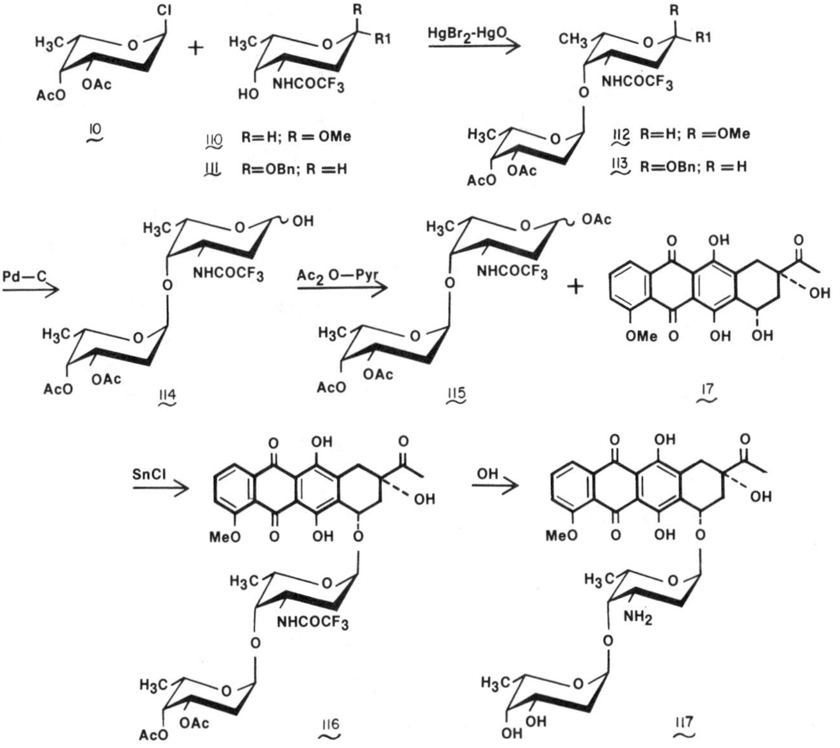

Figure 17. *Synthetic scheme for 2-deoxy-fucosyl daunosominyl daunomycinone*

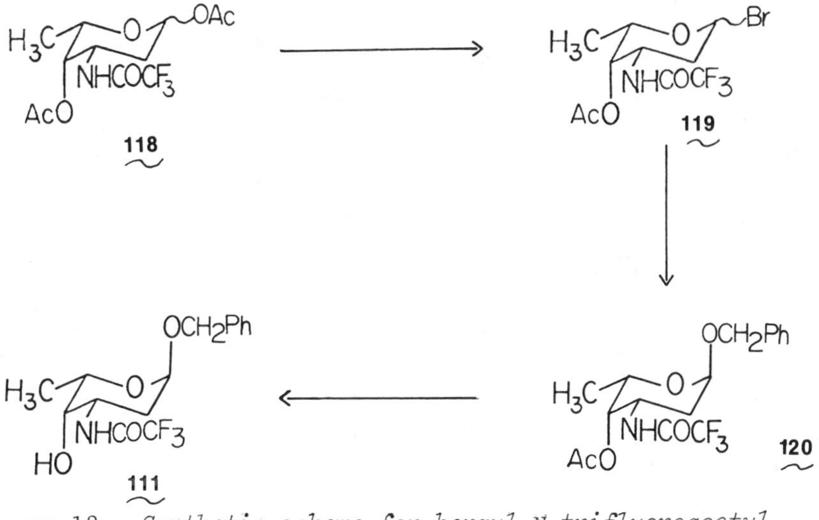

Figure 18. *Synthetic scheme for benzyl N-trifluoroacetyl-α-L-daunosaminide*

The synthesis of the target disaccharide started with
the synthesis of daunosaminyl bromide (119) by treating
fully acetylated *N*-trifluoroacetamido-L-daunosamine (118)
with trimethyl bromosilane in dichloroethane. The extremely
labile glycosyl bromide was reacted immediately without
characterization with excess benzyl alcohol in the presence
of mercuric bromide, yellow mercuric oxide and finely
powdered 4Å molecular sieves. The anomerically pure benzyl
4-*O*-acetyl-3-trifluoroacetamido-α-L-daunosaminide (120) was
obtained as a crystalline compound in 82% yield after
chromatographic separation and crystallization. This compound was treated with sodium methoxide in dry methanol to
afford compound 111 (see Figure 18), which was reacted with
2-deoxy-L-fucosyl chloride (10) under Koenigs–Knorr
conditions[53] in the presence of mercuric bromide, yellow
mercuric oxide and finely powdered 4Å molecular sieves. The
reaction was completed within 30 minutes and after chromatographic separation, the desired disaccharide (113) was
obtained in 72% yield.

Coupling of disaccharide (115) to daunomycinone presented
several difficulties. The Koenigs–Knorr condensation was the
primary choice because it was tried before on monosaccharides
and afforded the anthracyclines in high yields.[33] However,
all attempts to prepare glycosyl bromides from the
disaccharide acetate using trimethyl bromosilane as a brominating agent resulted in the splitting of the interglycosidic
bond. Trimethyl bromosilane[54] has been used as a mild
selective brominating agent to replace the anomeric acetyl
group with bromide, but the 2-deoxy-L-fucosyl bond seems to
be very labile. The next choice was to use the disaccharide
acetate (115) directly for coupling. One equivalent of
the disaccharide acetate (115) and daunomycinone were
reacted in the presence of tintetrachloride. After the
work-up, followed by chromatographic separation, the
disaccharide glycoside was obtained in 60% yield.[55] It was
deblocked and submitted for screening on P388 at the
National Cancer Institute. The results are shown in Table IV.
For a synthetic scheme, see Figure 17.

The above preparation constitutes the first successful
synthesis of a disaccharide anthracyclinone having part of
the sugar moiety of aclacinomycin linked to daunomycinone.
The same synthesis is presently being repeated on adriamycinone. In addition, some ten other disaccharides have been
prepared and linked to various anthracyclinones.

Table IV. Antitumor Screening Results[a]

tumor	dose, mg/kg	MST, days (% T/C)	av. wt. change	survivors, day 5
P388	36.00	123	-2.0	6/6
	18.00	126	-2.9	6/6
	9.00	123	-2.3	6/6
	4.50	113	-1.6	6/6
	2.25	113	-3.5	6/6

[a]Tests done on P388 were carried out in the NCI according to the protocol described in Instruction 14, Screening Data Summary Interpretation and Outline of Current Screen, Drug Evaluation Branch, Drug Research and Development Program Division of Cancer Treatment, National Cancer Institute, Bethesda, Md. Evaluation: MST = median survival time in days; % T/C = MST treated/MST control x 100. Criteria: % T/C = 125 considered significant antitumor effect.

REFERENCES

1   W. A. Remers, *The Chemistry of Antitumor Antibiotics*,
    Chapter 2, Anthracyclines, John Wiley and Sons, New York,
    63 (1979).

2   P. H. Wiermik, *Current Status of Adriamycin and Dauno-
    rubicin in Cancer Treatment in Anthracyclines: Current
    Status and New Developments*, S. T. Crooke and S. D. Reich
    (Editors), Academic Press, Inc., 273 (1980).

3   G. Bonadonna, S. Monfardini, Lancet 1969-1, 837 (1979).

4   F. P. Metller, D. M. Young and J. M. Ward, *Cancer Res.*, *37*,
    2705 (1977).

5   a. V. H. DuVernay, S. Mong, S. T. Crooke, *Molecular
    Pharmacology of Anthracyclines*, *Anthracyclines* (see
    Ref. 2), 61.

    b. T. W. Doyle, *Anthracycline Oligosaccharides*, Chapter 6,
    Anthracyclines (see Ref. 2), 61.

6   T. Oki, T. Takeuchi, S. Oka and H. Umezama, *Current Status
    of Japanese Studies with New Anthracycline Antibiotics
    Aclacinomycin A*, in Recent Results in Cancer Research,
    G. Mathé and F. M. Muggia (Editors), Springer-Verlog,
    Vol. 74, 207 (1980).

7   R. H. Thomson, *Naturally Occurring Quinones*, Academic
    Press, Inc., Chapter 6, *Anthracyclinones*, 536 (1971).

8   A. Grein, C. Spalla, A. Di Marco, and G. Canevazzi,
    Giorn, Microbial., *11*, 109 (1963).

9   M. Du Bost, P. Gauter, R. Maral, L. Ninet, S. Pinnert,
    J. Preúdhomme, and G. H. Werner, *C. R. Acad. Sci.*, Paris,
    257, 1813 (1963).

10 M. Blumauerora, J. Mateju, K. Stajiner and Z. Vanek,
    C. R. Acad. Sci., Paris, *257*, 1813 (1963).

11 M. G. Brazhnikova, N. V. Konstantinova, V. A. Pomaskova,
    and B. V. Zacharov, *Antibiotiki*, *11*, 763 (1963).

12 T. Komiyama, Y. Matsuzawa, T. Oki, T. Inui, Y. Takahashi,
    H. Naganawa, T. Takeucchi and H. Umezawa, *J. Antibiotics*,
    30, 619 (1977).

13 F. Arcamone, G. Franceschi, P. Orezzi, G. Cassinelli, W. Barbieri, and R. Mondelli, *J. Am. Chem. Soc.*, *86*, 5334 (1964).

14 F. Arcamone, G. Franceschi, P. Orezzi, S. Penco, and R. Mandelli, *Tetrahedron Lett.*, 3349 (1968).

15 F. Arcamone, G. Franceschi, P. Orezzi, G. Francheschi and R. Mandelli, *J. Am. Chem. Soc.*, *86*, 5335 (1964).

16 R. Angiuli, F. Foresti, L. Riva Di Sanserverino, N. W. Isaacs, O. Kennard, W. D. S. Motherwell, D. L. Wampler, and F. Arcamone, *Nature New Biol.*, *78*, 234 (1971).

17 a. F. Arcamone, G. Francheschi, S. Penco, and A. Seliva, *Tetrahedron Lett.*, 1007 (1969).

b. F. Arcamone, G. Cassinelli, G. Fantini, A. Grein, P. Orezzi, C. Pol, and C. Spalla, *Biotechnol. Bioeng.*, *11*, 1101 (1969), *A New Antitumor Antibiotic from S. Peucetius Var. Caesius.*, *Biotechnol. Bioeng.*, *11*, 1101 (1969).

18 G. F. Gauze, M. A. Sveshnikova, R. S. Vkholina, G. V. Gavrilina, V. A. Ponomarenko, N. P. Potapova, *Antibiotiki*, *18*, 675 (1973).

19 M. G. Brazhnikova, V. B. Abarskii, M. K. Kudinova, L. I. Murav'era, V. I. Pomomarenko, N. P. Potapova, *Antibiotiki*, *18*, 678 (1973).

20 M. G. Brazhikova, V. B. Zbarsky, V. I. Ponomarenko, and N. P. Potapova, *J. Antibiot.*, *27*, 254 (1974).

21 G. F. Gauze, M. G. Brazhnikova, and V. A. Shorin, *Cancer Chemotherapy Rep.*, *Part 2*, *58*, 255 (1974).

22 V. A. Shorin, V. S. Bazhanov, L. A. Averbukh, G. N. Lepeshikina, and A. M. Grinshtein, *Antitiotiki*, *18*, 681 (1973).

23 H. Brockmann und W. Lenk: Über Actinomyceten farbstoffe, *Chem. Ber.*, *92*, 1904 (1959).

24 H. Brockmann and B. Spohler, *Naturwissenschaften*, *48*, 716 (1961).

25 W. D. Ollis and I. O. Sutherland, *Chemistry of Natural Phenolic Compounds*, W. D. Ollis (Editor), Pergamon, London, 212 (1961).

26 L. Ettlinger, E. Gäumann, R. Hutter, W. Keller-Schierlein, F. Kradolfer, L. Neipp, V. Prelog, P. Reusser, and H. Zahner, *Chem. Berg.*, *92*, 1867 (1959).

27 W. Keller-Schierlein and W. Richle, *Antimicrob. Agents Chemotherapy*, 68 (1970).

28 W. Richle, E. K. Winkler, D. M. Howley, M. Dobler, and W. Keller-Schierlein, *Helv. Chem. Acta*, *55*, 467 (1972).

29 D. E. Nettleton, Jr., W. T. Bradner, J. A. Bush, A. B. Coon, J. E. Moseley, R. W. Myllymaki, F. A. O'Herron, R. H. Schreiber, and A. L. Vulcano, *J. Antibiot.*, Tokyo, *30*, 525 (1977).

30 T. W. Doyle, D. E. Nettleton, R. E. Grulich, D. M. Bolitz, D. L. Johnson and A. L. Vulcano, *J. Am. Chem. Soc.*, *101*, 7041 (1979).

31 T. Oki, *Japan J. Antibiotics 30 suppl.*, (1977), S-70, Reference cited herein.

32 F. Strelitz, H. Flan, U. Weiss and I. N. Asheshov, *J. Bacterial*, *27*, 90 (1956).

33 G. L. Tong, H. Y. Wu, T. H. Smith and D. W. Henry, *J. Med. Chem.*, *22*, 912 (1979).

34 H. S. El Khadem and D. L. Swartz, *J. Med. Chem.*, *24*, 11 (1981).

35 E. F. Fuchs, D. Horton, W. Weckerle and E. Winter-Mihaly, *J. Med. Chem.*, *22*, 406 (1979).

36 D. Horton, W. Priebe, and W. R. Turner, *Carbohydr. Res.*, *94*, 11 (1981).

37 H. S. El Khadem, D. L. Swartz and R. C. Cermak, *J. Med. Chem.*, *20*, 957 (1977).

38 Thomas S. Winowiski, *A Thesis for Master of Science*, Michigan Technological University, 1978.

39   A. M. Casazza, A. Di Marco, G. Bonadonna, V. Bonfante,
     C. Bertazzoli, O. Bellini, G. Pratesi, L. Sala and
     L. Ballerini, "Effects of Modifications in Position 4
     of the Chromophore or in position 4 of the Amino Sugar,
     on the Antitumor Activity and Toxicity of Daunorubicin
     and Doxorubicin", *Anthracyclines*, Chapter 2, 403.

40   H. S. El Khadem and R. C. Cermak, *Carbohydr. Res.*, *75*,
     335 (1979); R. C. Cermak, *A Doctoral Dissertation*,
     Michigan Technological University, 1980.

41   H. S. El Khadem and D. Matsuura, *Carbohydr. Res.*, *75*,
     331 (1979); D. Matsuura, *A Thesis for Master of Science*,
     Michigan Technological University, 1978.

42   Thomas S. Winowiski, *A Thesis for Master of Science*,
     Michigan Technological University, 1978.

43   F. Arcamone, "The Development of New Antitumor
     Anthracyclines", *Anticancer Agents Based on Natural
     Product Model, Medicinal Chemistry*, Vol. 16, Chapter 1,
     J. M. Cassady and J. D. Douros (Editors), Academic Press,
     1 (1980).

44   A. Di Marco, F. Arcamone and F. Zunino, Daunomycin
     (Daunorubicin) and Adriamycin and Structural Analogs:
     Biological Activity and Mechanism of Action,
     Antibiotics III, J. N. Corcoran and F. E. Hahn (Editors),
     Springer-Verlog, 102 (1975).

45   D. Matsuura, *A Doctoral Dissertation*, Michigan
     Technological University, 1981.

46   T. Oki, "Microbial Transformation of Anthracycline
     Antibiotics and Drug Development of New Anthracyclines",
     *182nd American Chemical Society National Meeting,
     New York*, (August 23-28, 1981).

47   T. Oki, A. Yoshimoto and Y. Matsuzawa, *J. Antibiotics*,
     33, 1331 (1980).

48   T. Komiyama, Y. Matsuzawa, T. Oki, T. Inui, Y. Takahashi,
     H. Naganawa, T. Takeuchi and H. Umezawa, *J. Antibiotics*,
     30, 619 (1977); T. Takahashi, H. Naganawa, T. Takeuchi,
     H. Umezawa, T. Komiyama, T. Oki and T. Inui,
     J. Antibiotics, *30*, 622 (1977).

49   H. Emezawa, Y. Takahashi, M. Kinoshita, H. Naganawa,
     T. Masuda, M. Ishizuka, K. Tatsuta and T. Takeuchi,
     J. Antibiotics, 32, 1082 (1979).

50   D. Dantcheu, M. Paintrand, M. Hayat, C. Bourut and
     G. Mathe, *J. Antibiotics, 32,* 1085 (1979).

51   E. M. Acton and G. L. Tong, *J. Med. Chem., 24,* 669 (1981).

52   H. S. El Khadem, D. L. Swartz, J. K. Nelson and
     L. A. Berry, *Carbohydr. Res., 74,* 199 (1979).

53   H. S. El Khadem and D. Matsuura, *Carbohydr. Res., 88,*
     332 (1981).

54   L. R. Schroeder and J. W. Green, *J. Chem. Soc.,* C,
     530 (1966); E. F. Fuchs, D. Horton and W. Weckerle,
     Carbohydr. Res., 57, c36 (1977).

55   J. W. Gillard and M. Israel, *Tetrahedron Letters, 22,*
     513 (1981).

56   H. S. El Khadem, D. L. Swartz, R. Cermak and D. Matsuura,
     Abstracts of the 182nd National ACS Meeting, Carbohydr. 13
     (1981).

Index